Atlas of Elastosonography

Dirk-André Clevert
Mirko D'Onofrio • Emilio Quaia
Editors

Atlas of Elastosonography

Clinical Applications with Imaging Correlations

Springer

Editors
Dirk-André Clevert
Interdisciplinary Ultrasound-Center
Department of Clinical Radiology
University of Munich-Grosshadern
Campus
Munich
Germany

Emilio Quaia
Clinical Research Imaging Centre
Queen's Medical Research Institute
Edinburgh
UK

Mirko D'Onofrio
Department of Radiology
University Hospital GB Rossi
University of Verona
Verona
Italy

ISBN 978-3-319-44199-3 ISBN 978-3-319-44201-3 (eBook)
DOI 10.1007/978-3-319-44201-3

Library of Congress Control Number: 2016959473

Printed on acid-free paper

This Springer imprint is published by Springer Nature
The registered company is Springer International Publishing AG
The registered company address is Gewerbestrasse 11, 6330 Cham, Switzerland

Foreword

In the past few years, elastosonography has recently been presented in clinical studies as a new technique applied to ultrasound imaging. This new technique evaluates noninvasively tissue-specific consistency.

Clinical experiences in elastosonography have been given promising results in the study of numerous organs. As for Doppler also, elastosonography improves the diagnostic capability of ultrasound imaging.

This book, titled *Atlas of Elastosonography* – clinical applications with imaging correlations – edited by Clevert, D'Onofrio, and Quaia, presents an extensive series of images which describe possible applications of elastosonography in the routine clinical practice. After a brief technical introduction, all applications of elastosonography in the superficial parts and abdomen are effectively described by representative cases, also with imaging correlations.

Due to the nowadays applications of elastosonography on most of body organs, this atlas is divided into nine chapters, starting with the technical and physical aspect of elastosonography moving to clinical applications in liver and spleen, pancreas, kidney, breast, musculoskeletal, thyroid, carotid artery, and testis.

Important editorial news lies on the rich illustrations of this book and especially on the presence of imaging correlations. In fact, a key concept presented in this book is that elastosonography is certainly innovative as Doppler ultrasound but evaluating only the tissue stiffness, this new technique needs to be supported by other imaging studies because of the overlap between pathological and normal values of tissue stiffness and the overlap between benign and malignant characteristics. Therefore, the information given by elastosonography is absolutely innovative and useful, sometime essential to reach the definitive diagnosis if correctly integrated with clinical and imaging findings.

Verona, Italy — Roberto Pozzi Mucelli

Preface

Elastography has recently been used in ultrasound clinical studies. Elastosonography is a new complementary technique applied to ultrasound imaging. Elastosonography is a powerful technique to assess noninvasively the elasticity of tissues.

Various tissue compression methods derived from two technical solutions, known as strain elastosonography and shear wave elastosonography, have been proposed in elastosonography. Elastosonography can also be based on the deformation generated by an imparted force on the target organ. This new technique allows to obtain a qualitative and/or quantitative evaluation of the stiffness of the lesion, target organ object of the study.

Applications of elastosonography have been proved to be clinical useful in the study of numerous organs, giving promising and exclusive results.

This atlas describes all the potential applications of elastosonography in studying the liver, spleen, pancreas, kidney, breast, thyroid, testis, musculo-skeletal system, and vascular system. Helpful correlations with other imaging studies, often essential for elastosonography, are presented.

Munich, Germany — Dirk-André Clevert
Verona, Italy — Mirko D'Onofrio
Trieste, Italy — Emilio Quaia

Contents

Contributors

Laura Bernardoni Department of Gastroenterology, GB Rossi University Hospital, University of Verona, Verona, Italy

Chandra Bortolotto Radiology Institute, IRCCS Policlinico San Matteo Foundation, University of Pavia, Pavia, Italy

Costanza Bruno Department of Radiology, Policlinico GB Rossi, Verona, Italy

Alessandra Bucci Department of Radiology, Policlinico GB Rossi, Verona, Italy

Fabrizio Calliada Department of Radiology, University Hospital S. Matteo, Pavia, Italy

Teresa Cammarota Department of Radiology, Azienda Ospedaliero-Universitaria Città della Salute e della Scienza di, Torino, Italy

Vito Cantisani Department of Radiological Sciences, Policlinico Umberto I, Sapienza University of Rome, Rome, Italy

Nicolò Cardobi Department of Radiology, GB Rossi University Hospital, University of Verona, Verona, Italy

Valentina Ciaravino Department of Radiology, GB Rossi University Hospital, University of Verona, Verona, Italy

Dirk-André Clevert Interdisciplinary Ultrasound-Center, Department of Clinical Radiology, University of Munich-Grosshadern Campus, Munich, Germany

Stefano Francesco Crino Department of Gastroenterology, GB Rossi University Hospital, University of Verona, Verona, Italy

Ferdinando D'Ambrosio Department of Radiological Sciences, Policlinico Umberto I, Sapienza University of Rome, Rome, Italy

Mirko D'Onofrio Department of Radiology, GB Rossi University Hospital, University of Verona, Verona, Italy

Emanuele David Department of Biomedical Sciences and Morphological and Functional Imaging, University of Messina, Messina, Italy

Armanda De Marchi Azienda Ospedaliero-Universitaria Città della Salute e della Scienza, Torino, Italy

Riccardo De Robertis Department of Radiology, GB Rossi University Hospital, University of Verona, Verona, Italy

Christoph Frank Dietrich Department of Internal Medicine 2, Caritas Krankenhaus, Bad Mergentheim, Germany

Antonio Giulio Gennari Department of Radiology, Cattinara Hospital, University of Trieste, Trieste, Italy

Hektor Grazhdani Associazione dei Cavalieri Italiani, Sovrano Militare Ordine di Malta, Poliambulatorio Roma Eur, Rome, Italy

Antonio Pio Masciotra Casa di Cura Villa Maria, Campobasso, Italy

Simona Pozza Ospedaliero-Universitaria Città della Salute e della Scienza, Torino, Italy

Emilio Quaia Clinical Research Imaging Centre, Queen's Medical Research Institute, Edinburgh, UK

Maija Radzina Diagnostic Radiology Institute, Paula Stradins Clinical University Hospital, Riga, Latvia

Alessandro Sarno Department of Radiology, GB Rossi University Hospital, University of Verona, Verona, Italy

Anita Spezzacatene Department of Radiology, Cattinara Hospital, University of Trieste, Trieste, Italy

Giorgia Tedesco Department of Radiology, GB Rossi University Hospital, University of Verona, Verona, Italy

Giulia Tremolada Department of Radiology, GB Rossi University Hospital, University of Verona, Verona, Italy

Irene Zorzenon Department of Radiology, Cattinara Hospital, University of Trieste, Trieste, Italy

Part I

Introduction

Technical and Physical Aspects

1

Emilio Quaia and Antonio Giulio Gennari

Physical examination (PE) and medical history are the fundamental steps of medical approach to patients and help to define differential diagnosis, further medical tests, and treatments. PE is composed of four actions: inspection, palpation, percussion, and auscultation. Palpation defines tissue characteristics, which are closely connected to pathological modifications; however, palpation is subjective and limited by depth. Elastography is a relatively new diagnostic tool which provides diagnostic information on tissue stiffness, thus overcoming palpation. Since the first release in 2003, elastography has been implemented in the standard ultrasonography equipment [1].

1.1 Mechanical Tissue Properties and Basic Elastography Principles

Stiffness is defined on how much a substance resists to a deformation produced by an external force. Nowadays there are three different elastographic techniques available to analyze tissue stiffness:

1. Manual compression which exploits the compression applied to the tissue by the sonographer through the probe or the compression produced by cardiovascular pulsation or respiratory motion
2. Acoustic radiation force impulse (ARFI)
3. External mechanical vibration [2]

Elastographic images rely on two different physical approaches: the assessment of the strain produced in the tissue by external compression (strain imaging) or the evaluation of the shear waves' (SW) speed propagation in the medium (shear wave imaging). Both methods aim to evaluate qualitatively (display contrast) and quantitatively (measure) the Young's modulus (YM). Despite the YM does not take into account the system size and the amount of material, it is considered the physical parameter corresponding to stiffness [3]. The quantification of YM allows excellent tissue characterization based on different values of YM [4].

In biological tissues two different mechanical properties act against any type of deformation (shear): elasticity and viscosity [1, 5]. With the application of a slow external force on a tissue,

E. Quaia (✉)
Clinical Research Imaging Centre, Queen's Medical Research Institute, 47 Little France Crescent, Edinburgh EH16 4TJ, UK
e-mail: equaia@ed.ac.uk

A.G. Gennari
Department of Radiology, Cattinara Hospital, University of Trieste, Strada di Fiume 447, 34149 Trieste, Italy

D.-A. Clevert et al. (eds.), *Atlas of Elastosonography*, DOI 10.1007/978-3-319-44201-3_1

such as the probe compression (strain imaging), the effect of viscosity can be disregarded. Conversely, if a high-frequency vibration is applied as in SW imaging, the viscous component will have a major effect which is proportional to the vibration frequency [1].

1.1.1 Strain Compression Imaging

In strain imaging compression (stress) could theoretically be applied in three different ways: on the whole surface, peripherally on a surface, or homogeneously on a volume. Each of them is described by his own modulus: YM, shear modulus, and bulk modulus, respectively. In order to simplify the comprehension, we will focus our discussion on the two-dimensional model avoiding a detailed explanation of the bulk modulus.

As previously said a simple shearing force can be applied to a single portion of an object causing a deformation without volume modification (shear stress, SS). Contrary a deformation could be the result of a compressive force on the whole surface of the body (YM) [5];

- YM evaluation model: if an imaginary rectangular shape of a homogeneous material is rigidly bound along one face and further compressed by a parallel plate on the other, its form will be modified and expanded along the axis perpendicular to the one of the compression force, but its volume will be maintained [6]. Imaging before and after displacement (t_0,…t_n) permits to determine the response of the material to the compression force, and its intrinsic characteristics, until sufficient relaxation has occurred. This theoretical model is more complex in inhomogeneous materials in which different stiffness materials are present within the same medium. In the former model, the compression may be graphically represented as a straight line. Conversely in the latter one, the presence of the inhomogeneity varies the material characteristics and produces a local deviation from the linear slope [6] which depends on the different characteristics of the other materials.
- SS evaluation model: applying the same force but on a different direction (perpendicular to the former and on one edge) to the same imaginary rectangular-shaped model, the block will again modify its form without any volume variation. Once again images will be obtained at different times, previous and during material modification, and the presence of inclusions will perturb the graphical representation in the same way as explained before.

In the purely elastic module described above, stress and strain are linked through the Hook's law. The equation which explains this relation is $\sigma = E \cdot \varepsilon$, where σ is the stress applied, *E* the YM, and $\varepsilon = \Delta L/L$ the longitudinal strain. The deformations occurring in human tissues are far more complex than what explained here, but these two ideal cases approximate the basis of the two imaging modalities: SS exemplifies ARFI imaging, whereas YM describes those produced by transducer compression.

1.1.2 Shear Wave Imaging

In SW imaging, a time-varying force is applied to the tissue. This force can be a limited transient mechanical force or a fixed frequency oscillatory one [3]. After wave generation two types of plane waves propagate independently in the material: SW and pressure waves (PW) [6]. PWs cannot be used in imaging due to the high wave speed which is orders of magnitude faster compared to the SW one [6]. Therefore, SW imaging is based on the propagation of SWs which propagate in the tissues perpendicularly to the ordinal pulse echo longitudinal waves.

SWs are slow transverse waves which attenuate rapidly compared to the diagnostic longitudinal waves and disappear in the MHz ultrasound band, with a propagation frequency below 1 KHz in vivo. Their velocity is 1000 times slower (i.e., $c_s = 1–10$ m/s) compared to longitudinal waves ($c_L = 1540$ m/s) [1, 5]. Maps of YM are derived from the SW propagation speed in order to display material stiffness. Due to the high water content, biological tissues are considered incompressible and, as a consequence, the YM is three times the shear modulus ($E = 2[\nu + 1] \cdot G \approx 3G$, where ν is the Poisson's ratio which is equal to 0.5 in incompressible media and G is the shear modulus) [1, 3]. Another rudiment that a sonographer must kept in mind is that SW does not propagate in nonviscous pure fluid [5].

When the free face of the rectangular shape described above is displaced repetitively, the behavior of the medium obeys to classic wave equation [6]. The displacement can occur at low and high frequencies. At low frequencies the response of the medium will peak at specific natural frequencies typical for each material. At high frequencies the response is different in biological tissues due to the irregular shape of organs and imperfect boundaries [6]. Therefore, in high frequencies of displacement imaging techniques, a multiharmonic excitation model, which will produce a uniform vibration without null point, is necessary [6]. The presence of an inhomogeneity within the medium produces a variation in the vibration pattern which is easily identifiable using multifrequency excitations [6].

All these physical theories and models allowed the development of multiple methods, which have been integrated in clinical practice:

1. Strain elastography (SE)
2. Transient elastography (TE)
3. ARFI
4. SW speed measurement and imaging

Strain elastography Tissue displacement is produced by tissue compression with the probe. Since static compression is subjectively achieved, only strain (ε) is displayed; as a consequence, this type of imaging is only qualitative. Alternatively, pseudo-quantitative methods such as the strain ratio [7] or the comparison of lesion size to the size of the stiffer portion have been used [8].

Transient elastography A controlled vibrating external piston (which acts as a "punch") mounted on a probe with a fixed focal spot is used to either generate or evaluate the SW which has been produced. This type of SW quantification is used essentially by FibroScan™ to evaluate tissue stiffness.

ARFI A focused acoustic radiation force "pushing" pulse is used to deform tissues within a defined region. The probe works as a generator of the push and to monitor tissue displacement sending an imaging pulse prior and after the push impulse. The evaluation of multiple beam lines allows the creation of an image, which displays the intrinsic differences of the tissue.

SW speed measurement and imaging Using ARFI excitation SW are produced in a preselected point of the organ and then the centrifugal propagation of SW from the pushing pulse location is measured [2]. As previously described for ARFI, the probe generates the SW but also images its spread. The application of ARFI at multiple focal zone configuration, in which each one is interrogated in rapid succession, leads to a more complex tissue-SW interaction with a cylindrically shaped SW extending over a larger depth and enabling real-time SW imaging [2]. This multiple focal zone approach has been termed "supersonic shear imaging" (SSI) [9].

1.1.3 Display Methods

Small lesion detection and also the discrimination of multiple discrete small lesions are the major concerns of elastographic imaging.

Strain imaging is now implemented in the majority of ultrasound equipment; however every manufacturer has its own method to measure the displacement, leading to differences in image characteristics (temporal and spatial resolution) and measurement conditions. Several methods are available to image tissue displacement:

1. Spatial correlation method (or speckle tracking method) provides images by tracking the movement of image patterns [1, 2]. If the strain is extremely slight, patterns move while maintaining their speckle pattern. Therefore, setting a region of interest (ROI) and

calculating the spatial correlation of the ROI before and after compression, the quantity of movement is easily calculated [1, 2]. This is the simplest method to measure the 1 direction (D) displacement along the beam axis. In reality, a thorough definition of tissue displacement needs a 2D search, both in the range and in the azimuthal direction, due to the movement that each ROI covers in azimuthal direction in the cross section [1, 2]. The advantages of the speckle tracking method are the ability to measure large displacement, even the one that exceeds the wavelength, and the capability of tracking the ROI movement in 2D and in 3D. On the other hand, this technique has drawbacks as the noise effect susceptibility and the lost of real-time capability when the calculation of correlation requires enormous computational power [1, 2]. In addition the accuracy of this method is limited when the speckle patterns are not clear.

2. Phase difference detection method uses the same technique of color Doppler and tissue Doppler [10]. The phase difference of echo signals created by transmitting repeated pulse is received by an autocorrelation method, which permits the displacement calculation [1, 2]. An excellent real-time capability and the relative robustness to noise are the main advantages of the Doppler methods. Conversely the disadvantages are the capability to measure the only 1D displacement in the beam direction due to the angle dependence and moreover the aliasing errors which may occur measuring a large displacement that exceeds half the wavelength [1, 2].
3. Combined method combines the phase difference detection method and the spatial correlation technique [11, 12]. This technique is nowadays the most common between vendors.

In strain imaging inclusions will be displayed as a local region of lower or higher strain (hard or soft inclusion, respectively). However it is obvious that any inclusion must be larger than the resolution scale of the imaging system or it is not doable to estimate displacements [6]. The definition of multiple inclusions as separate small lesions is similarly related to the imaging system resolution and to any localized effects of stress concentration [6]. In everyday practice additional issues complicate practical considerations as noise, decorrelation, and displacement estimation [13]. To date most vendors propose a translucent, colored, elastogram image which is superimposed on a B-mode image [2] . Although some authors have proposed color scales to characterize pathological findings [14–16], currently different equipment exploits different colors and gray displays. In addition users can modify the color scale as they prefer [2].

SW propagation, which is directly connected to tissue elasticity, is determined in SW elastography to derive tissue elasticity [17]. There are some methods used such as the conventional algorithm time-of-flight (TOF) measurement [18], inversion of the wave equation [19], and estimation of the phase gradient from propagating SW [20]. TOF typically employs a linear regression of the wave arrival time versus position data [1, 2]. Some a priori assumptions to determine the SW speed are adopted such as local homogeneity and known direction of wave propagation, i.e., the arrival time of the wave at the adjacent positions [1, 2]. Anyhow, a systematic description and explanation of the other methods is beyond the purpose of this book. In SW elastography detectability and resolution are all related to wave equation. In fact a small elastic inhomogeneity acts as a source of scattered SW. The degree of this source strength is directly proportional to its elastic contrast, times wave number squared, times the strength of the incident shear wave [6]. Conceptually this overcomes one of the main drawbacks of strain imaging, the inability to image inclusion smaller than wavelength. Even a small inhomogeneity, even one below the resolution possibilities of the imaging system, can be detected as a localized disturbance [6]. Stimulations and experiments have demonstrated that, with increasing of frequencies, the contrast of lesions increases [21] until other frequency-dependent effects, such as lossy behavior, present a practical upper frequency limitation [22]. However the scattered wave pattern due to inherent type of blur, which adds coherently when the two lesions are closely spaced, limits the possibility of differentiation [6]. Moreover, there is an inverse correlation between precision and spatial resolution in SW estimation methods. The use of large propagation distances to compute the wave speed presumes a large homogeneous region. It is typically associated with higher precision and accuracy but lower spatial resolution [23]. Conversely, in everyday practice smaller propagation distances are employed to obtain higher spatial resolution; however, decreasing the distance over which the SW is calculated increases the variance of the estimation at each pixel [2].

It is also mandatory to understand which parameter could be displayed:

- Strain imaging: strain elastography helps the evaluation of strain or normalized strain, geometric measures (size and shape of the altered strain area), strain ratio (defined as the ratio of the lesion strain versus the normal tissue strain, at the same depth), and *E*/*B* size ratio (represented by the ratio of the size of a lesion in the strain image to the size in normal B-mode image). Similarly ARFI imaging shows displacement or normalized displacement, geometric measures, displacement ratio, and *E*/*B* size ratio.
- SW imaging: SW speed, YM converted from SW speed when the assumptions of constant density, homogeneity, isotropy, and incompressibility are fulfilled [2].

In general, strain images have higher spatial resolution, while SW images provide higher contrast resolution: however, when the assumptions used to derive the images do not accurately reflect tissue behaviors, differences between images from different techniques can be anticipated [2].

1.1.4 Artifacts

Even though a comprehensive and systematic review of all artifacts of elastographic imaging is beyond the purpose of this book, a sonographer should be aware of at least some of them.

In strain imaging stress is not homogeneously distributed within tissues; moreover the relatively small surface of the probe produces poor penetration and homogeneity of stress and strain [5]. A footprint extended compressor seemed to overcome those issues [24], but similar results are guaranteed positioning two fingers, of the free hand, in front of, and posteriorly to the probe reaching a deeper and more homogeneous strain [5]. Furthermore soft tissues adjacent to hard tissues strain more after compression creating "edge-enhancement" effects [5]. Other sources of artifacts are out-of-plane structures that modify in-plane strain and slippery boundaries [25, 26]. The thorough knowledge of artifacts improve comprehension of images displayed and ease their understanding.

SW imaging counts both transient elastography, ARFI imaging, and SSI. The Quantitative Imaging Biomarker Alliance of the Radiology Society of North America (RSNA) performed an interlaboratory study comparing SW speeds from four different elastography machines (FibroScan, Philips, ACUSON S2000, and Aixplorer) in 2013 [27]. The study demonstrated the presence of variation of SW velocity values using different machines and at different depths [27]. Moreover, SW velocities vary according to the patient's position, number of measurements, acquisition depth, and the representative values such as median or mean values [27–29]. Other studies demonstrated the effects of transducers on evaluation of SW velocities between different machines and depths [30]. In conclusion cautious evaluation and usage of quantitative-derived data of SW velocities and YM values should be applied, particularly in comparing values between vendors, acquisition depths, and usage of different transducers.

1.2 Image Gallery

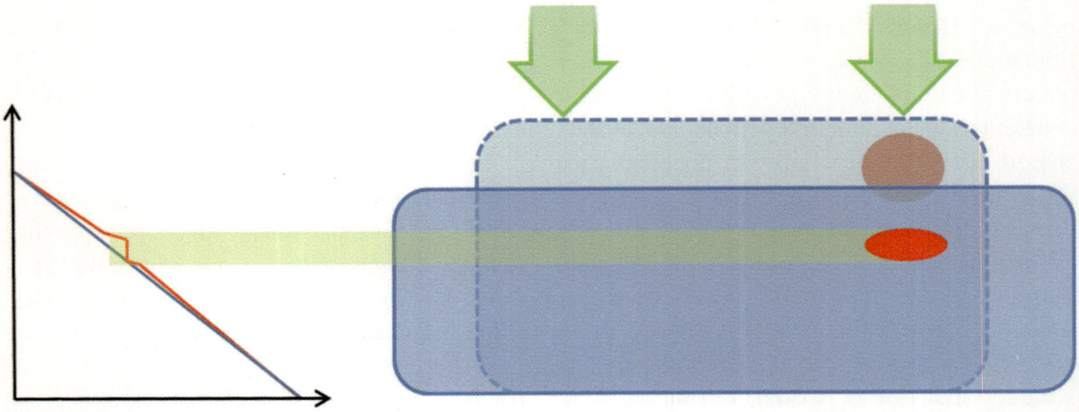

Fig. 1.1 Exemplification of the pure stress (*arrows*) applied on the surface of a rectangular shaped homogeneous medium, which deforms it maintaining its volume. The *blue line* on the diagram represents the graphic correlation, whereas the *red line* depicts the modification related to the presence of an inhomogeneity within the same material

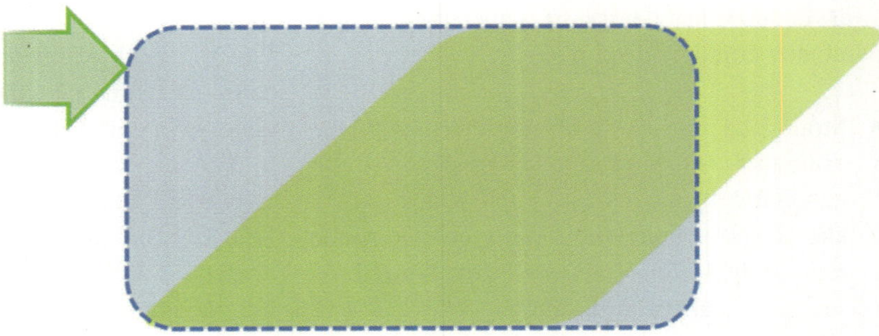

Fig. 1.2 Exemplification of a shear stress (*arrow*) applied on an edge of the rectangular shaped homogeneous medium deforms it maintaining its volume

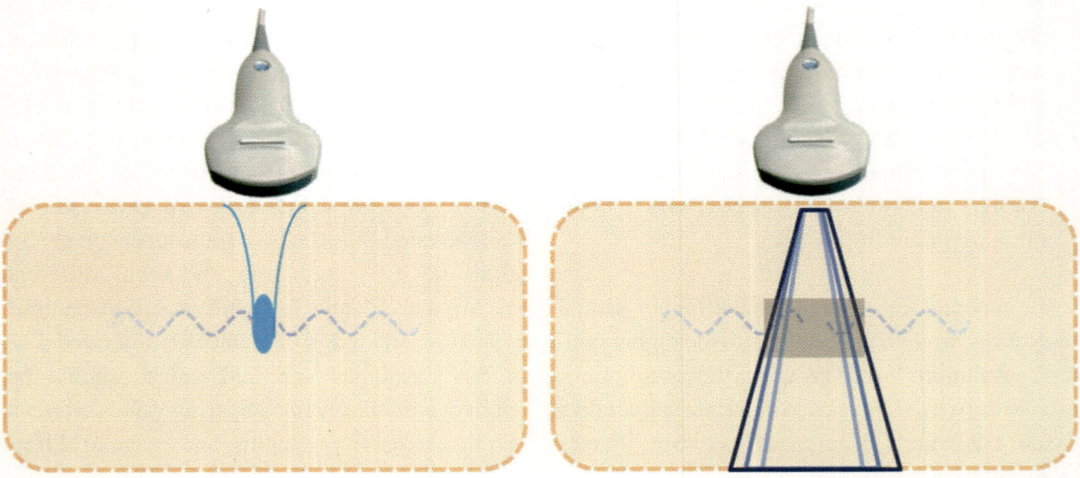

Fig. 1.3 An ARFI model in which the probe initially produces the push pulse (*blue oval shaped figure*) at a defined spot. After that the SW generated travel away from it. The probe is then switched to imaging modality and the progression of the SW is read at different times within a predefined area

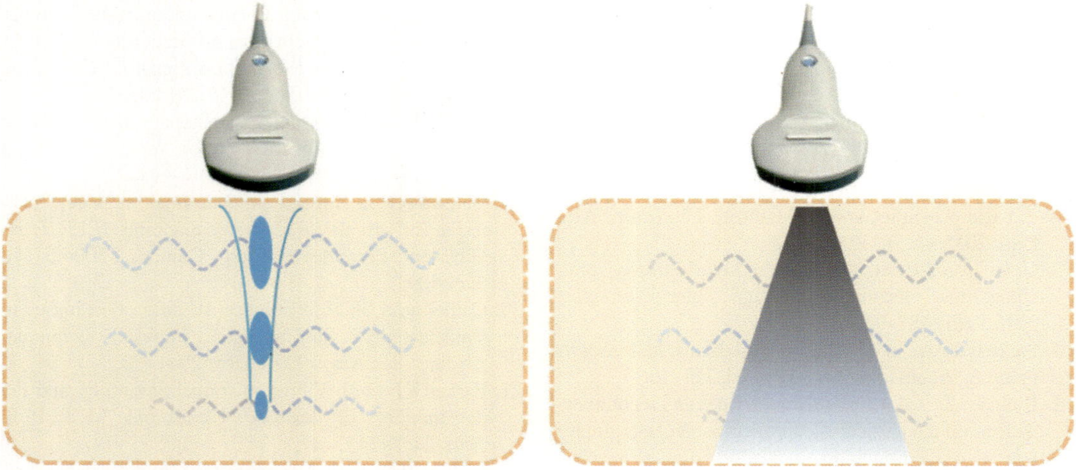

Fig. 1.4 The SSI produces different push pulse at various depths producing a cylindrically shaped SW extending over a larger depth. The high-frequency probe then permits a real-time SW imaging of large areas

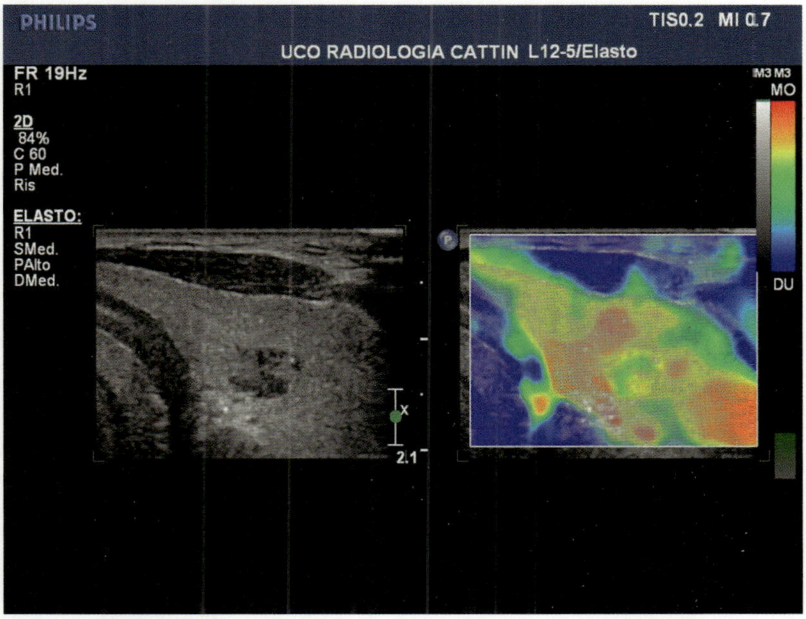

Fig. 1.5 A translucent, colored, elastogram image is superimposed on a B-mode image of a nodule within thyroid gland

References

1. Shiina T. JSUM ultrasound elastography practice guidelines: basics and terminology. J Med Ultrason. 2013;40(4):309–23.
2. Shiina T, et al. WFUMB guidelines and recommendations for clinical use of ultrasound elastography: part 1: basic principles and terminology. Ultrasound Med Biol. 2015;41(5):1126–47.
3. Gennisson J-L, et al. Ultrasound elastography: principles and techniques. Diagn Interv Imaging. 2013;94(5):487–95.
4. Sarvazyan A, et al. Biophysical bases of elasticity imaging. Acoust Imaging. 1995;21:223–40.
5. Bambers J, et al. EFSUMB guidelines and recommendations on the clinical use of ultrasound elastography. Part 1: basic principles and technology. Ultraschall Med. 2013;34(2):169–84.
6. Parker KJ, et al. A unified view of imaging the elastic properties of tissues. J Acoust Soc Am. 2005;117(5):2705–12.
7. Ueno E, et al. New quantitative method in breast elastography: fat lesion ratio (FLR). RSNA 2007 Scientific Assembly and Annual Meeting, 25–30 Nov. Chicago. p. 25–30.
8. Garra BS, et al. Elastography of breast lesions: initial clinical result. Radiology. 1997;202(1):79–86.
9. Bercoff J, et al. Monitoring thermally-induced lesions with supersonic shear imaging. Ultrason Imaging. 2004;26(2):71–84.
10. Thomas A. Doppler and strain imaging for evaluating tissue elasticity of breast lesions. Acad Radiol. 2007;14(5):522–9.
11. Shiina T. Strain imaging using combined RF and envelope autocorrection processing. In: Proceedings of the 1996 IEEE Int Ultrasonocs Symposium; 1996. p. 1331–6.
12. Shiina T, et al. Real time elasticity imaging using the combined autocorrelation method. J Med Ultrason. 2002;29(3):119–28.
13. Srinivasan S, et al. Tradeoff between axial resolution and signal-to-noise ratio in elastography. Ultrasound Med Biol. 2003;29(6):847–66.
14. Itoh A, et al. Breast disease: clinical application of US elastography for diagnosis. Radiology. 2006;239(2):341–50.
15. Rago T, et al. Elastography: new developments in ultrasound for predicting malignancy in thyroid nodules. J Clin Endocrinol Metab. 2007;92(8):2917–22.
16. Asteria C, et al. US-elastography in the differential diagnosis of benign and malignant thyroid nodules. Thyroid. 2008;18(5):523–31.
17. Engel AJ, et al. Enabling real-time ultrasound imaging of soft tissue mechanical properties by simplification of the shear wave motion equation. Conf Proc IEEE Eng Med Biol Soc. 2015;2015:3831–4.
18. Palmeri ML, et al. Quantifying hepatic shear modulus in vivo using acoustic radiation force. Ultrasound Med Biol. 2008;34(4):546–58.
19. Bercoff J, et al. Supersonic shear imaging: a new technique for soft tissue elasticity mapping. IEEE Trans Ultrason Ferroelectr Freq Control. 2004;51(4):396–409.
20. Catheline S, et al. A solution of diffraction biases in sonoelasticity: the acoustic impulse technique. J Acoust Soc Am. 1999;105(5):2941–50.
21. Parker KJ, et al. Vibration sonoelastography and the detectability of lesions. Ultrasound Med Biol. 1998;24(9):1437–47.
22. Walker WF, et al. A fundamental limit on delay estimation using partially correlated speckle signals. IEEE Trans Ultrason Ferroelectr Freq Control. 1995;42(2):301–8.
23. Rouze NC, et al. Parameters affecting the resolution and accuracy of 2-D quantitative shear wave images. IEEE Trans Ultrason Ferroelectr Freq Control. 2012;59(8):1729–40.
24. Doyley MM, et al. A freehand approach elastographic imaging approach for clinical breast imaging: system development and performance evaluation. Ultrasound Med Biol. 2001;27(10):1347–57.
25. Thitaikumar A, et al. Effect of lesion boundary conditions in axial strain elastogram: a parametric study. Ultrasound Med Biol. 2007;33(9):1463–7.
26. Chakraborty A, et al. Slip elastography: a novel method for visualizing and characterizing adherence between two surface in contact. Ultrasonics. 2012;52(3):364–76.
27. Carlsen JF, et al. A comparative study of strain and shear wave elastography in an elasticity phantom. AJR Am J Roentgenol. 2015;204(3):W236–42.
28. Wang CZ, et al. Influence of measurement depth on the stiffness assessment of healthy liver with real-time shear wave elastography. Ultrasound Med Biol. 2014;40(3):461–9.
29. Tozaki M, et al. Ultrasonographic tissue quantification of the breast using acoustic radiation force impulse technology: phantom study and clinical application. Jpn J Radiol. 2011;29(8):598–603.
30. Shin HJ, et al. Comparison of shear wave velocities on ultrasound elastography between different machines, transducers, and depths: a phantom study. Eur Radiol. 2016;26(10):3361–7. doi: 10.1007/s00330-016-4212-y. Epub 2016 Jan 26.

Part II

Clinical Applications

Liver and Spleen

2

Emilio Quaia, Anita Spezzacatene, Irene Zorzenon, Valentina Ciaravino, Alessandro Sarno, Giorgia Tedesco, Dirk-André Clevert, and Mirko D'Onofrio

2.1 Liver

2.1.1 Introduction

Liver diseases represent an important health problem, diffuse worldwide. The diagnosis of liver fibrosis is crucial in order to make decisions about treatment, evaluate treatment efficacy and assess patient prognosis.

At present both invasive and non-invasive techniques are available for the diagnosis of liver fibrosis. Liver biopsy is an invasive technique that has been considered for a long time the gold standard to assess liver fibrosis [1], but it has some intrinsic limitations, mainly related to complications due to its invasive approach [2], possible sampling errors and interobserver variability [3]. In the last years, ultrasonographic (US) elastography techniques have been developed in order to replace liver biopsy for the evaluation of liver fibrosis, and at present they are considered valid diagnostic and prognostic tools in this field [4]. Transient elastography (TE), performed with the Fibroscan® device, is considered the best and most widely used non-invasive method to assess liver fibrosis, even though also shear-wave elastography (SWE) using acoustic radiation force impulse (ARFI) with point SWE (pSWE) (Virtual Touch Quantification (VTQ, Siemens Healthcare, Mountain View, Calif) and ElastPQ (Philips Healthcare, Bothell, Wash)), two-dimensional SWE (2D-SWE) (SuperSonic Imagine (Aix-en-Provence, France), Siemens Healthcare (Mountain View, Calif), Toshiba Medical Systems (Tochigi Otawara, Japan) and GE (Waukesha, Wis)) and three-dimensional SWE (3D-SWE) have recently shown promising results. US elastography is largely in use in clinical practice and is applied for the diagnosis of liver fibrosis in a wide range of liver diseases, such as chronic hepatitis C (also in recurrent forms after liver transplantation), chronic hepatitis B, alcoholic liver disease, non-alcoholic fatty liver disease (NAFLD), non-alcoholic steatohepatitis (NASH) and liver cirrhosis.

E. Quaia, (✉)
Clinical Research Imaging Centre, Queen's Medical Research Institute, 47 Little France Crescent, Edinburgh EH16 4TJ, UK
e-mail: equaia@ed.ac.uk

A. Spezzacatene • I. Zorzenon
Department of Radiology, Cattinara Hospital, University of Trieste, Strada di Fiume 447, 34149 Trieste, Italy

V. Ciaravino • A. Sarno • G. Tedesco • M. D'Onofrio
Department of Radiology, GB Rossi University Hospital, University of Verona, Verona, Italy

D.-A. Clevert
Interdisciplinary Ultrasound-Center
Department of Clinical Radiology, University of Munich-Grosshadern Campus, Marchioninistr. 15, 81377 Munich, Germany

D.-A. Clevert et al. (eds.), *Atlas of Elastosonography*, DOI 10.1007/978-3-319-44201-3_2

2.1.2 Chronic Hepatitis C

Chronic hepatitis C is a long-course disease characterized by progressive hepatic fibrosis, which very often leads to cirrhosis, hepatocellular carcinoma and the need for liver transplantation. Evaluation of liver fibrosis is of great relevance in the follow-up of affected patients, and hepatic ultrasound elastography represents a valid option to liver biopsy, a more invasive approach. Transient elastography (TE) was the first ultrasound-based elastographic technique introduced in 2003 for the study of hepatic diseases, and it was extensively validated in patients with chronic hepatitis C [5]. TE has a high diagnostic accuracy for the detection of early cirrhosis in chronic HCV-infected patients (mean AUROC of 0.94) [6–8], and it is useful to stratify these patients for treatment [9]. However, some studies showed that it is more accurate in the differentiation between absence or mild fibrosis and significant fibrosis or cirrhosis rather than distinguish contiguous stages of fibrosis [4, 6, 7]. TE is also accurate in the diagnosis of liver fibrosis in patients with HCV/HIV co-infection [10] and in patients with recurrence of HCV after liver transplantation [11]. Other ultrasound elastography techniques have been developed and tested for the study of hepatic fibrosis in patients with chronic hepatitis C, such as pSWE using acoustic radiation force impulse (ARFI) and 2D-SWE. The accuracy of ARFI for the diagnosis of liver fibrosis is considered similar to TE [12], even though it is still dependent on different shear wave methodologies and different brand of scanners. Real-time 2D-SWE is considered an accurate method for the assessment of fibrosis in many liver diseases, including chronic viral hepatitis. Indeed, it is able to distinguish not only different stages of liver fibrosis but also liver fibrosis from cirrhosis and compensated from decompensated cirrhosis [13], with an accuracy even better than TE [14–16].

2.1.3 Chronic Hepatitis B

Patients with chronic hepatitis B can be divided in two groups: patients with inactive state of disease and those with active hepatitis, who are more likely to develop liver fibrosis and eventually cirrhosis. Elastography is a useful and validated tool developed to evaluate liver fibrosis in order to differentiate patients with inactive HBV infection (absence of fibrosis) from those with active hepatitis (significant fibrosis) [9]. Despite the elevated accuracy of TE, confounding factors such as elevated transaminases (particularly alanine transaminase (ALT) levels) may affect liver stiffness measurements, and therefore they should always be taken in consideration. For this reason it has been suggested to adapt cut-off values of liver stiffness to different levels of ALT [17] or, as an alternative, to correct measurements for the ALT levels in probability scores [18].

2.1.4 Non-alcoholic Fatty Liver Disease (NAFLD)

NAFLD represents the most common liver disorder in developed countries [19]. It includes a wide range of diseases, from steatosis to non-alcoholic steatohepatitis (NASH) and potentially cirrhosis, complicated by hepatocellular carcinoma (HCC). Diagnosis and differentiation of different stages of fibrosis are therefore crucial in the management of patients, in particular to decide treatment, predict prognosis and evaluate response to treatment [9]. Compared to liver biopsy, TE shows high sensitivity and specificity in the diagnosis of liver fibrosis, in particular in the evaluation of higher stages ($>F3$) of fibrosis, with a moderate accuracy for stage $F2$ or higher [20].

Among other ultrasound elastography techniques, pSWE with ARFI showed promising results in patients with NAFLD and NASH. Specifically, it is considered not inferior to TE, with a significant correlation between median velocity measured by using ARFI and severity of liver fibrosis [21].

2.1.5 Alcoholic Liver Disease

The presence of fibrosis, and in particular its progression to cirrhosis, is an important predictor of prognosis in patients with alcoholic liver disease.

Currently, transient elastography using Fibroscan® is considered the most reliable non-invasive test to diagnose advanced liver fibrosis and cirrhosis in patients with alcoholic liver disease [22].

It represents an important diagnostic tool to rule out liver cirrhosis (*F*4) in these patients, provided that the pretest probability is about 51 %, and it may also help in ruling out severe fibrosis (*F*3 or worse) [23]. pSWE with ARFI and SWE Supersonic Imaging represents valid alternatives to TE to stage liver fibrosis in alcoholic liver disease, with comparable accuracy [24]. However, when there is still doubt on the stage of liver fibrosis by non-invasive techniques, liver biopsy remains the alternative option.

2.1.6 Liver Cirrhosis

Liver cirrhosis is a chronic pathologic condition, representing the end stage of many liver diseases, and it is frequently the substrate for the development of severe complications such as portal hypertension and hepatocellular carcinoma. Liver cirrhosis is the result of progressive subverting of liver architecture, with fibrotic deposition, vascular alterations and regenerative nodule formation. It is very important to recognize liver fibrosis in order to monitor the progression of disease and make early decisions. US elastography techniques such as TE and pSWE (ARFI) represent reliable and non-invasive methods in the non-invasive assessment of liver stiffness. It is recommended to obtain ten stiffness measurements in the same location with at least 60 % of valid shots and an interquartile range (IQR) ≤30 % of the median liver stiffness measurement value [25]. In a recent meta-analysis, Tsochatzis et al. proposed the following cut-offs to discriminate between different stages of fibrosis by TE: 6 kPa for $F \geq 1$, 7.2 kPa for $F \geq 2$, 9.6 kPa for $F \geq 3$ and 14.5 kPa for $F = 4$ [26]. Sporea et al. found a high significant correlation between TE and 2D-SWE measurements, with 2D-SWE cut-offs ranging from 7.1 kPa (presence of fibrosis) to 11.5 kPa (liver cirrhosis) [16]. According to a recent meta-analysis by Bota et al., ARFI elastography is considered a valid method to assess liver fibrosis, with a higher rate of reliable measurements and similar predictive value to TE for significant fibrosis and cirrhosis [27].

However, TE is the most largely used technique currently, and in particular its role in the prediction of portal hypertension (in correlation with liver stiffness measurements) and development of oesophageal varices in patients with liver cirrhosis has been largely investigated, as long as in the screening for the risk of hepatocellular carcinoma (HCC) [8, 28–30].

2.1.7 Liver Steatosis

Fatty liver represents a condition wherein large vacuoles of triglycerides accumulate in liver cells via the process called steatosis. Liver steatosis is commonly associated to excessive alcohol intake (alcoholic liver disease) or non-alcoholic causes (NAFLD) such as obesity and metabolic syndrome.

TE has been demonstrated to be reliable for the non-invasive prediction of fibrosis in NAFLD patients, and, simultaneously with liver stiffness measurement, it is also possible to assess the degree of liver steatosis, thanks to a novel controlled attenuation parameter (CAP) developed for Fibroscan® [31].

2.1.8 Focal Liver Masses and HCC

Liver elastography provides additional information for the differential diagnosis of focal liver masses. Recent studies demonstrate that hepatocellular carcinomas (HCCs) generally appear softer (lower ARFI values) than the surrounding liver, whereas metastases, cholangiocellular carcinomas (CCC) and haemangiomas generally appear harder (higher ARFI values) than that of the surrounding liver despite some controversies among studies [32, 33]. Because haemangiomas, CCC and metastases were evaluated in patients without chronic liver disease in most studies [34, 35], ARFI values seemed consistently higher than those of a background liver. In contrast, because HCCs were evaluated in patients with chronic liver disease and diverse degrees of background liver fibrosis, the comparative results between ARFI values of HCCs and those of background liver differed among studies based on the characteristics of each study cohort [32, 34, 35]. Some researchers have attempted to suggest a cut-off ARFI value for distinguishing malignant liver masses from benign masses, but results are discordant, and further research is needed to prevent potential bias due to heterogeneity of the masses and to confirm the clinically applicable cut-off values for ARFI elastography [33].

A recent meta-analysis of 17 prospective cohort studies on 7058 patients with chronic liver disease (CLD) shows that non-invasive measurement of liver stiffness may be a useful tool in identifying patients with CLD at risk for progression to clinical events. In particular, a high liver stiffness measurement is able to predict future risk of hepatic decompensation, overall mortality and HCC in a dose-dependent manner: each unit of liver stiffness measurement is associated with an incremental 11 % increased risk of HCC [36]. In CLD patients, the diagnosis of less than 2 cm in diameter tumour may be more difficult with contrast imaging techniques due to the risk of false negative. Fifty-six to 64 % of cirrhotic patients with small nodules are hypovascular, and in these small nodules, 2D real-time elastography (RTE) with Supersonic Imaging may be a better alternative to contrast-enhanced US (CEUS) and can eliminate the need for liver biopsy, which cannot be done due to contraindications and which is also prone to sample errors and false-negative results [37]. Another study demonstrated that also in HBV patients receiving antiviral therapy, the prognostic value of TE may be better than that of histological information in assessing the risk of HCC development [38]. Therefore, liver stiffness measurement may evolve from its role as a diagnostic test to a surveillance procedure that actively helps in the management of patients at the highest need for vigilance, but further high-quality, prospective cohort studies in patients at similar (early) stages of CLD receiving similar treatment are needed. Some studies have proposed using ARFI technique to assess the outcome of radio frequency ablation (RFA) treatment in liver carcinoma as one alternative technique in respect to contrast-enhanced ultrasound (CEUS), showing discordant results: on one hand virtual touch tissue imaging (VTI) technique cannot demonstrate residual tumour post RFA [39], and on the other, recurrent HCCs were found to be softer [40].

2.2 Spleen

The main application of elastography in the spleen is the evaluation of patients affected by chronic liver disease in order to determine the risk of portal hypertension. Recent studies have shown that spleen stiffness correlates with hepatic fibrosis, portal hypertension and the risk of oesophageal varices in patients with chronic liver disease.

Portal hypertension is a common consequence of chronic liver disease, leading to the formation of oesophageal and gastric varices and other severe complications, such as portosystemic encephalopathy, ascites, sepsis and liver failure [41].

The gold standard for the evaluation of portal hypertension is the hepatic venous pressure gradient (HVPG), which, unfortunately, is an invasive and expensive procedure and is not routinely available in clinical practice. Therefore spleen elastography has been proposed as one of the possible non-invasive methods for determining portal venous pressure [42]. Portal hypertension determinates histological changes in the spleen such as hyperplasia among splenic histiocytes, arterial terminal lengthening, increased white pulp volume and even fibrosis between splenic trabeculae. These changes result in increased splenic elasticity and may be quantified by transient elastography (TE) or ARFI [43–46].

One recent study has demonstrated that the spleen and liver stiffness measurements obtained by TE were more accurate than other parameters and suggested their use as a non-invasive assessment and in monitoring portal hypertension and oesophageal varices. Although TE is widely applied to stage chronic liver disease, there is mounting evidence that its diagnostic accuracy is far from being optimal, owing to several confounders such as liver cell inflammation, cholestasis and steatosis which may overcome the correct assessment of liver fibrosis. The measurement of spleen stiffness may therefore represent an attractive as well as a challenging opportunity to elude these liver TE confounders, thereby improving the non-invasive assessment of disease severity [47].

Splenic elasticity has a close linear relationship with HVPG and can help predict the presence of oesophageal varices in patients with chronic liver disease [48]. Oesophageal varices are present in 40 % of patients with compensated and 60 % of those with decompensated liver cirrhosis, and the major risk is represented by massive haemorrhage (the mortality rate of the first bleeding episode in these patients reaching up to 40 %). Performing an esophagogastroduodenoscopy (EGD) still remains the best way to diagnose and evaluate oesophageal and gastric varices and the risk of variceal bleeding; however, it is expensive for the health system and unpleasant for the patient. Therefore, identification of alternative, non-invasive parameters for surveillance of oesophageal varices in patients with liver cirrhosis would restrict its use only to those cases that necessarily need it, resulting in an increased compliance of the patients to surveillance protocol and a decreased risk of procedure-related complications [42]. Recent studies demonstrate that spleen stiffness is superior to liver stiffness, spleen length and Child-Pugh score in predicting variceal haemorrhage [49], showing an excellent sensitivity (96 %) and specificity (88 %) and a 96 % negative predictive value with ARFI measurements [50].

However, these studies show that the reproducibility of spleen stiffness measurements in different populations depends on the expertise of the operator, and in order to achieve a good agreement between measurements, a training period is required. Another disadvantage includes the relativeness of the indirect evaluation. Further studies with larger series of patients should be performed to compare the elasticity values of normal and pathologic tissues to determine the diagnostic role of those techniques. Finally, sonographic spleen stiffness may be used for surveillance of transjugular intrahepatic portosystemic shunt (TIPS) function in chronic liver disease patients. Spleen stiffness has been demonstrated to be altered after TIPS placement, and this change can be a useful surrogate for evaluating functional changes in the TIPS [51]. There is minimal information available for the use of elastography in focal splenic masses.

2.3 Image Gallery

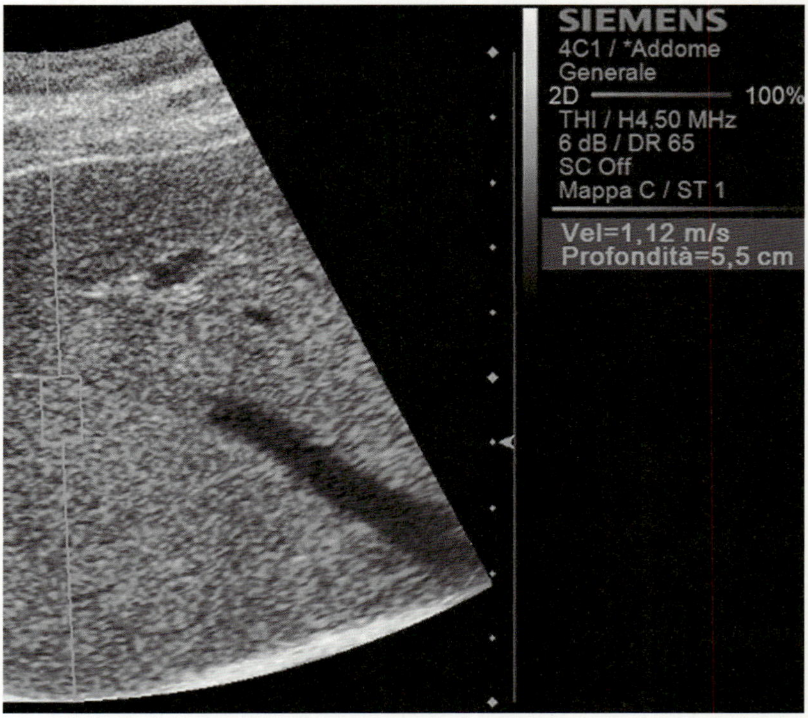

Fig. 2.1 ARFI liver. Normal value in healthy liver

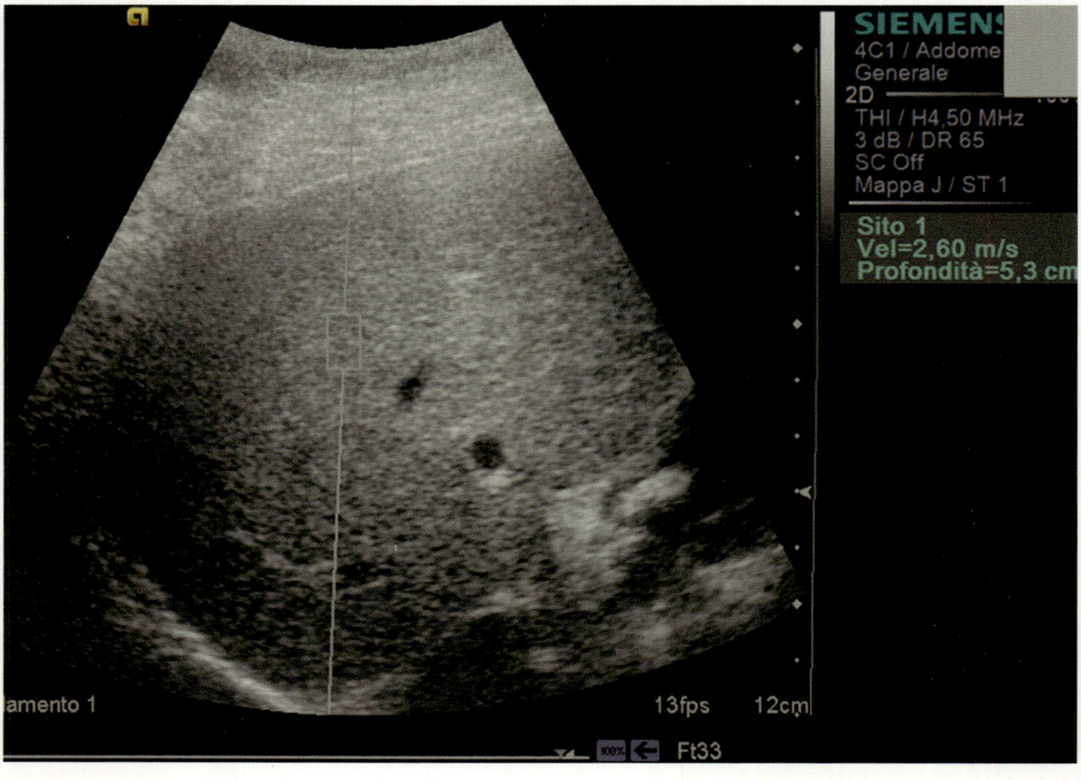

Fig. 2.2 ARFI liver. High value in cirrhotic liver

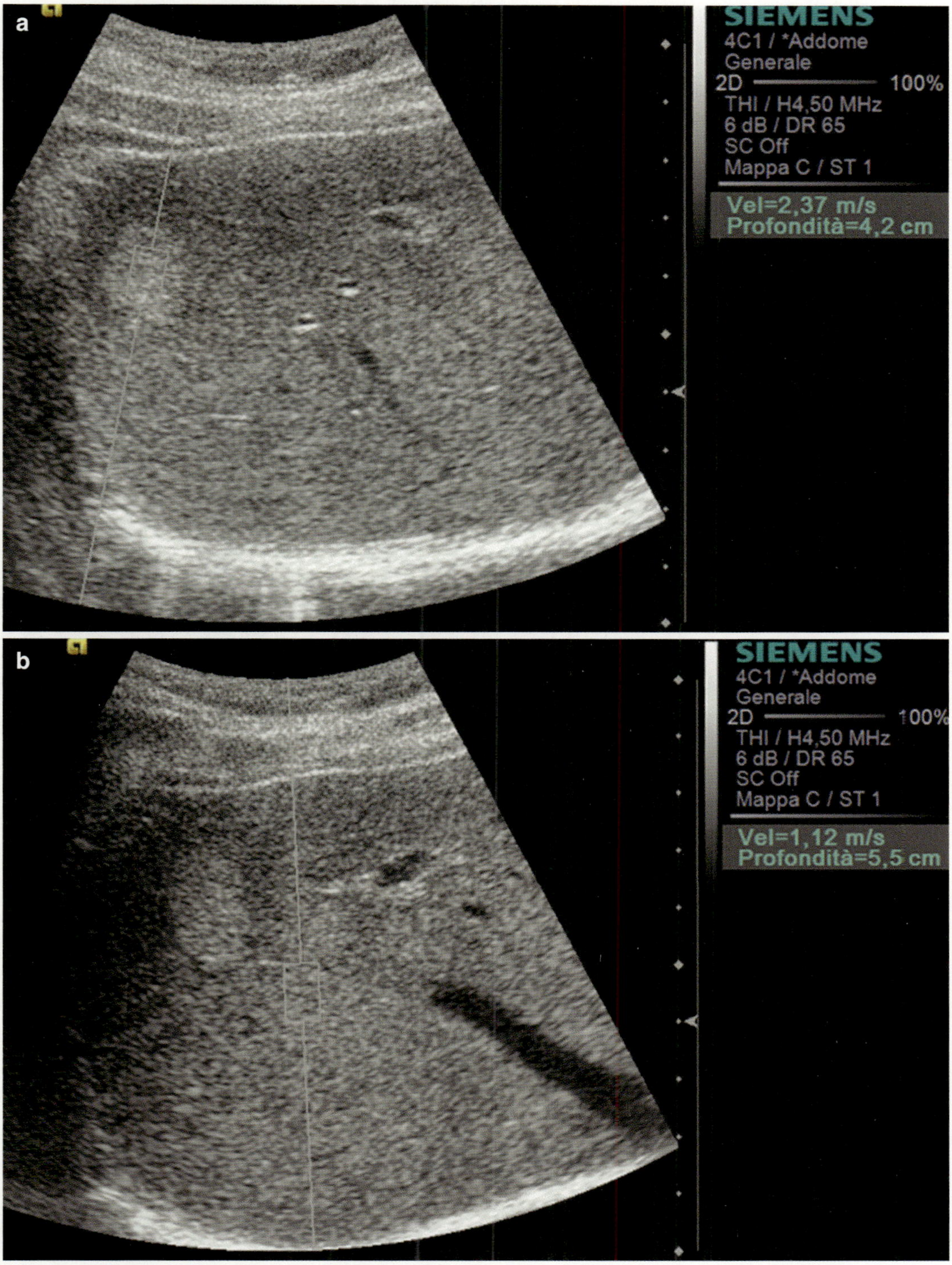

Fig. 2.3 Haemangioma. Higher value in the focal hyperechoic liver lesion (**a**) in respect to the adjacent liver parenchyma (**b**)

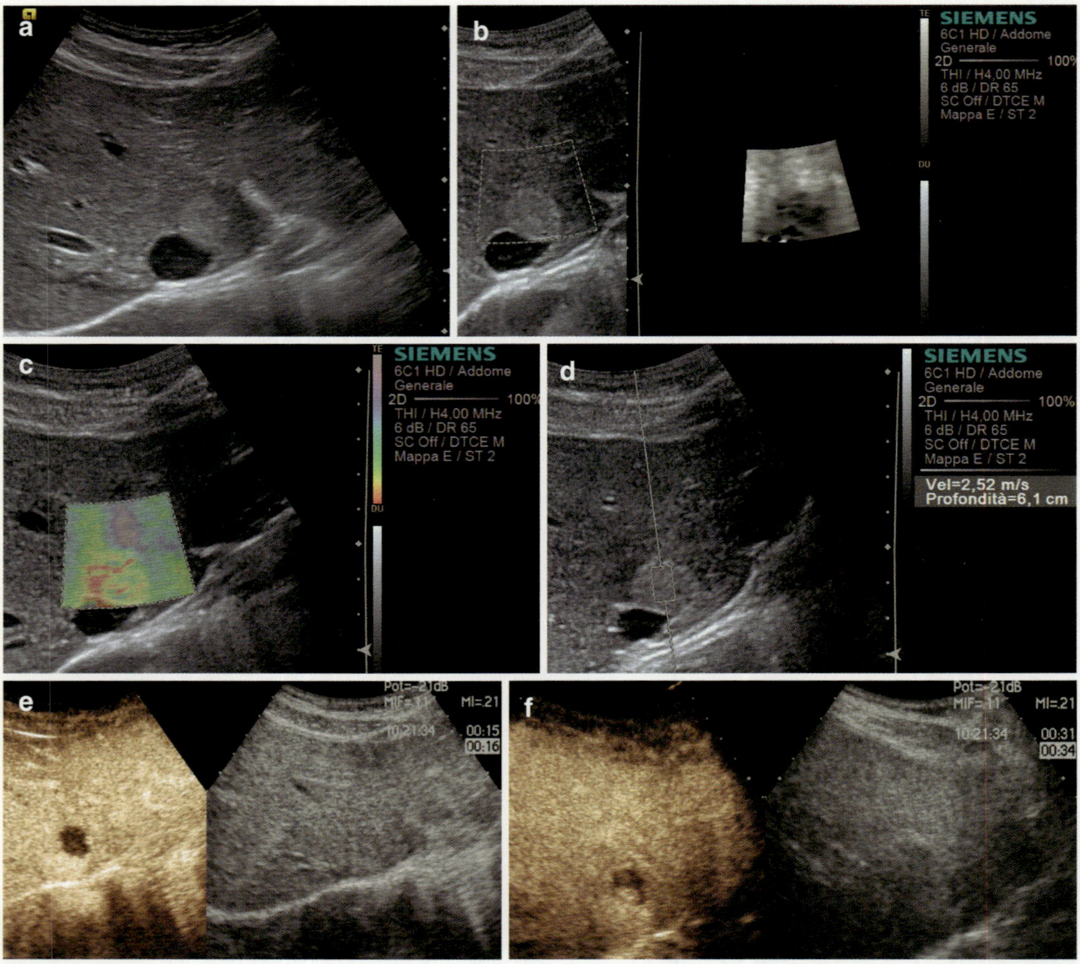

Fig. 2.4 Haemangioma (**a**–**f**) complete US study: round-shaped hyperechoic mass (**a**) resulting stiff (*green*, *yellow and red* in **c** and *dark* in **b**) due to sclerosis in the elastogram. At the quantitative ARFI elastography, a velocity value of 2,52 m/s is detected (**d**). At CEUS the lesion typically shows a globular enhancement in the peripheral area of the lesion in the arterial phase with progressive centripetal fill-in (**e** and **f**)

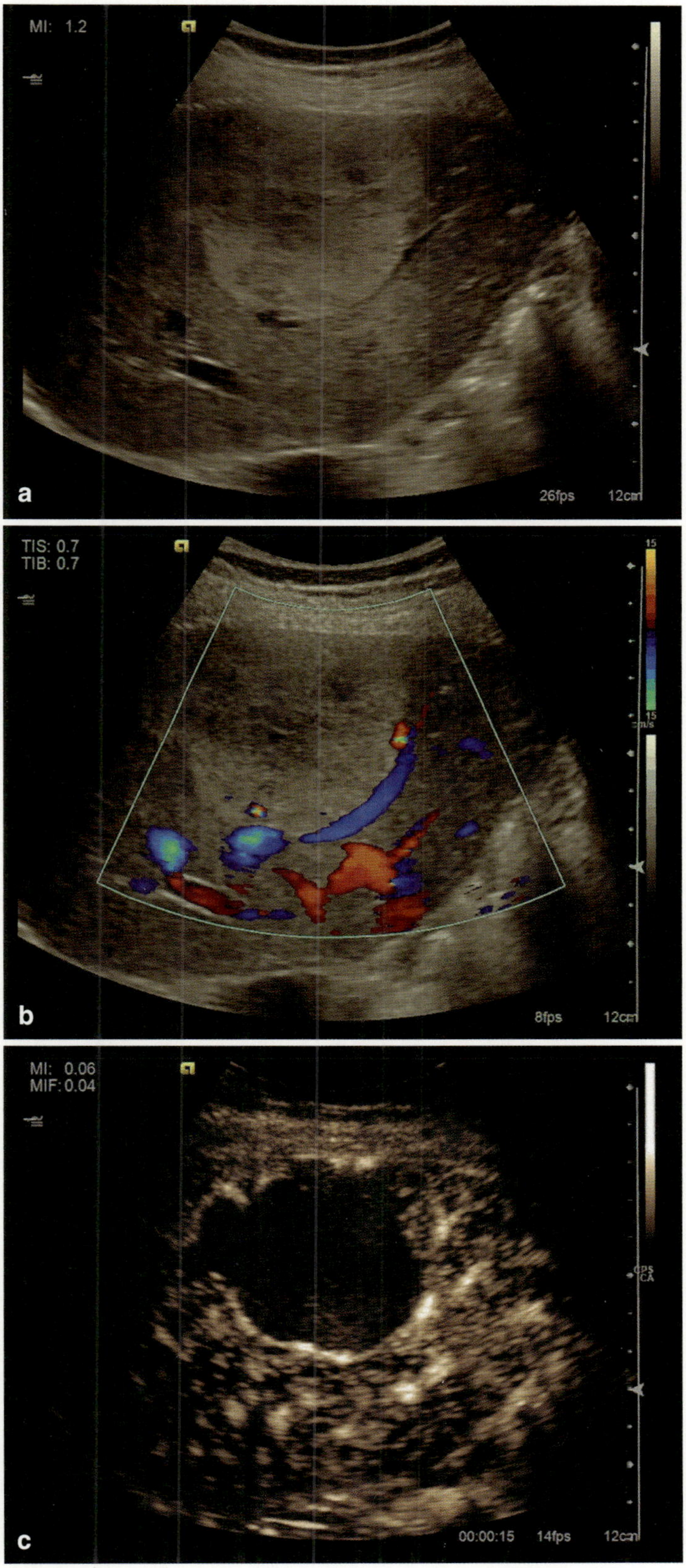

Fig. 2.5 Haemangioma. (**a**) B-mode ultrasound demonstrates a hyperechoic liver lesion. (**b**) Colour Doppler ultrasound demonstrates no increased vascularity of the liver lesion in comparison to the surrounding tissue. (**c**) Contrast-enhanced ultrasound depicted a peripheral nodular enhancement of the tumour in the arterial phases. (**d**) Contrast-enhanced ultrasound depicted a growing of the peripheral nodular enhancement of the tumour in the portal venous phase. (**e**) In the late phase, there is still the peripheral nodular enhancement of the tumour visible which matches with a haemangioma with central thrombotic changes. (**f**) In VTI mode elastography, the haemangioma appears in dark grey indicating a stiff lesion in comparison to the surrounding liver tissue. (**g**) In VTQ mode, the shear wave velocity was measured in the haemangioma with a velocity of $v = 3.30$ m/s. (**h**) In VTQ mode, the shear wave velocity was measured in the liver tissue with a velocity of $v = 1.84$ m/s. (**i**) In sonoelastography, the haemangioma appears in *red* as an indicator for a very stiff tissue. The border of the lesions is displayed well in this technique

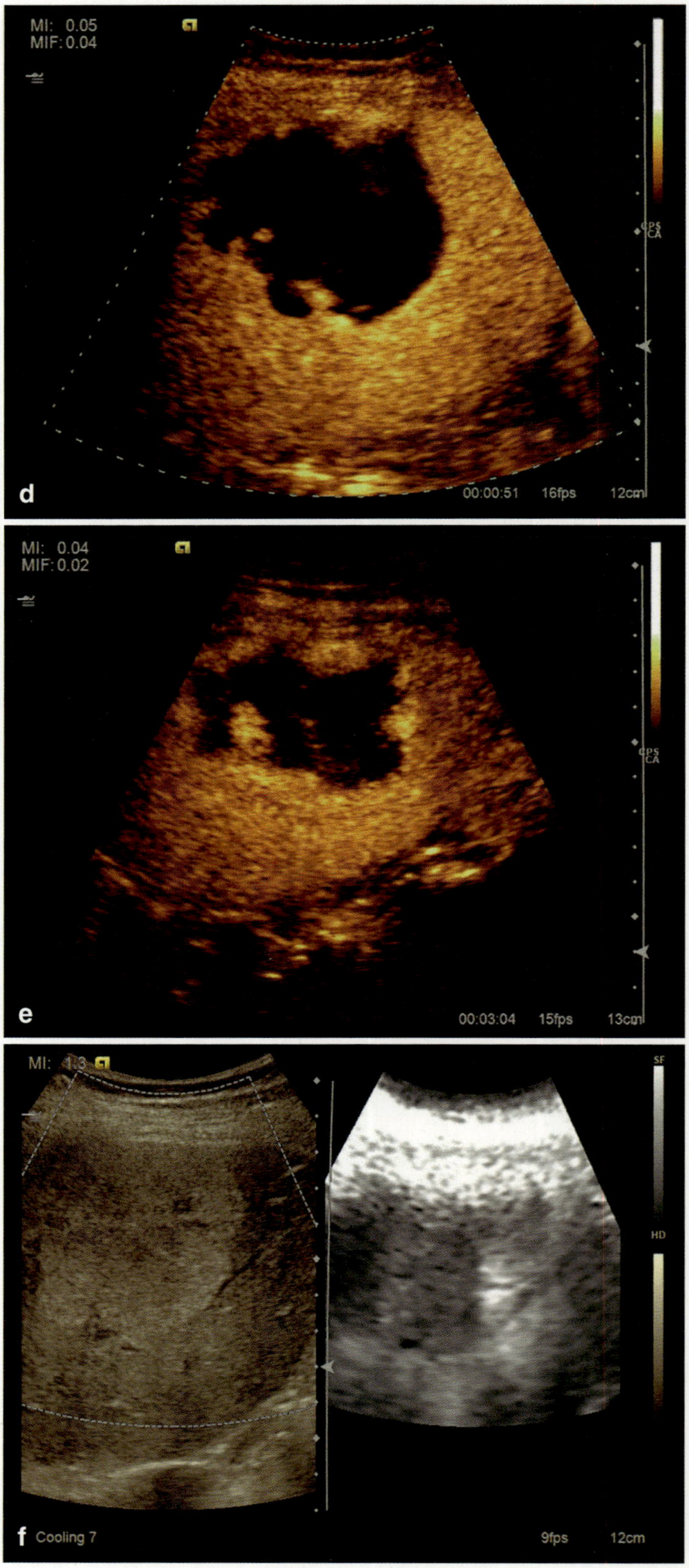

Fig. 2.5 (continued)

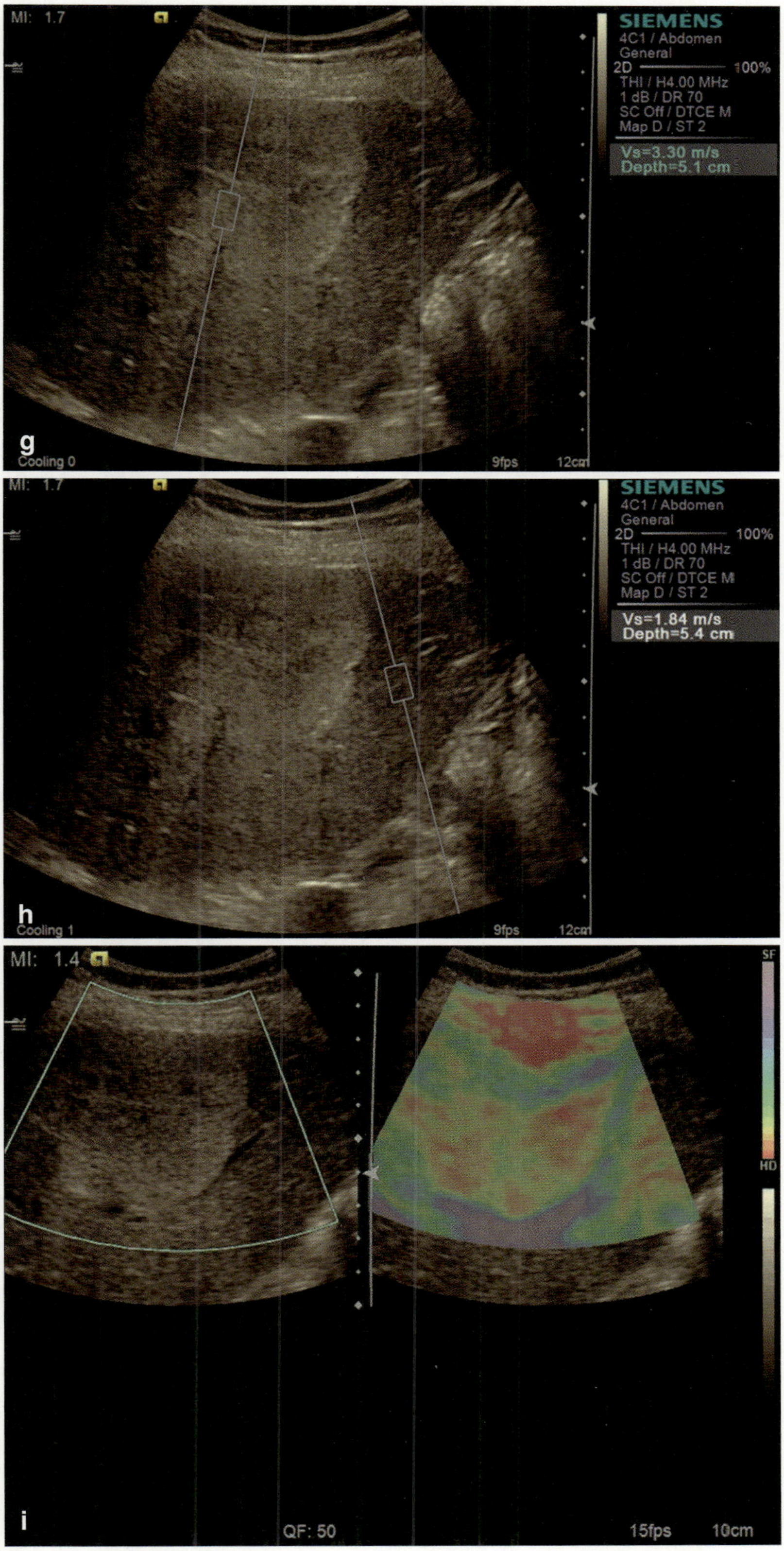

Fig. 2.5 (continued)

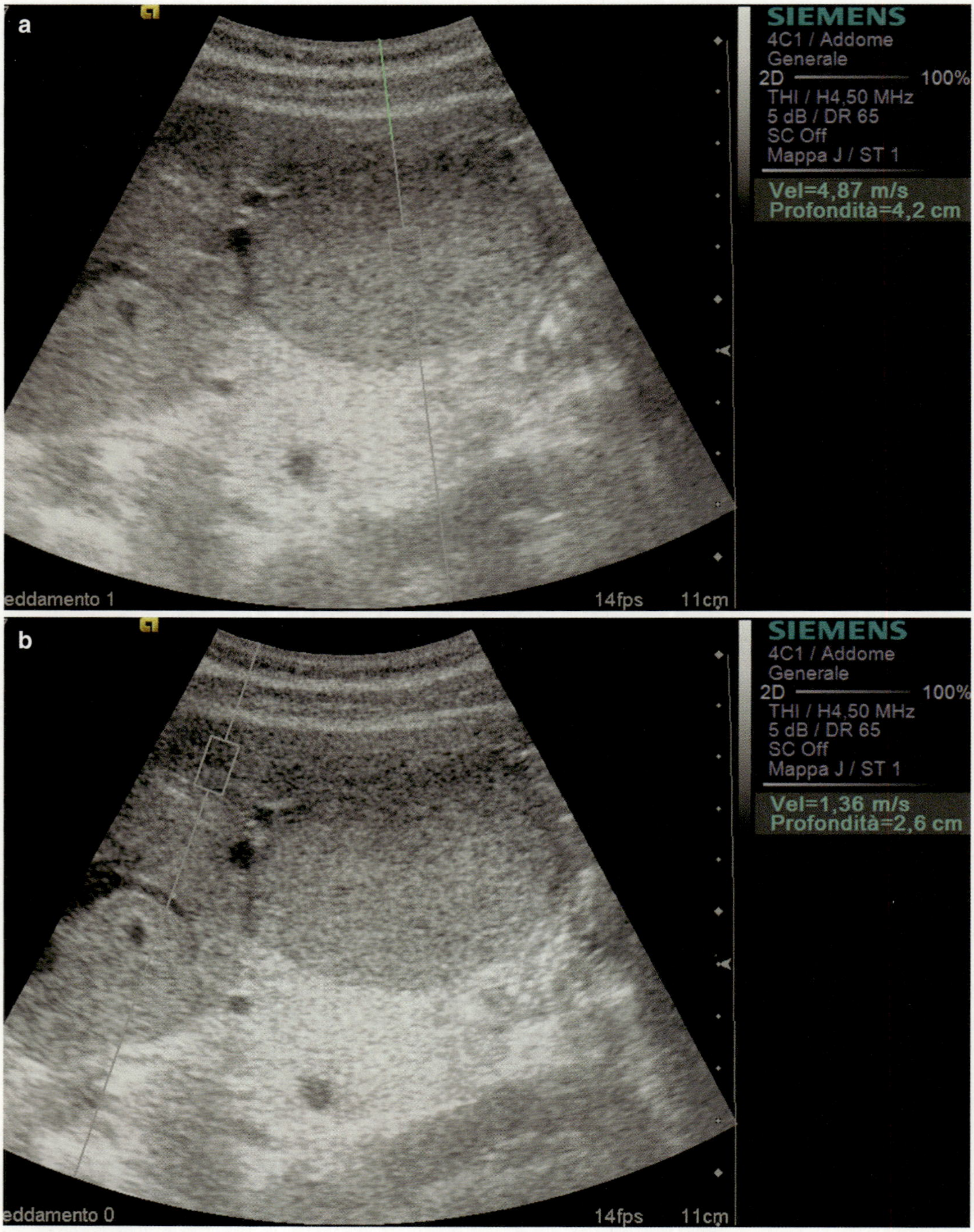

Fig. 2.6 Focal nodular hyperplasia. Higher value in the focal liver mass (**a**) in respect to the adjacent liver parenchyma (**b**)

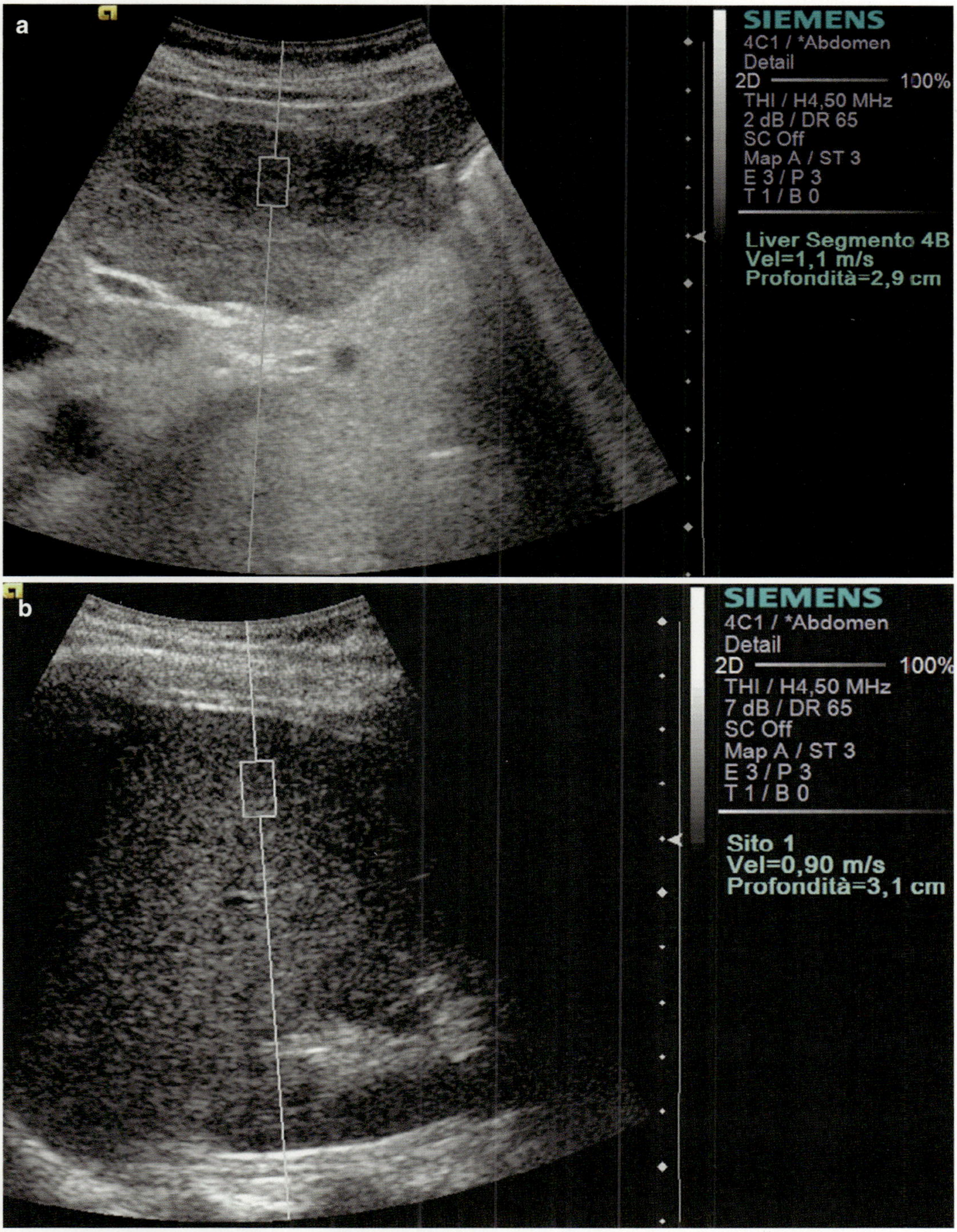

Fig. 2.7 Adenoma. In the focal liver mass (**a**) resulted quite the same values of the adjacent liver parenchyma (**b**)

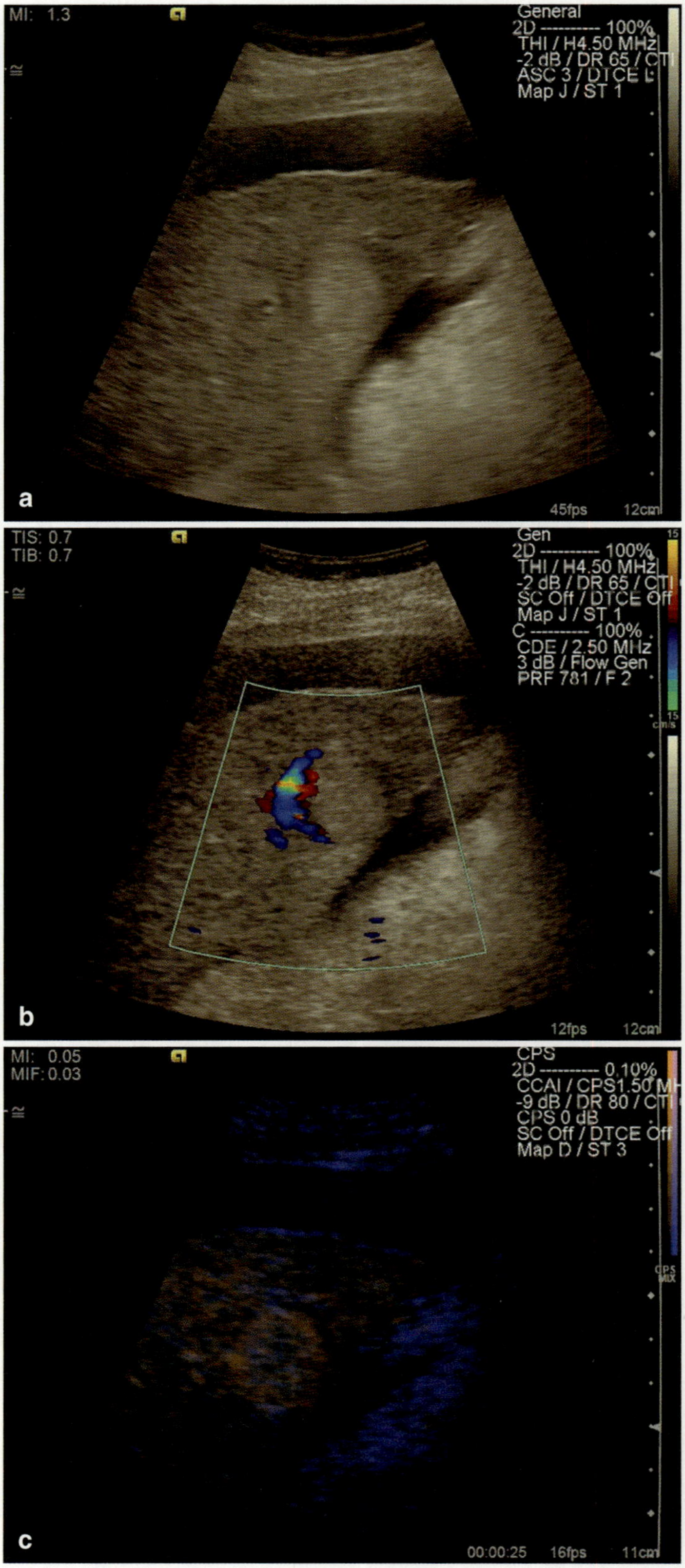

Fig. 2.8 HCC. (**a**) B-mode ultrasound demonstrates a hyperechoic liver lesion in a cirrhotic liver. (**b**) Colour Doppler ultrasound demonstrates some peripheral vessels adjacent to the lesion but no increased vascularity inside the liver lesion. (**c**) Contrast-enhanced ultrasound depicted an intense enhancement of the tumour in the arterial phases. (**d**) Contrast-enhanced ultrasound depicted a washout of the lesion in the late phase and confirmed the suspicion of an HCC. (**e**) In VTI mode elastography, the tumour appears slightly bright to the surrounding liver tissue. (**f**) In VTQ mode, the shear wave velocity was measured in HCC with a velocity of $v = 2.58$ m/s. (**g**) In VTQ mode, the shear wave velocity was measured in the cirrhotic liver with a velocity of $v = 2.19$ m/s

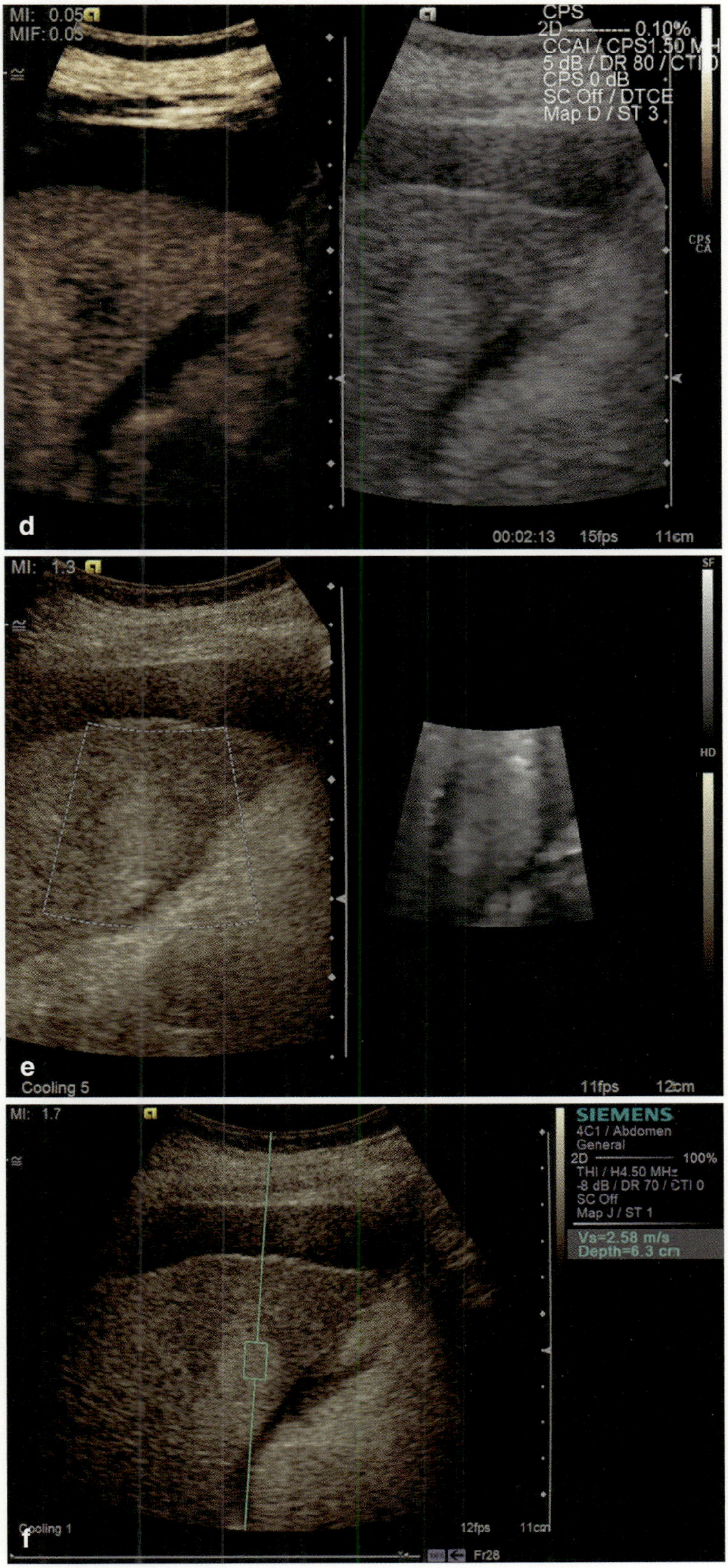

Fig. 2.8 (continued)

Fig. 2.8 (continued)

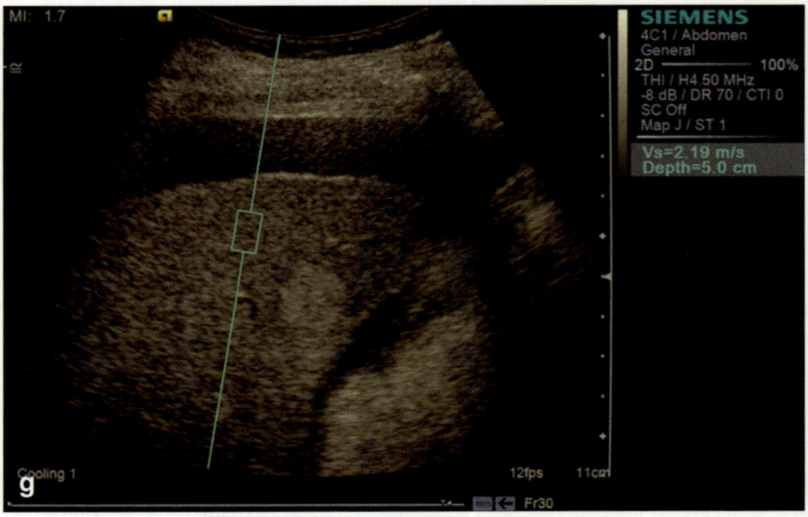

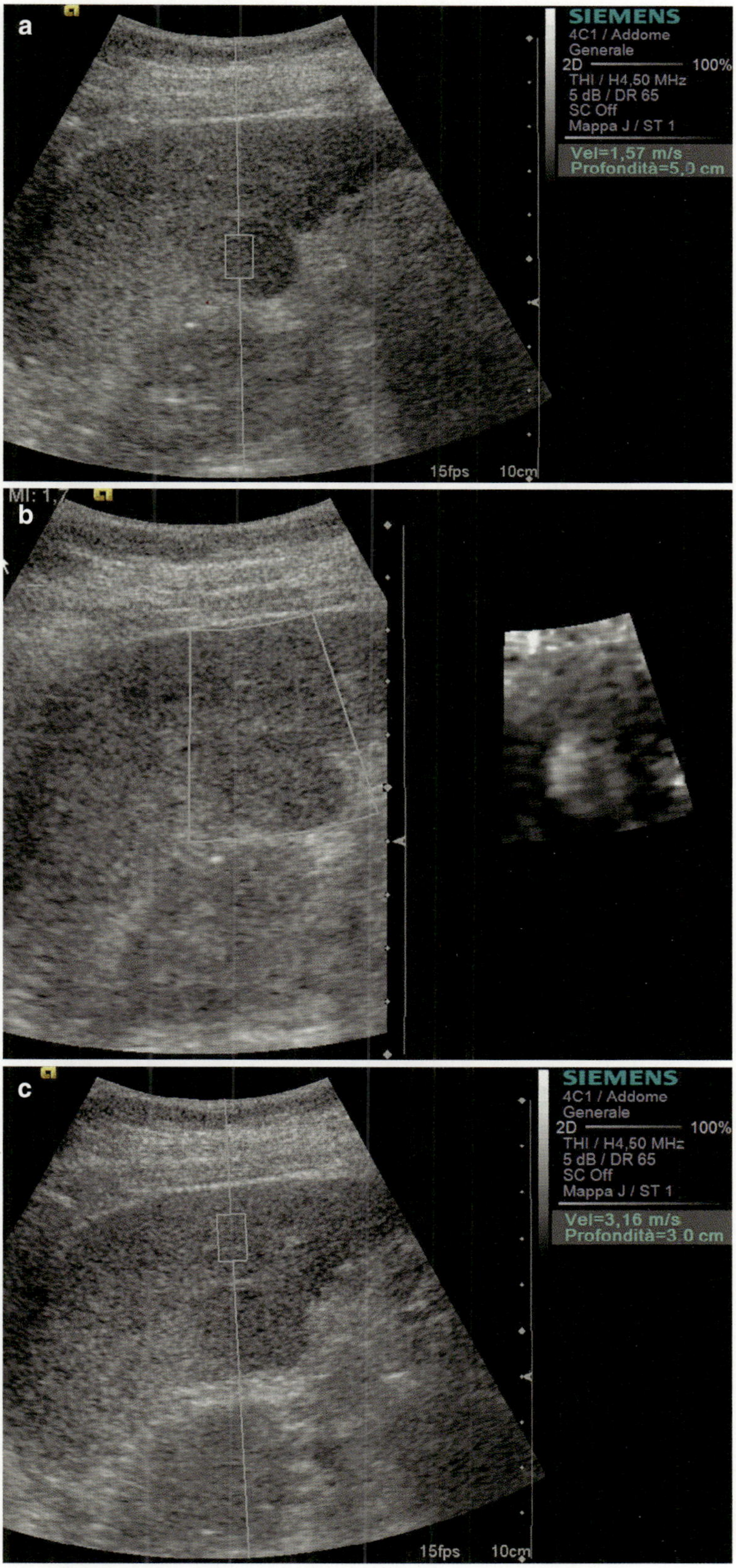

Fig. 2.9 HCC in the focal liver nodule is softer (**a**) and brighter (**b**) at elastography in respect to the stiff liver cirrhotic parenchyma (**c**)

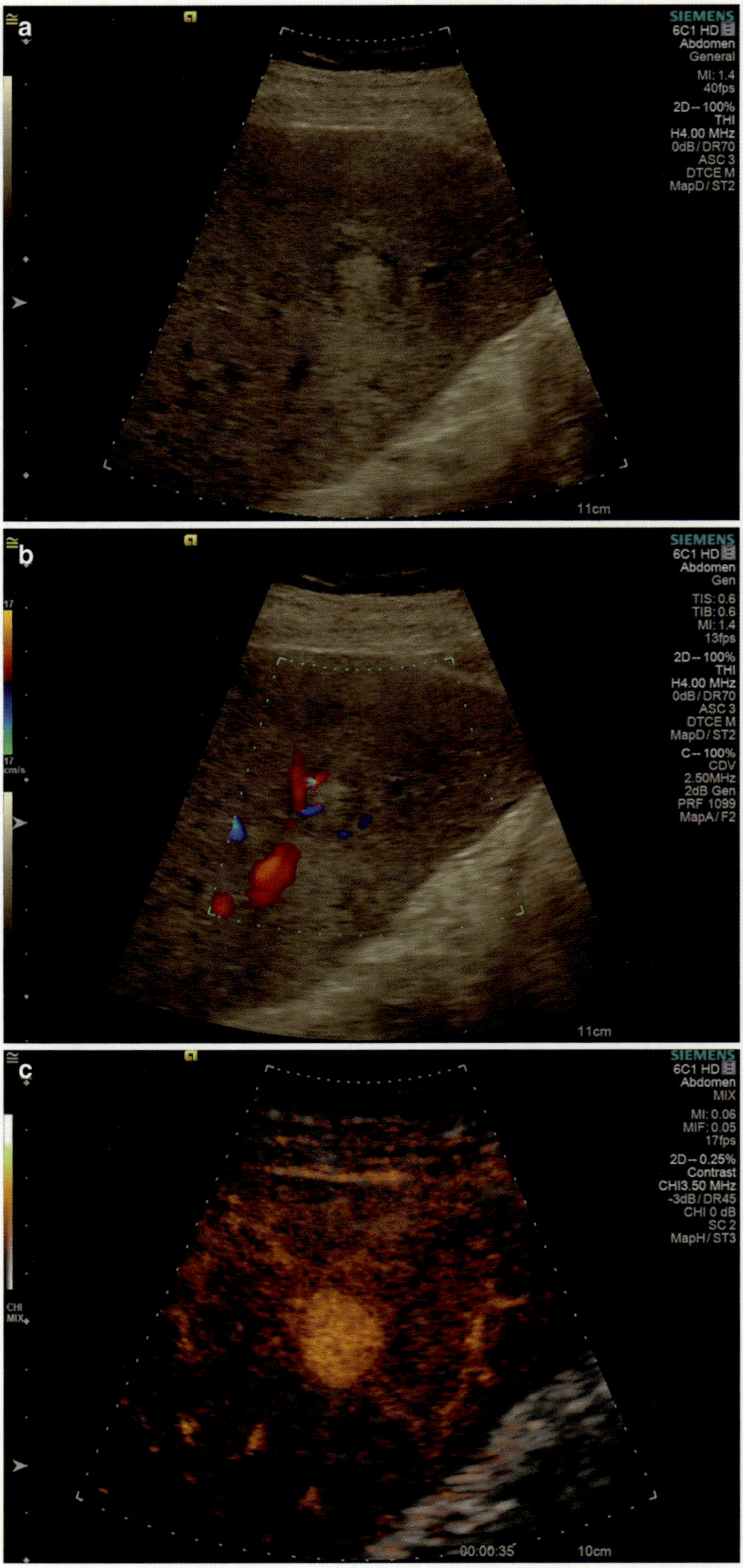

Fig. 2.10 HCC. (**a**) B-mode ultrasound demonstrates a hyper- until isoechoic liver lesion. (**b**) Colour Doppler ultrasound demonstrates some peripheral and central vessels inside the liver lesion. (**c**) Contrast-enhanced ultrasound depicted an intense enhancement of the tumour in the arterial phases, in comparison to the surrounding liver tissue. (**d**) Contrast-enhanced ultrasound depicted a moderate washout of the lesion in the late phase and confirmed the suspicion of an HCC. The histological diagnosis proven by surgery was an HCC. (**e**) In VTI mode elastography, HCC appears in yellow indicating a less stiffness of the lesion in comparison to the cirrhotic liver tissue. (**f**) In VTQ mode, the shear wave velocity was measured in HCC with a velocity of $v = 1.68$ m/s. (**g**) In sonoelastography, the lesion appears in green as an indicator for a less stiff tissue in comparison to the surrounding cirrhotic liver tissue. The border of the lesions is displayed well in this technique

Fig. 2.10 (continued)

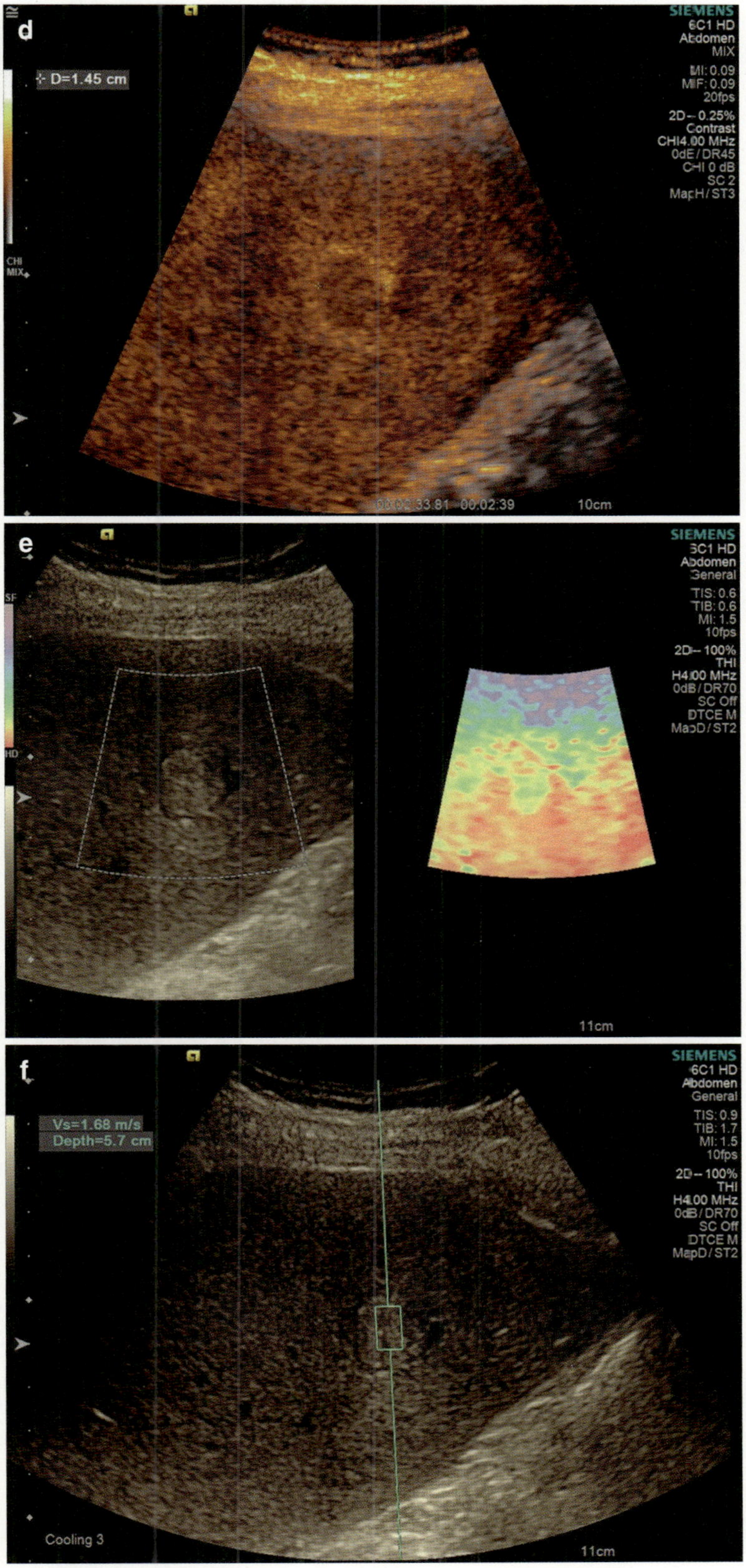

Fig. 2.10 (continued)

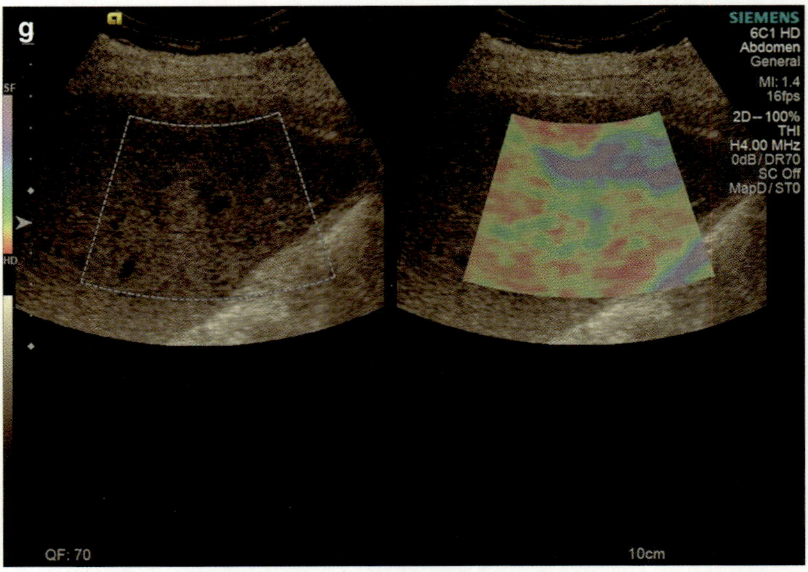

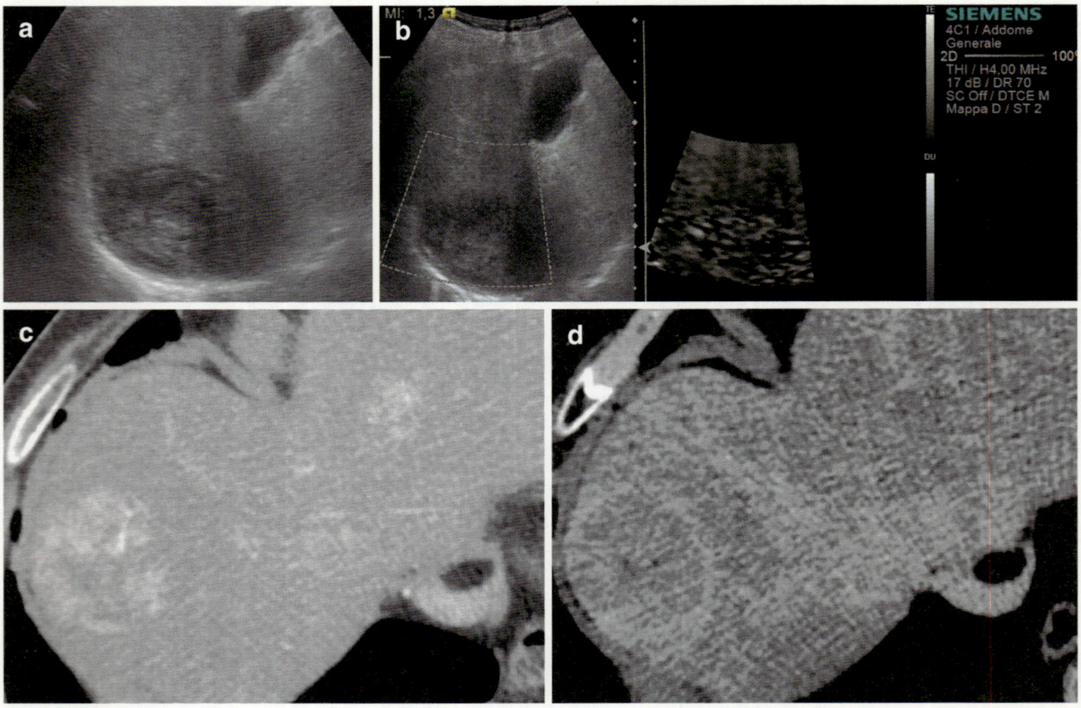

Fig. 2.11 Hepatocellular carcinoma (**a**, **b**) US study: round-shaped hypoechoic liver mass (**a**) resulting stiff in the centre and inhomogeneously soft in the periphery at elastography (**b**) due to presence of fibrotic tissue and vessels. (**c**, **d**) CT study: typical appearance of a hepatocellular carcinoma, presenting as a hypervascular (**c**) lesion with washout resulting hypodense with capsule (**d**) in the late phase

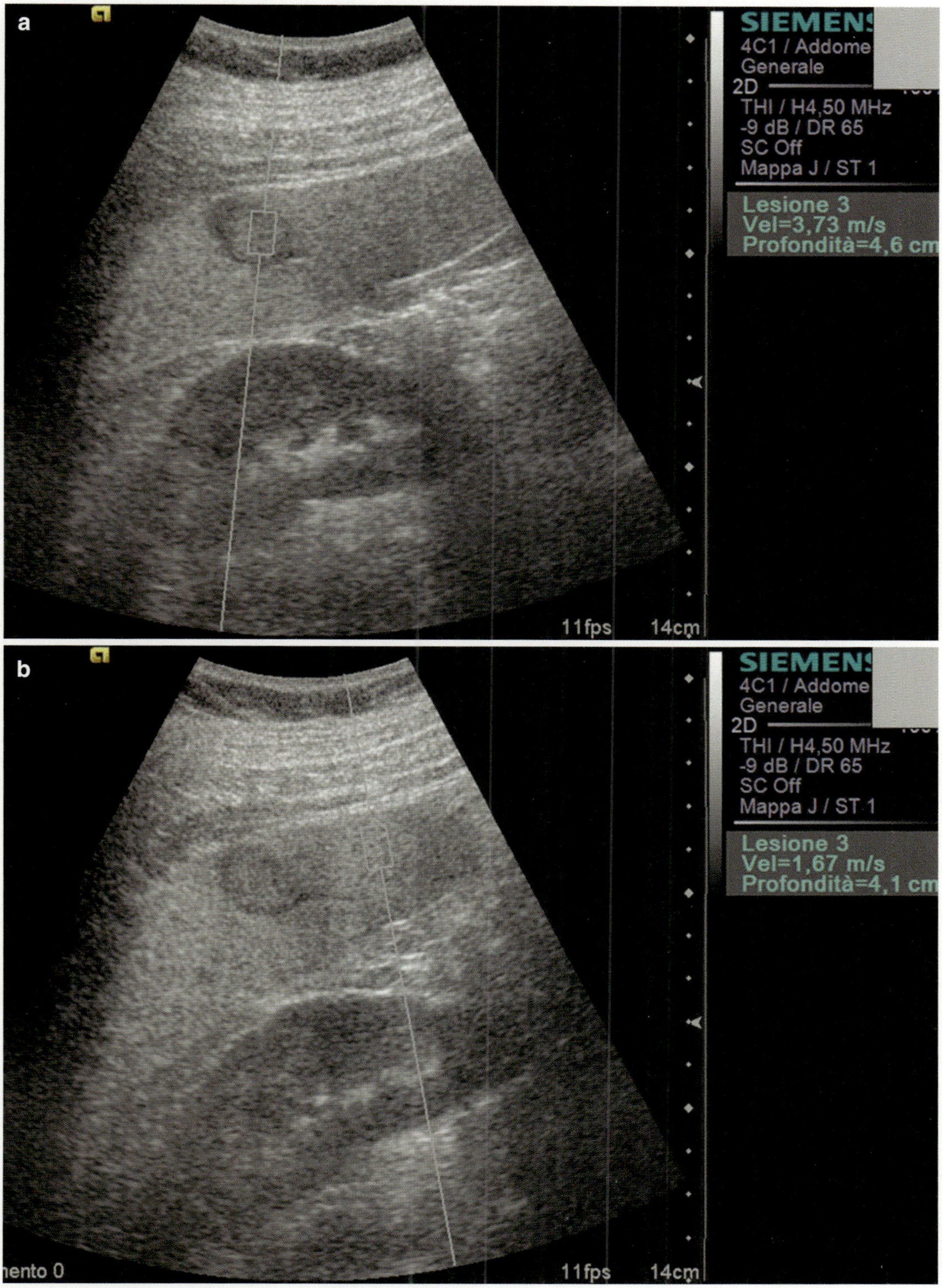

Fig. 2.12 Liver metastasis. Liver nodule is stiffer (**a**) in respect to the liver parenchyma (**b**)

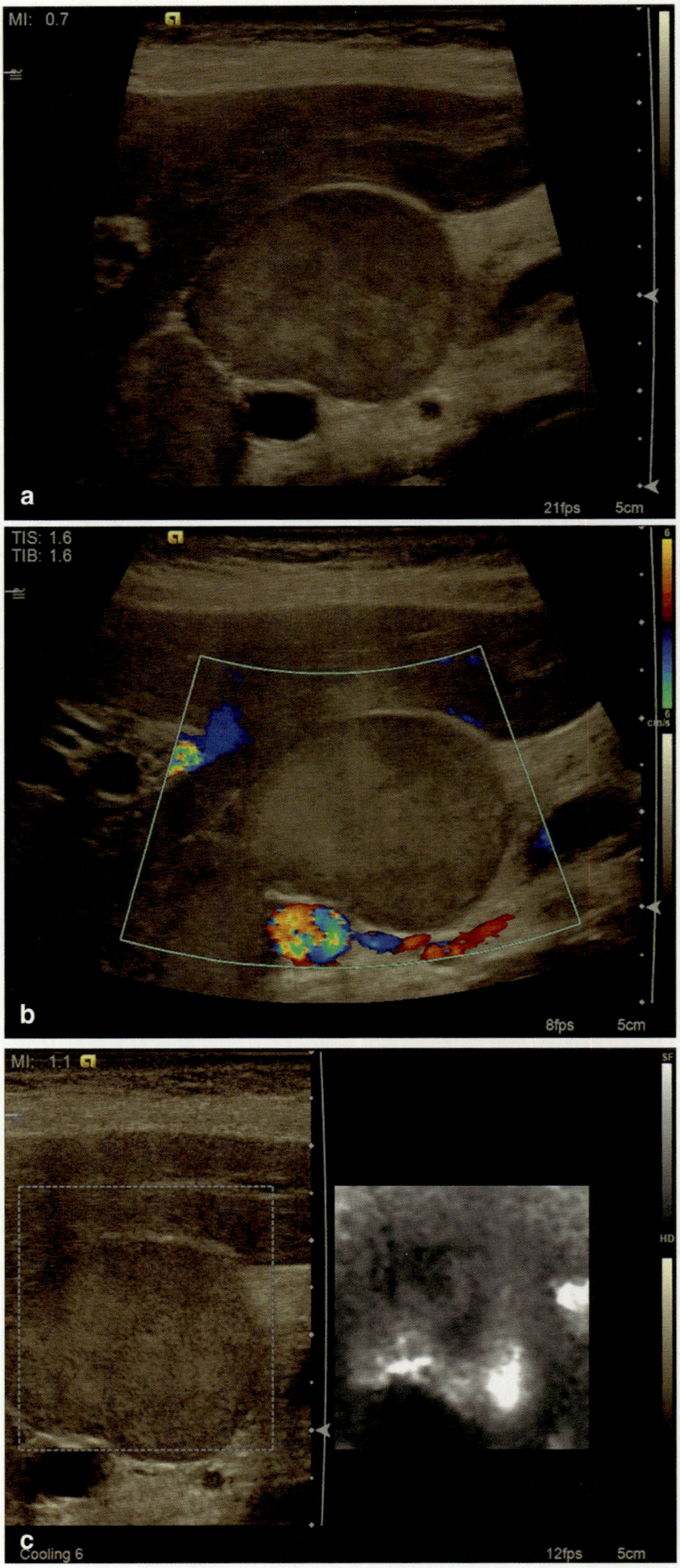

Fig. 2.13 Metastatic lymph node at hepatic hilum. (**a**) A 75-year-old woman with intestine cancer and suspicion of a lymph node metastasis in ultrasound examination. B-mode ultrasound demonstrates an isoechoic lesion adjacent to the liver tissue. (**b**) Colour Doppler ultrasound demonstrates no increased vascularity of the lymph node metastasis. (**c**) In VTI mode elastography, the capsular tumour appears in dark grey indicating a stiff tissue, and the centre appears in white as an indicator for soft tissue. (**d**) In VTQ mode, the shear wave velocity was measured in the liver tissue with a velocity of $v = 2.58$ m/s. (**e**) In VTQ mode, the shear wave velocity was measured in the lymph node metastasis with a velocity of $v = 2.44$ m/s. (**f**) In sonoelastography, the lesion appears in dark grey as an indicator for a stiff tissue. The border of the lesions is displayed well in this technique

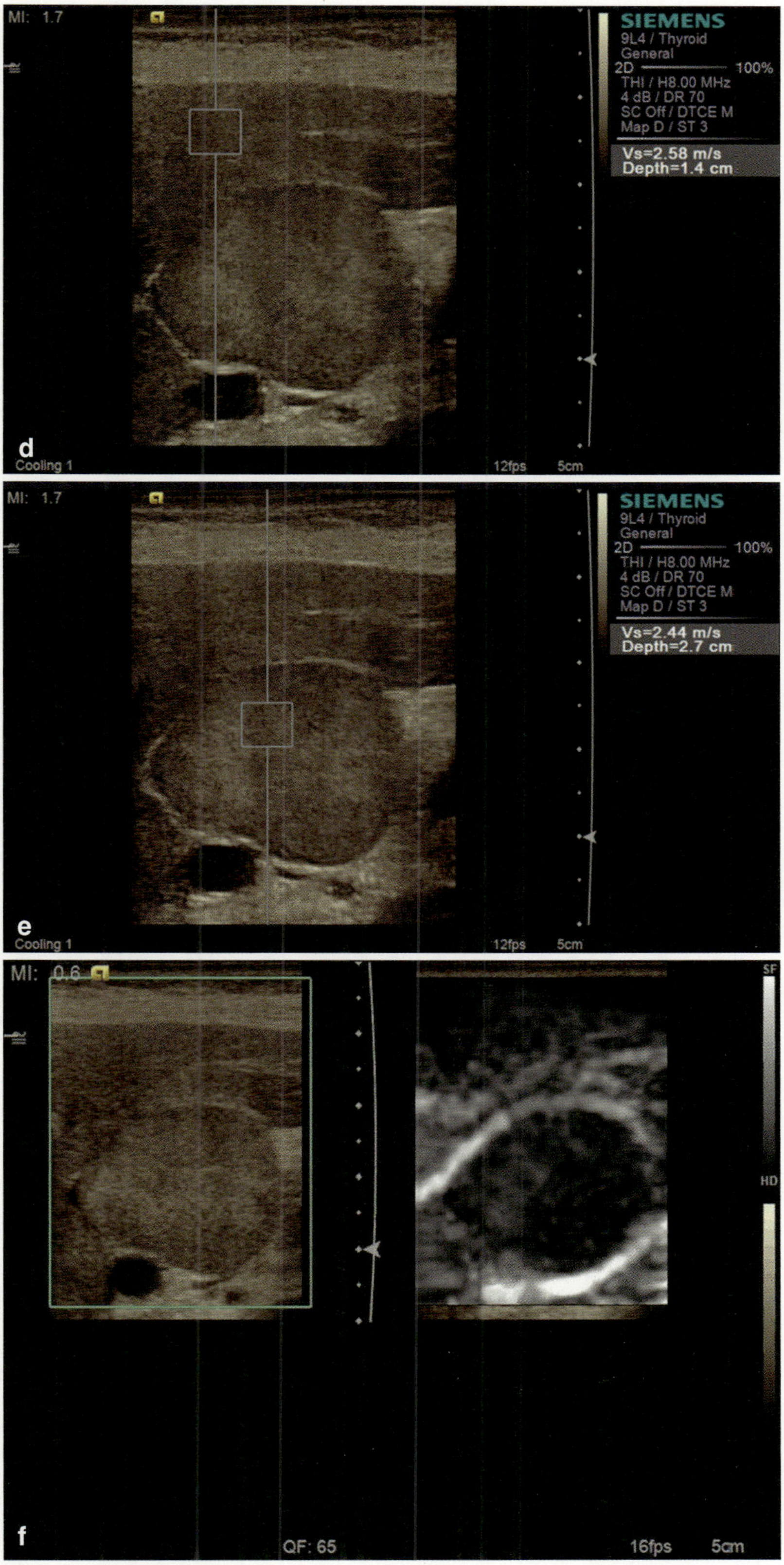

Fig. 2.13 (continued)

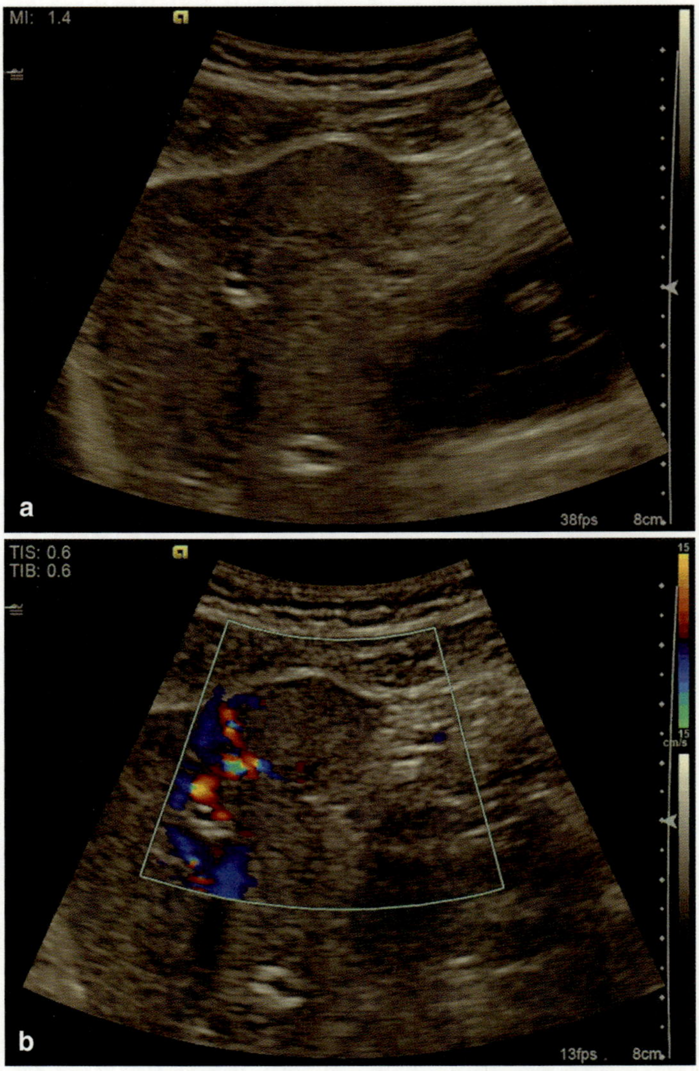

Fig. 2.14 Liver neuroendocrine metastasis. (**a**) A 55-year-old man with known neuroendocrine tumour of the pancreas and an unclear liver lesion depicted in ultrasound examination. B-mode ultrasound demonstrates a slight hyper- until isoechoic liver lesion. (**b**) Colour Doppler ultrasound demonstrates some peripheral vessels of the tumour. (**c**) In VTI mode elastography, the tumour appears in *dark grey* indicating a stiff lesion in comparison to the surrounding liver tissue. (**d**) In VTQ mode, the shear wave velocity was measured in the liver tissue with a velocity of $v=1.41$ m/s. (**e**) In VTQ mode, the shear wave velocity was measured in the tumour tissue with a velocity of $v=3.28$ m/s. (**f**) In sonoelastography, the lesion appears in *dark grey* as an indicator for a very stiff tissue. The border of the lesions is displayed well in this technique. (**g**) Same patient as Fig. 30–35. High-resolution B-mode ultrasound (9 MHz) demonstrates a slight hyper- until isoechoic liver lesion. (**h**) Colour Doppler ultrasound demonstrates some peripheral and central vessels of the tumour. (**i**) Contrast-enhanced ultrasound depicted an intense enhancement of the tumour in the arterial phases, in comparison to the surrounding liver tissue. (**j**) Contrast-enhanced ultrasound depicted a clear washout of the lesion in the late phase and confirmed the suspicion of a liver metastasis. The histological diagnosis proven by surgery was a metastasis from neuroendocrine tumour. (**k**) VTIQ velocity colour overlay displayed relative shear wave velocities according to the adjacent colour spectrum, *red* areas corresponding to higher values and blue areas corresponding to lower values. Shear wave velocity was measured in the metastasis between $v=1.50$ and 3.45 m/s and in the surrounding tissue between $v=0.85$ and 1.08 m/s. (**l**) In VTI mode elastography, the tumour appears in *dark grey* indicating of a stiff lesion in comparison to the normal tissue. (**m**) In VTQ mode, the shear wave velocity was measured in the metastasis with a velocity of $v=4.04$ m/s. (**n**) In VTQ mode, the shear wave velocity was measured in the liver tissue with a velocity of $v=1.92$ m/s. (**o**) In sonoelastography, the lesion appears in *dark grey* as an indicator for a very stiff tissue. The border of the lesions is displayed well in this technique

Fig. 2.14 (continued)

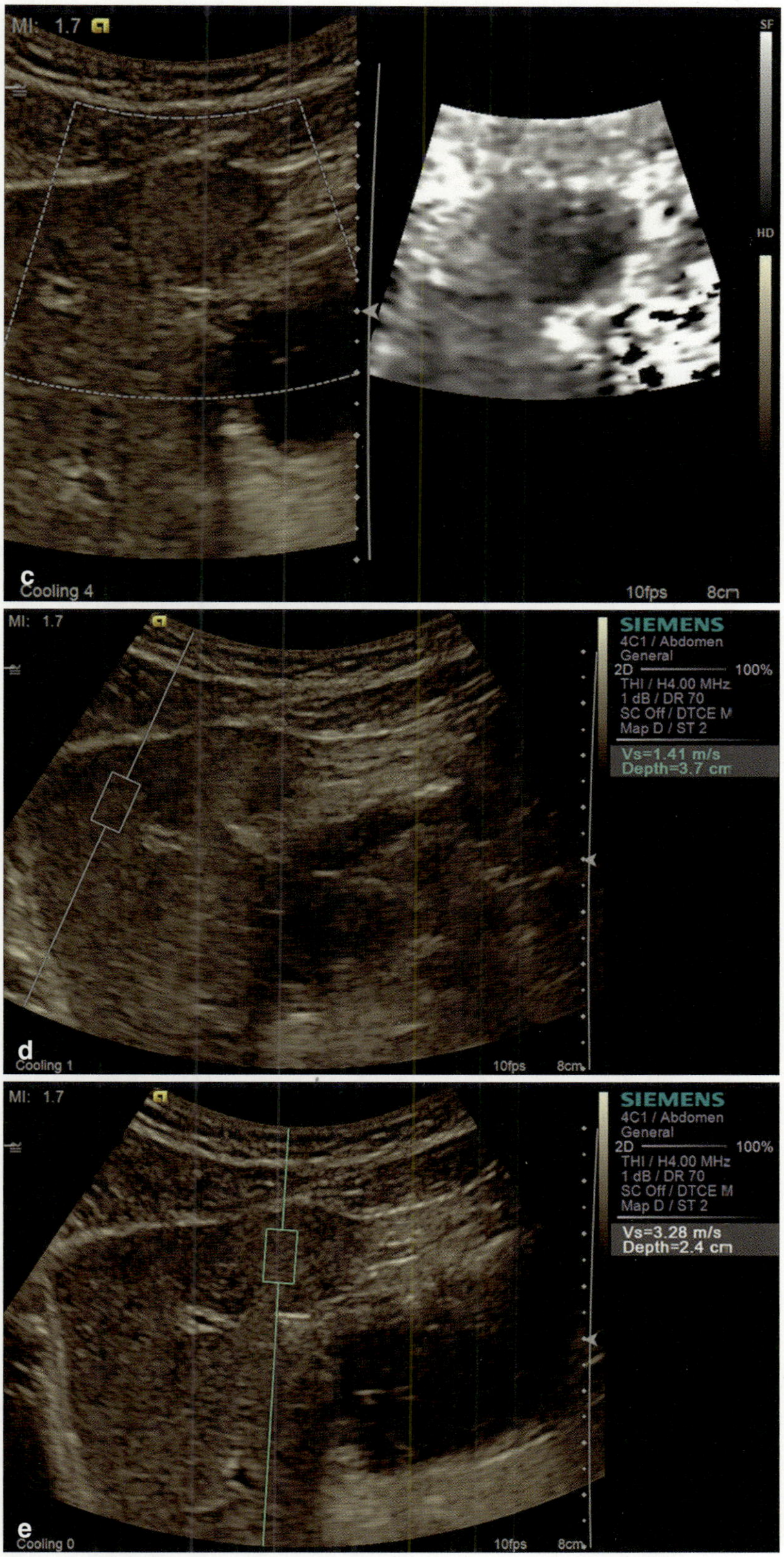

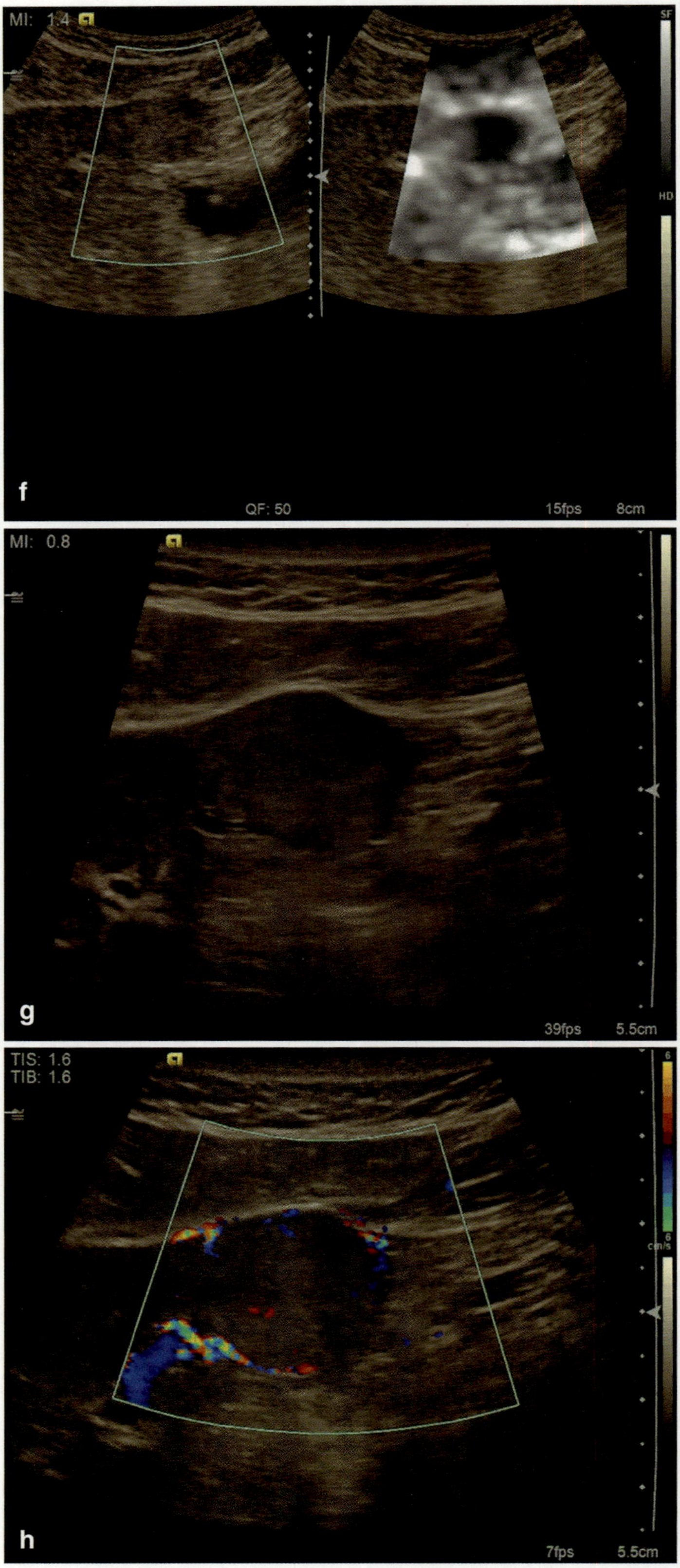

Fig. 2.14 (continued)

Fig. 2.14 (continued)

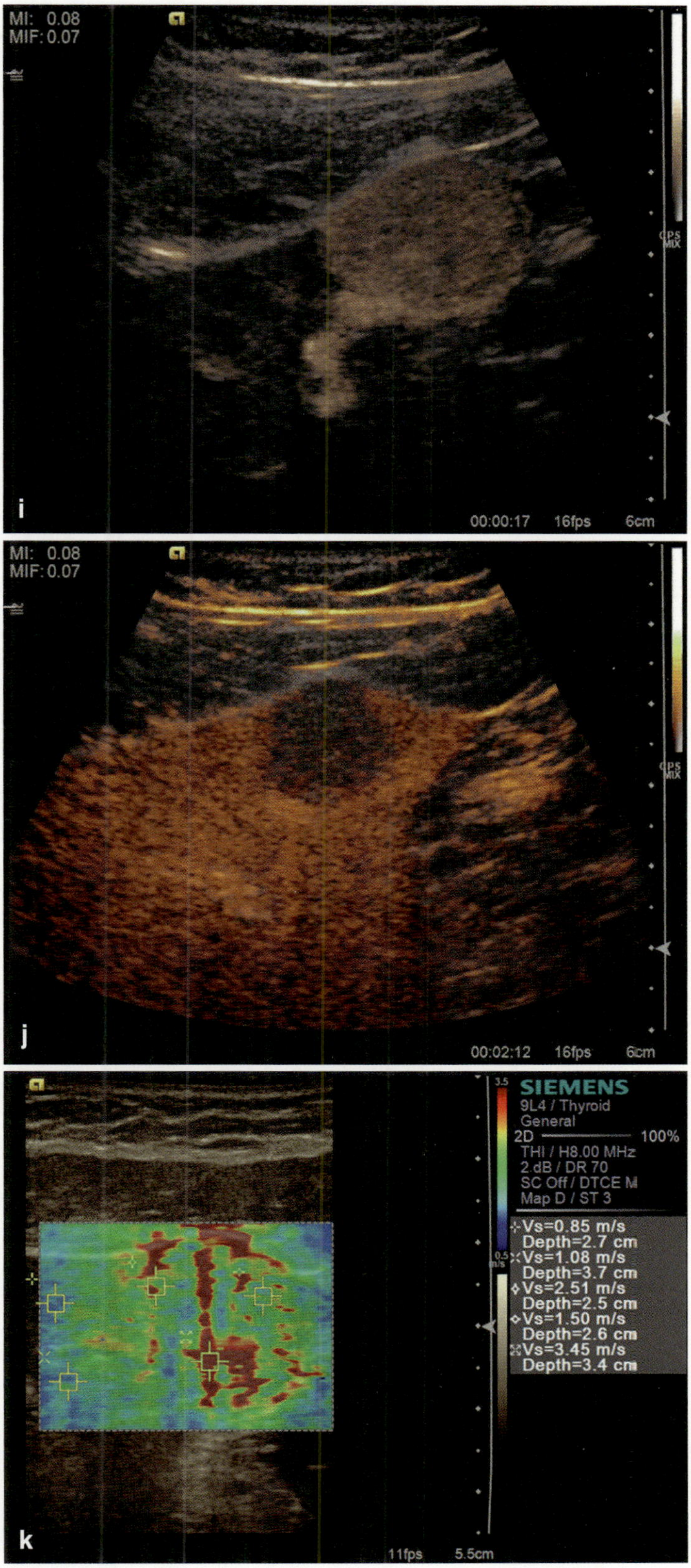

Fig. 2.14 (continued)

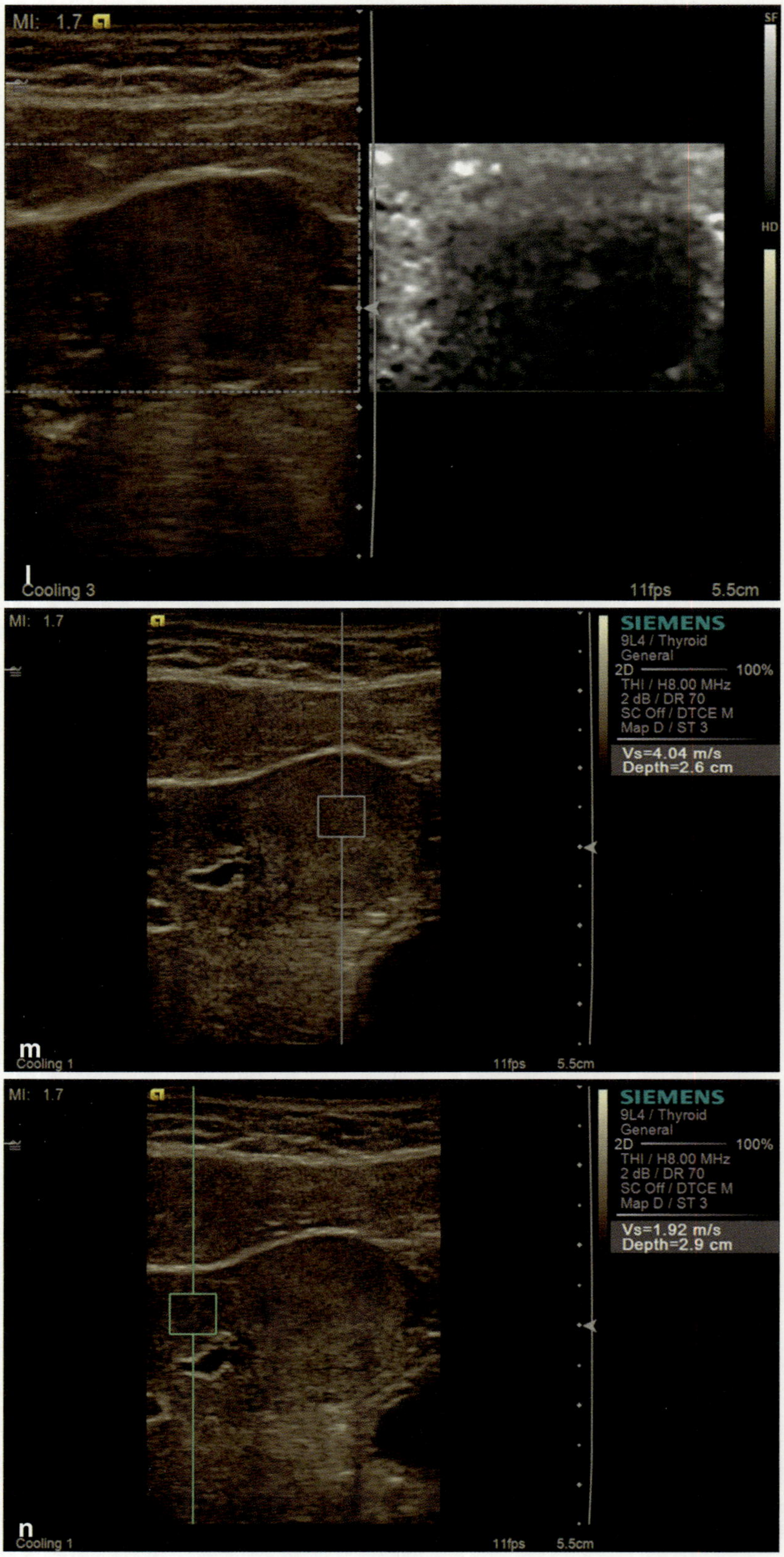

Fig. 2.14 (continued)

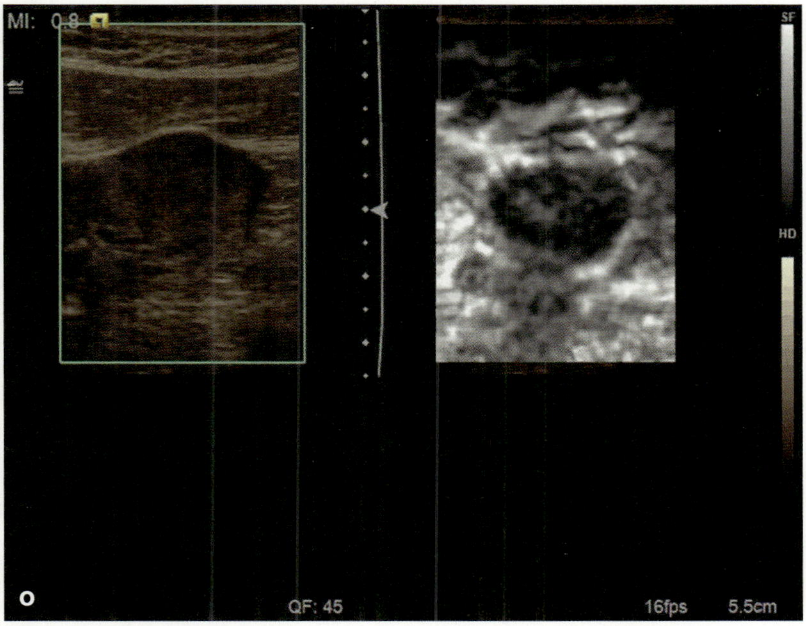

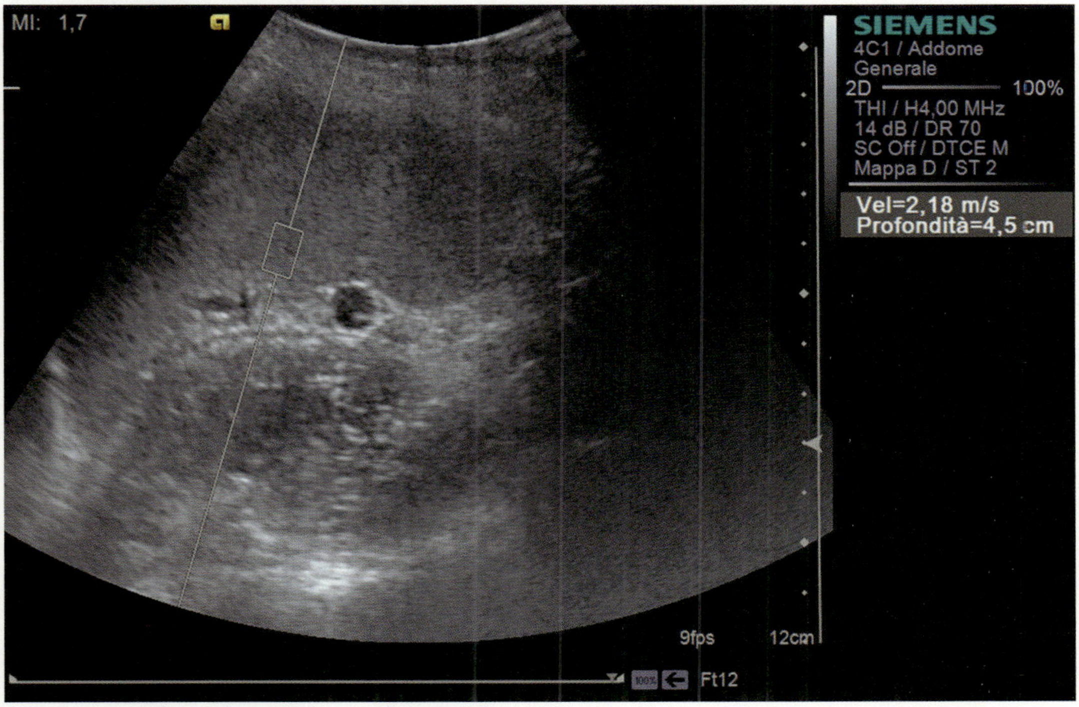

Fig 2.15 Spleen. Normal value of the spleen that result superior to the liver in healthy subjects

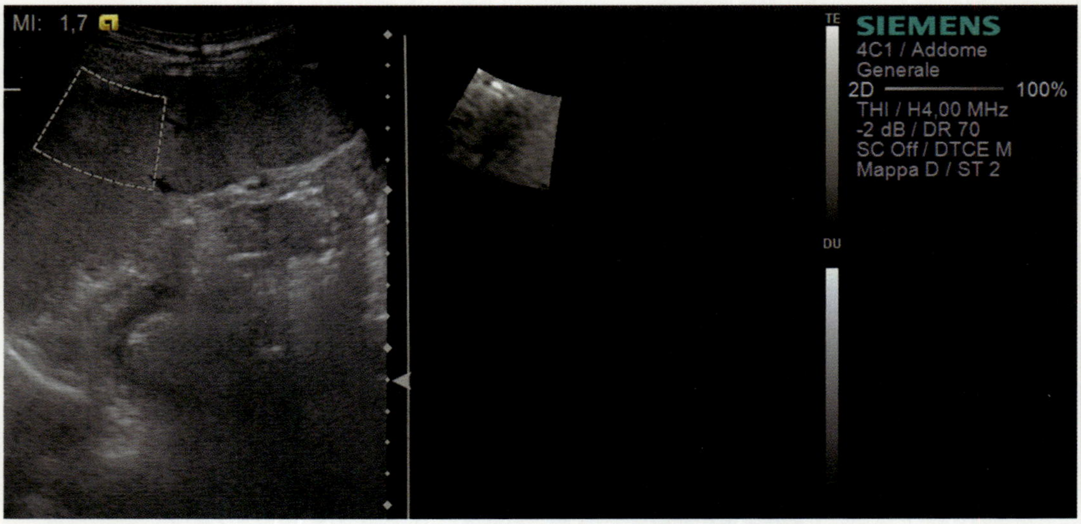

Fig 2.16 Spleen nodule. Mainly isoechoic focal splenic lesion absolutely better visible as black because stiffer in respect to the adjacent parenchyma on elastogram

References

1. Gebo KA, Herlong HF, Torbenson MS, Jenckes MW, Chander G, Ghanem KG, El-Kamary SS, Sulkowski M, Bass EB. Role of liver biopsy in management of chronic hepatitis C: a systematic review. Hepatology. 2002;36:S161–72.
2. Seeff LB, Everson GT, Morgan TR, Curto TM, Lee WM, Ghany MG, Shiffman ML, Fontana RJ, Di Bisceglie AM, Bonkovsky HL, Dienstag JL, HALT–C Trial Group. Complication rate of percutaneous liver biopsies among persons with advanced chronic liver disease in the HALT-C trial. Clin Gastroenterol Hepatol Off Clin Pract J Am Gastroenterol Assoc. 2010;8:877–83.
3. Regev A, Berho M, Jeffers LJ, Milikowski C, Molina EG, Pyrsopoulos NT, Feng ZZ, Reddy KR, Schiff ER. Sampling error and intraobserver variation in liver biopsy in patients with chronic HCV infection. Am J Gastroenterol. 2002;97:2614–8.
4. Cosgrove D, Piscaglia F, Bamber J, Bojunga J, Correas JM, Gilja OH, Klauser AS, Sporea I, Calliada F, Cantisani V, D'Onofrio M, Drakonaki EE, Fink M, Friedrich-Rust M, Fromageau J, Havre RF, Jenssen C, Ohlinger R, Saftoiu A, Schaefer F, Dietrich CF, EFSUMB. EFSUMB guidelines and recommendations on the clinical use of ultrasound elastography. Part 2: clinical applications. Ultraschall Med. 2013;34:238–53.
5. Sandrin L, Fourquet B, Hasquenoph JM, Yon S, Fournier C, Mal F, Christidis C, Ziol M, Poulet B, Kazemi F, Beaugrand M, Palau R. Transient elastography: a new noninvasive method for assessment of hepatic fibrosis. Ultrasound Med Biol. 2003;29:1705–13.
6. Friedrich-Rust M, Ong MF, Martens S, Sarrazin C, Bojunga J, Zeuzem S, Herrmann E. Performance of transient elastography for the staging of liver fibrosis: a meta-analysis. Gastroenterology. 2008;134:960–74.
7. Talwalkar JA, Kurtz DM, Schoenleber SJ, West CP, Montori VM. Ultrasound-based transient elastography for the detection of hepatic fibrosis: systematic review and meta-analysis. Clin Gastroenterol Hepatol Off Clin Pract J Am Gastroenterol Assoc. 2007;5:1214–20.
8. Castera L, Le Bail B, Roudot-Thoraval F, Bernard PH, Foucher J, Merrouche W, Couzigou P, de Ledinghen V. Early detection in routine clinical practice of cirrhosis and oesophageal varices in chronic hepatitis C: comparison of transient elastography (fibroscan) with standard laboratory tests and non-invasive scores. J Hepatol. 2009;50:59–68.
9. Chang PE, Goh GB, Ngu JH, Tan HK, Tan CK. Clinical applications, limitations and future role of transient elastography in the management of liver disease. World J Gastrointest Pharmacol Ther. 2016;7:91–106.
10. Vergara S, Macias J, Rivero A, Gutierrez-Valencia A, Gonzalez-Serrano M, Merino D, Rios MJ, Garcia-Garcia JA, Camacho A, Lopez-Cortes L, Ruiz J, de la Torre J, Viciana P, Pineda JA, Grupo para el Estudio de las Hepatitis Viricas de la S. The use of transient elastometry for assessing liver fibrosis in patients with HIV and hepatitis C virus coinfection. Clin Infect Dis Off Pub Infect Dis Soc Am. 2007;45:969–74.
11. Rigamonti C, Donato MF, Fraquelli M, Agnelli F, Ronchi G, Casazza G, Rossi G, Colombo M. Transient elastography predicts fibrosis progression in patients with recurrent hepatitis C after liver transplantation. Gut. 2008;57:821–7.
12. Rizzo L, Calvaruso V, Cacopardo B, Alessi N, Attanasio M, Petta S, Fatuzzo F, Montineri A, Mazzola A, L'Abbate L, Nunnari G, Bronte F, Di Marco V, Craxi A, Camma C. Comparison of transient elastography and acoustic radiation force impulse for non-invasive staging of liver fibrosis in patients with chronic hepatitis C. Am J Gastroenterol. 2011;106:2112–20.
13. Grgurevic I, Puljiz Z, Brnic D, Bokun T, Heinzl R, Lukic A, Luksic B, Kujundzic M, Brkljacic B. Liver and spleen stiffness and their ratio assessed by real-time two dimensional-shear wave elastography in patients with liver fibrosis and cirrhosis due to chronic viral hepatitis. Eur Radiol. 2015;25:3214–21.
14. Bavu E, Gennisson JL, Couade M, Bercoff J, Mallet V, Fink M, Badel A, Vallet-Pichard A, Nalpas B, Tanter M, Pol S. Noninvasive in vivo liver fibrosis evaluation using supersonic shear imaging: a clinical study on 113 hepatitis C virus patients. Ultrasound Med Biol. 2011;37:1361–73.
15. Ferraioli G, Tinelli C, Dal Bello B, Zicchetti M, Filice G, Filice C, Liver Fibrosis Study G. Accuracy of real-time shear wave elastography for assessing liver fibrosis in chronic hepatitis C: a pilot study. Hepatology. 2012;56:2125–33.
16. Sporea I, Bota S, Gradinaru-Tascau O, Sirli R, Popescu A, Jurchis A. Which are the cut-off values of 2d-shear wave elastography (2d-swe) liver stiffness measurements predicting different stages of liver fibrosis, considering transient elastography (te) as the reference method? Eur J Radiol. 2014;83:e118–22.
17. Chan HL, Wong GL, Choi PC, Chan AW, Chim AM, Yiu KK, Chan FK, Sung JJ, Wong VW. Alanine aminotransferase-based algorithms of liver stiffness measurement by transient elastography (fibroscan) for liver fibrosis in chronic hepatitis B. J Viral Hepat. 2009;16:36–44.
18. Wong VW, Lampertico P, de Ledinghen V, Chang PE, Kim SU, Chen Y, Chan HL, Mangia G, Foucher J, Chow WC, Ahn SH, Hou J. Probability-based interpretation of liver stiffness measurement in untreated chronic hepatitis B patients. Dig Dis Sci. 2015;60:1448–56.
19. Rinella ME. Nonalcoholic fatty liver disease: a systematic review. JAMA. 2015;313:2263–73.
20. Kwok R, Tse YK, Wong GL, Ha Y, Lee AU, Ngu MC, Chan HL, Wong VW. Systematic review with meta-analysis: Non-invasive assessment of non-alcoholic fatty liver disease–the role of transient elastography and plasma cytokeratin-18 fragments. Aliment Pharmacol Ther. 2014;39:254–69.

21. Yoneda M, Suzuki K, Kato S, Fujita K, Nozaki Y, Hosono K, Saito S, Nakajima A. Nonalcoholic fatty liver disease: us-based acoustic radiation force impulse elastography. Radiology. 2010;256:640–7.
22. Fernandez M, Trepo E, Degre D, Gustot T, Verset L, Demetter P, Deviere J, Adler M, Moreno C. Transient elastography using fibroscan is the most reliable non-invasive method for the diagnosis of advanced fibrosis and cirrhosis in alcoholic liver disease. Eur J Gastroenterol Hepatol. 2015;27:1074–9.
23. Pavlov CS, Casazza G, Nikolova D, Tsochatzis E, Burroughs AK, Ivashkin VT, Gluud C. Transient elastography for diagnosis of stages of hepatic fibrosis and cirrhosis in people with alcoholic liver disease. Cochrane Database Syst Rev. 2015;(1):CD010542
24. Mueller S, Seitz HK, Rausch V. Non-invasive diagnosis of alcoholic liver disease. World J Gastroenterol. 2014;20:14626–41.
25. Barr RG, Ferraioli G, Palmeri ML, Goodman ZD, Garcia-Tsao G, Rubin J, Garra B, Myers RP, Wilson SR, Rubens D, Levine D. Elastography assessment of liver fibrosis: society of radiologists in ultrasound consensus conference statement. Radiology. 2015;276:845–61.
26. Tsochatzis EA, Gurusamy KS, Ntaoula S, Cholongitas E, Davidson BR, Burroughs AK. Elastography for the diagnosis of severity of fibrosis in chronic liver disease: a meta-analysis of diagnostic accuracy. J Hepatol. 2011;54:650–9.
27. Bota S, Herkner H, Sporea I, Salzl P, Sirli R, Neghina AM, Peck-Radosavljevic M. Meta-analysis: ARFI elastography versus transient elastography for the evaluation of liver fibrosis. Liver Int Off J Int Assoc Study Liver. 2013;33:1138–47.
28. Vizzutti F, Arena U, Romanelli RG, Rega L, Foschi M, Colagrande S, Petrarca A, Moscarella S, Belli G, Zignego AL, Marra F, Laffi G, Pinzani M. Liver stiffness measurement predicts severe portal hypertension in patients with HCV-related cirrhosis. Hepatology. 2007;45:1290–7.
29. Bureau C, Metivier S, Peron JM, Selves J, Robic MA, Gourraud PA, Rouquet O, Dupuis E, Alric L, Vinel JP. Transient elastography accurately predicts presence of significant portal hypertension in patients with chronic liver disease. Aliment Pharmacol Ther. 2008;27:1261–8.
30. Masuzaki R, Tateishi R, Yoshida H, Goto E, Sato T, Ohki T, Imamura J, Goto T, Kanai F, Kato N, Ikeda H, Shiina S, Kawabe T, Omata M. Prospective risk assessment for hepatocellular carcinoma development in patients with chronic hepatitis C by transient elastography. Hepatology. 2009;49:1954–61.
31. Sasso M, Tengher-Barna I, Ziol M, Miette V, Fournier C, Sandrin L, Poupon R, Cardoso AC, Marcellin P, Douvin C, de Ledinghen V, Trinchet JC, Beaugrand M. Novel controlled attenuation parameter for noninvasive assessment of steatosis using fibroscan((r)): Validation in chronic hepatitis C. J Viral Hepat. 2012;19:244–53.
32. Fahey BJ, Nelson RC, Bradway DP, Hsu SJ, Dumont DM, Trahey GE. In vivo visualization of abdominal malignancies with acoustic radiation force elastography. Phys Med Biol. 2008;53:279–93.
33. Park H, Park JY, do Kim Y, Ahn SH, Chon CY, Han KH, Kim SU. Characterization of focal liver masses using acoustic radiation force impulse elastography. World J Gastroenterol. 2013;19:219–26.
34. Gallotti A, D'Onofrio M, Romanini L, Cantisani V, Pozzi MR. Acoustic radiation force impulse (ARFI) ultrasound imaging of solid focal liver lesions. Eur J Radiol. 2012;81:451–5.
35. Shuang-Ming T, Ping Z, Ying Q, Li-Rong C, Ping Z, Rui-Zhen L. Usefulness of acoustic radiation force impulse imaging in the differential diagnosis of benign and malignant liver lesions. Acad Radiol. 2011;18:810–5.
36. Singh S, Fujii LL, Murad MH, Wang Z, Asrani SK, Ehman RL, Kamath PS, Talwalkar JA. Liver stiffness is associated with risk of decompensation, liver cancer, and death in patients with chronic liver diseases: a systematic review and meta-analysis. Clin Gastroenterol Hepatol Off Clin Pract J Am Gastroenterol Assoc. 2013;11:1573–84. e1571–2; quiz e1588–9.
37. Gheorghe L, Iacob S, Iacob R, Dumbrava M, Becheanu G, Herlea V, Gheorghe C, Lupescu I, Popescu I. Real time elastography – a non-invasive diagnostic method of small hepatocellular carcinoma in cirrhosis. J Gastrointestin Liver Dis JGLD. 2009;18:439–46.
38. Seo YS, Kim MN, Kim SU, Kim SG, Um SH, Han KH, Kim YS. Risk assessment of hepatocellular carcinoma using transient elastography vs. Liver biopsy in chronic hepatitis B patients receiving antiviral therapy. Med. 2016;95:e2985.
39. Xu X, Luo L, Chen J, Wang J, Zhou H, Li M, Jin Z, Chen N, Miao H, Lin M, Dai W, Ahuja AT, Wang YX. Acoustic radiation force impulse elastography for efficacy evaluation after hepatocellular carcinoma radiofrequency ablation: a comparative study with contrast-enhanced ultrasound. Biomed Res Int. 2014;2014:901642.
40. Kwon HJ, Kang MJ, Cho JH, Oh JY, Nam KJ, Han SY, Lee SW. Acoustic radiation force impulse elastography for hepatocellular carcinoma-associated radiofrequency ablation. World J Gastroenterol. 2011;17:1874–8.
41. Merli M, Nicolini G, Angeloni S, Rinaldi V, De Santis A, Merkel C, Attili AF, Riggio O. Incidence and natural history of small esophageal varices in cirrhotic patients. J Hepatol. 2003;38:266–72.
42. Bintintan A, Chira RI, Mircea PA. Non-invasive ultrasound-based diagnosis and staging of esophageal varices in liver cirrhosis. A systematic review of the literature published in the third millennium. Med Ultrason. 2013;15:116–24.
43. Colecchia A, Montrone L, Scaioli E, Bacchi-Reggiani ML, Colli A, Casazza G, Schiumerini R, Turco L, Di

Biase AR, Mazzella G, Marzi L, Arena U, Pinzani M, Festi D. Measurement of spleen stiffness to evaluate portal hypertension and the presence of esophageal varices in patients with HCV-related cirrhosis. Gastroenterology. 2012;143:646–54.
44. Bota S, Sporea I, Sirli R, Focsa M, Popescu A, Danila M, Strain M. Can arfi elastography predict the presence of significant esophageal varices in newly diagnosed cirrhotic patients? Ann Hepatol. 2012;11:519–25.
45. Vermehren J, Polta A, Zimmermann O, Herrmann E, Poynard T, Hofmann WP, Bojunga J, Sarrazin C, Zeuzem S, Friedrich-Rust M. Comparison of acoustic radiation force impulse imaging with transient elastography for the detection of complications in patients with cirrhosis. Liver Int Off J Int Assoc Study Liver. 2012;32:852–8.
46. Takuma Y, Nouso K, Morimoto Y, Tomokuni J, Sahara A, Toshikuni N, Takabatake H, Shimomura H, Doi A, Sakakibara I, Matsueda K, Yamamoto H. Measurement of spleen stiffness by acoustic radiation force impulse imaging identifies cirrhotic patients with esophageal varices. Gastroenterology. 2013;144:92–101.e102.
47. Fraquelli M, Giunta M, Pozzi R, Rigamonti C, Della Valle S, Massironi S, Conti CB, Aghemo A, Ronchi G, Iurlo A, Primignani M, Conte D, Colombo M. Feasibility and reproducibility of spleen transient elastography and its role in combination with liver transient elastography for predicting the severity of chronic viral hepatitis. J Viral Hepat. 2014;21:90–8.
48. Hirooka M, Ochi H, Koizumi Y, Kisaka Y, Abe M, Ikeda Y, Matsuura B, Hiasa Y, Onji M. Splenic elasticity measured with real-time tissue elastography is a marker of portal hypertension. Radiology. 2011 261:960–8.
49. Kim HY, Jin EH, Kim W, Lee JY, Woo H, Oh S, Seo JY, Oh HS, Chung KH, Jung YJ, Kim D, Kim BG, Lee KL. The role of spleen stiffness in determining the severity and bleeding risk of esophageal varices in cirrhotic patients. Medicine. 2015;94:e1031.
50. Rizzo L, Attanasio M, Pinzone MR, Berretta M, Malaguarnera M, Morra A, L'Abbate L, Balestreri L, Nunnari G, Cacopardo B. A new sampling method for spleen stiffness measurement based on quantitative acoustic radiation force impulse elastography for non-invasive assessment of esophageal varices in newly diagnosed HCV-related cirrhosis. Biomed Res Int. 2014;2014:365982.
51. Novelli PM, Cho K, Rubin JM. Sonographic assessment of spleen stiffness before and after transjugular intrahepatic portosystemic shunt placement with or without concurrent embolization of portal systemic collateral veins in patients with cirrhosis and portal hypertension: a feasibility study. J Ultrasound Med Off J Am Inst Ultrasound Med. 2015;34:443–9.

3 Pancreas

Valentina Ciaravino, Giulia Tremolada,
Laura Bernardoni, Stefano Francesco Crino,
Alessandro Sarno, Giorgia Tedesco,
Nicolò Cardobi, Riccardo De Robertis,
and Mirko D'Onofrio

Elastography of the pancreas is a new useful technique that completes and improves the accuracy of transcutaneous or endoscopic pancreatic ultrasound study, giving important information on tissue under examination.

The accuracy of ultrasonography has been increased in last decades by techniques able to evaluate mechanical strain properties of tissues. This innovative and not invasive method of analyzing tissue stiffness immediately received an increasing interest during the last years owing to a revolutionary approach of studying diffuse and focal diseases, thus providing a new important diagnostic tool for making diagnosis. Tissue stiffness has ever been evaluated by clinicians and surgeons through physical palpation to detect pathological conditions. So the possibility to evaluate tissue stiffness became a new useful implement, complementary to the other traditional imaging features to reach a diagnosis [1]. The challenge of elastography is to distinguish different tissues on the basis of their specific consistency: usually malignant neoplasms tend to be stiffer than healthy parenchyma of different organs. First organs and diseases studied with elastography were the breast, thyroid, and prostate nodules. In the last years, pancreatic ultrasound elastography became more relevant.

3.1 Examination Technique

Elastography of the pancreas can be obtained by using two main imaging techniques: first is strain elastography (SE); second is shear wave elastography (SWE), which includes transient elastography (TE), point SWE, 2D-SWE and 3D-SWE, and acoustic radiation force impulse (ARFI).

In strain elastography, a continuous external mechanical compression done with the probe is required, or the compressions are given by the respiratory movements and the cardiac pulsations. The deformation degree is calculated by measuring variations in the US frequency before and after compression. A dedicated software calculates the tissue elasticity in a defined ROI. This type of elastography obviously supplies compressions that cannot be quantified, and moreover the site compressed cannot be restricted to specific areas. Strain elastography provides a qualitative study with the creation of an area where a color map pattern is superimposed, according to the color scale in the monitor side basing on tissue stiffness. The color elastogram is superimposed to the US image [2–5], and it consists in a color map (stiffer areas are coded in blue or in red

V. Ciaravino • G. Tremolada • A. Sarno • G. Tedesco
N. Cardobi • R. De Robertis • M. D'Onofrio (✉)
Department of Radiology, GB Rossi University
Hospital, University of Verona, Verona, Italy
e-mail: mirko.donofrio@univr.it

L. Bernardoni • S.F. Crino
Department of Gastroenterology, GB Rossi
University Hospital, University of Verona,
Verona, Italy

D.-A. Clevert et al. (eds.), *Atlas of Elastosonography*, DOI 10.1007/978-3-319-44201-3_3

usually, softer areas are red or blue, and green indicates intermediate levels of elasticity). Some types of US equipment display a gray scale, with stiffer tissues represented as darker. Elastography by compression gives only qualitative and not quantitative information because it is impossible to precisely define the intensity of the force exerted on the tissues. Moreover, the relative elasticity representation may change according to the tissues in the studied area, with the size of the box and with the intensity of the exerted pressure [2]. Information given by this study are relative, and not absolute, because it is always necessary a comparison between the studied lesion or interested area and the adjacent parenchyma, so the region of interest (ROI) that it will be choose must to be bigger than the lesion or the area that we want to study, comparing in this way different stiffness of different parenchyma areas [2].

Shear wave elastography provides a real-time evaluation of the shear wave propagation in the tissues: a conventional US probe generates pressure waves and registers in turn the tissue motion by a sequence of multiple images per second. The results can be both qualitative and quantitative: it is possible to create a chromatic two-dimensional map of the tissue viscoelastic properties, both in a gray scale or in a color scale (usually areas of great stiffness are black or red, respectively, softer areas are blue or light gray, green and different gray grades indicate an intermediate level of elasticity). Moreover the values of tissue stiffness are also expressed in kilopascals (kPa), giving absolute quantitative information about tissue properties [2, 6]. So shear wave imaging allows both qualitative and quantitative evaluations. In contrast with strain elastography, that is, qualitative, shear wave imaging leads to an absolute, quantitative, measure of tissue mechanical properties. Acoustic radiation force impulse (ARFI) imaging, being part of shear wave elastography imaging, can give information qualitatively and quantitatively about tissue stiffness with no need of external compression. It takes advantage of a short-duration acoustic radiation forces (<1 ms) to create a localized tissue displacements through a preliminary identified ROI, selected in the target tissue on a conventional US image-based anatomical location, that are then registered by the ultrasonographer scanner: the tissue displacements are obviously related to the viscoelastic local soft tissue properties [2, 7].

As previously said, ARFI can be used both in a qualitative and in a quantitative way. In the qualitative one a short acoustic impulse of high intensity is employed to deform tissue elements and create a static map (elastogram) of the relative stiffness of the tissues included in the region of interest (ROI). In the quantitative one a primary acoustic impulse focused on a ROI (a box with fixed dimensions) is used to generate pressure perpendicular waves able to deform the tissue. The speed of the wave through the tissue is calculated in m/s. The stiffer the tissue is, the greater the shear wave velocity [2, 8].

The ARFI method has positive sides, such as that it reduce interobserver variability and an external compression is not needed, but it provides only static information and not dynamic ones as a contrary of elastography by compression [2].

Pancreatic elastography can be performed by using two different approaches: the endoscopic and the percutaneous. The endoscopic approach still now is the most widely studied, whereas the percutaneous one, even though easily and immediately practicable, can be affected by the same intrinsic limitations that can compromise the ultrasound study of the pancreatic region.

3.1.1 Endoscopic Elastography

Endoscopic ultrasonography is the most frequent approach used for the elastographic study of the pancreas. The area that has to be evaluated is defined by a region of interest (ROI, color window). The pressure applied on the studied region can be modified by manipulating the probe, even if usually very little additional compression is required, because the pressure difference from the pulsation of adjacent vessels is normally sufficient. So with the endoscopic technique, the method used is the strain elastography. Elastographic and B-mode images are displayed simultaneously.

The ROI has to be sufficiently large to contain the area that has to be examined and enough surrounding tissue for comparison of relative tissue stiffness. Moreover, it is possible to have a semiquantitative value comparing two different areas of tissue within the ROI, calculating the strain ratio between a suspicious mass lesion and reference surrounding tissue [2].

3.1.2 Transabdominal Elastography

Transabdominal ultrasound elastography of the pancreas requires obviously a correct visualization of the pancreatic gland by means of ultrasound. Transcutaneous ultrasound elastography study can be performed both by using strain elastography, with qualitative and semiquantitative information, and share wave elastography with qualitative and quantitative data [2].

3.2 Clinical Applications

3.2.1 Normal Findings in Healthy Pancreas

A healthy pancreas appears as iso- to hyperechoic compared to the liver parenchyma, with echogenicity that however may increase with advancing age, due to a fibro-adipose involution. The normal pancreas appears as intermediately soft tissue, characterized by a homogeneous soft tissue green area at elastographic imaging [9–14].

Then, with the fat accumulation and fibrosis degeneration of the parenchyma, the elastographic image becomes heterogeneous, due to different color areas inside the gland.

At endoscopic ultrasound, pancreatic qualitative elastosonographic results about healthy parenchyma are univocally reported as soft tissue, as previously mentioned, represented by homogeneous green pattern in each published studies [2, 9–14].

Elastographic study consists of images that use chromatic maps with gray or color scale. In this hue chromatic (gray scale or red-green-blue) map, hard tissue areas are colored in black or dark blue or red (depending on the scale used), soft tissue areas are in white or red or blue (depending on the scale used), and intermediate stiffness tissues are characterized by different gray shadows or yellow or green. An important limitation of this elastographic technique is that the complete color spectrum from blue to red encoding is applied to each different elastographic record and it indicates the graduation of relative elasticity within the area sampled; as a consequence there is not an absolute scale of tissue stiffness [2].

Percutaneous ultrasound ARFI elastography has the capability of reading share waves velocity with a transabdominal probe: the stiffer a tissue is, the greater the mechanical wave speed will be. As reported in Literature, the mean wave velocity value obtained in a healthy pancreas with ARFI technique is about 1.40 m/s [1, 15, 16].

3.2.2 Inflammatory Diseases

3.2.2.1 Acute Pancreatitis

Acute pancreatitis is an inflammatory disease of the pancreas that can be divided, thanks to Atlanta classification 2012 revised [17], into edematous pancreatitis or necrotizing pancreatitis. In the edematous pancreatitis, interstitial edema causes a diffuse or a focalized enlargement of the gland due to inflammatory infiltrated cells, with preservation of microcirculation and of pancreatic perfusion. In the necrotizing pancreatitis, a microcirculation damage is present with tissue destruction and necrosis appearance that gets involved or only the pancreatic parenchyma, or only the peripancreatic tissue, or both.

As a consequence of pathology changes, the consistency of the pancreatic parenchyma becomes softer than the healthy pancreas, and it could be identified with strain elastography and with share wave elastography, including ARFI. Necrosis can be identified at elastography, both transabdominal and endoscopic, as soft areas for the presence of damaged tissue with specific colors linked to softness, such as blue or red, depending on the specific color scale of the utilized echographer [18]. Goya et al. compared in their prospective study the efficiencies of transabdominal ARFI imaging (both Virtual Touch Imaging (VTI) and Virtual Touch Quantification (VTQ)) with B-mode ultrasonography and CT at hospital admission for diagnosis of acute pancreatitis, conversely to other studies that did not have any comparison [19–21]. In this study, elastography disclosed changes in pancreatic parenchyma in all patients with diagnosis of acute pancreatitis compared with the ones in the control group. These results displayed the high success rate of ARFI elastography in the diagnosis of acute pancreatitis and its superiority compared to B-mode ultrasonography and CT. Furthermore ARFI elastography can successfully detect pancreatic inflammation both visually and quantitatively even in cases of mild pancreatitis, opposed to CT and ultrasonography, because all patients included in the study had a diagnosis of acute pancreatitis by ARFI imaging. ARFI-VTQ (Virtual Touch Quantification) has sensitivity and specificity of 100 % and 98 %, respectively, in diagnosis of acute pancreatitis, with a cutoff value of 1.63 m/s, specifying that the mean SWS value in patients with acute pancreatitis is significantly higher (values in pancreatic parenchyma of patients with pancreatitis ranged from 1.1 to 4.47 m/s) than the value found in the control group (value in normal pancreatic parenchyma ranged from 0.6 to 1.63 m/s), with a differential statistically significant, $p<0.001$. In case of necrosis, Virtual Touch Imaging (VTI) elastograms of the necrotic areas showed reduced stiffness compared with non-necrotic pancreatic tissue, due to the colliquation, and the Virtual Touch Quantification (VTQ) values seen by elastography ranged from 0.5 to 1.2 m/s. In case of segmental involvement, the VTQ values were higher for inflamed tissue areas than those of non-inflamed or less inflamed, showing that ARFI elastography can be used to visualize the location of inflammation in the pancreas, helping in case of segmental inflammation. Moreover sometimes acute inflammation can be focal, occurring mostly in the pancreatic head, and it presents as a hypoechoic mass, being difficult to be differentiated from a tumor: in these cases elastography can be useful in the differential diagnosis between these two diseases. Ultimately Goya et al. concluded that ARFI elastography is a noninvasive, radiation-free, rapid, and reproducible imaging method that can efficiently diagnose acute pancreatitis at hospital admission, providing reliable results and visualizing distribution of inflammation in parenchyma glands, in peripancreatic tissue, and necrosis distribution. Moreover, very important help is done by the positive diagnosis yielded by elastography in patients with negative CT [22]. Data regarding ARFI Virtual Touch Quantification are however controversial in patients with acute pancreatitis [21].

3.2.2.2 Chronic Pancreatitis

Chronic pancreatitis is a chronic fibrotic inflammatory process of the pancreas that causes permanent morphologic changes with function reduction. At the end in chronic pancreatitis, the pancreas is atrophic, with calcifications and dilation and irregularity of both principal pancreatic duct and secondary ducts; at pathology the normal lobular architecture of the gland is preserved with irregular loss of acinar and ductal tissues, combined with various degrees of chronic inflammation, duct alterations, and fibrosis. Due to these pathologic changes, the pancreatic tissue strain properties are different in respect to the healthy pancreas, but a pancreas with chronic pancreatitis may show a wide range of tissue strain due to inhomogeneity of the distribution of the alterations. At endoscopic ultrasound elastography, this benign pancreatic disease could appear as a honeycomb predominantly blue pattern, or a heterogeneous mixed colored pattern with prevalent soft tissues, or a homogeneously green pattern [2, 9, 11, 12]. Basically the elastogram shows harder pancreatic tissue (depending of course with the color scale of the echographer) [23]. At qualitative elastography, both transabdominal and endoscopic, chronic pancreatitis is shown with heterogeneous mixed colored pattern or honeycombed pattern, with predominantly hard strands [2, 9, 11, 12, 24]. Differently to solid pancreatic tumors, the elastographic appearance of chronic pancreatitis varies to some degree, probably caused by the inhomogeneous affection of the organs and the different stages of the chronic disease [9]. Elastography can therefore help in diagnosis of chronic pancreatitis, added to the standard Rosemont criteria [24–26], and it could be helpful in diagnosing early chronic pancreatitis cases [9, 24, 27]. Nevertheless, differential diagnosis between chronic pancreatitis and pancreatic cancer could be very difficult at elastography because these two diseases on EUS or transabdominal elastography have similar hardness. Furthermore, stones and calcifications, frequently associated with chronic pancreatitis, produce a homogeneously hard pattern comparable with malignant diseases [2, 9, 28]. Different studies on this topic show different conclusions. Janssen et al. assert that EUS elastography is not able to distinguish chronic pancreatitis from malignant tumors [9] and reported low specificity and positive predictive value for elastographic diagnosis of chronic pancreatitis (56.9 % and 46.6 %, respectively) and pancreatic neoplasms (65.4 % and 51.7 %). Itokawa et al. [11] affirmed that the specificity of EUS elastography in distinguishing benign from malignant pancreatic lesions is low (64.3 %), demonstrating that hard lesions may not always be malignant and soft lesions may not always be benign in pancreatic pathology. An important concept introduced by Itokawa et al. [11] is the strain ratio (SR), a semi-quantitative method to objectively evaluate tissue hardness: stress applied to two areas of pancreatic tissue (areas considered to be malignant and areas not malignant) at the same time, each strain increases in proportion to the stress. Thanks to this semiquantitative method, it is possible to see as SR of pancreatic cancer is usually significantly higher than SR for mass-forming pancreatitis and chronic pancreatitis, indicating that this new approach could be a useful method for the differential diagnosis between pancreatic cancer and chronic pancreatitis. Regarding the acoustic radiation force impulse, in literature it is reported that the pancreatic stiffness measured by ARFI used to be high in patients with chronic pancreatitis, more than cutoff value of 1.40 m/s [2, 29]. In both techniques, it could be useful to study also the adjacent parenchyma, in case of focal chronic pancreatitis mass, because at the elastogram and at the ARFI values, both chronic pancreatitis and ductal adenocarcinoma can be hard. The relative stiffness of a lesion compared to the adjacent parenchyma could help in differential diagnosis: fibrosis and calcification that developed also in the surrounding parenchyma and not only in the lesion implicate a higher stiffness than would be found in the adjacent parenchyma, so the relative stiffness of a lesion compared to its adjacent parenchyma can be expected to provide more accurate information than the absolute ARFI value of a lesion in the differential diagnosis between chronic pancreatitis and ductal adenocarcinoma [30]. In conclusion, share wave velocity (SWV) in patients with chronic pancreatitis used to be significantly higher than the one in healthy pancreas, making ARFI elastography a feasible modality for the diagnosis of chronic pancreatitis, showing in chronic pancreatitis high elasticity compared to findings in the normal pancreas [29].

3.2.2.3 Autoimmune Pancreatitis

Autoimmune pancreatitis (AIP) is a chronic pancreatitis caused by an autoimmune inflammatory process that at pathology has predominant lymphocytic peri-ductal inflammation and fibrosis. Often, this kind of chronic pancreatitis gets involved only a gland portion, and this can cause problems in the differential diagnosis with pancreatic ductal adenocarcinoma. Usually patients with autoimmune pancreatitis do not have calcifications and dilation of principal pancreatic duct. Dietrich et al. showed [31] that all patients with proved autoimmune pancreatitis that they enrolled in a study presented with a unique pattern of small spotted, mainly blue color signals that were evenly spread over the head and the body of the pancreas. So they concluded that elastography might be helpful in identifying patients with AIP, because the elastographic pattern of AIP was enough characteristic to allow it to be distinguished from all other pathological entities and from normal pancreatic tissue: in fact the characteristic stiff elastographic pattern in patients with AIP is visible both in the mass lesion and in the adjacent pancreatic parenchyma [24].

3.2.3 Pancreatic Solid Neoplasms

3.2.3.1 Pancreatic Ductal Adenocarcinoma

Pancreatic ductal adenocarcinoma is the most frequent solid pancreatic tumor, accounting for about 80 % of malignant pancreatic neoplasms. It is a malignant epithelial neoplasm with glandular differentiation, composed by neoplastic glands, with different degrees of differentiation, implanted in abundant desmoplastic stroma, that give to it a hard consistency, with low vascularization. As a consequence, pancreatic ductal adenocarcinoma is a hard hypovascular mass [12, 15, 32, 33]. Usually, keeping in mind tissue pathology, malignant pancreatic neoplasms have harder stiffness than adjacent pancreatic parenchyma, allowing elastographic technique to be a reliable tool for the differentiation of solid pancreatic masses with high sensitivity (95–97 %) and middle to high specificity (67–76 %), as said in some meta-analysis about endoscopic ultrasound elastography [34–37]. However, EUS elastography cannot substitute the histology confirmation in differential diagnosis between malignant and benign lesions, because often the difference in stiffness between these two entities is very little, so EUS elastography can be a very useful tool and an added value, but it should not be used as a first-line examination alone in the evaluation of focal pancreatic lesions [12]. Regarding endoscopic ultrasound elastography, at qualitative imaging, pancreatic ductal adenocarcinoma usually appears as a hard tissue, blue or red depending on the specific instrument color map, but it could also be characterized by a homogeneously green pattern (middle color in the stiffness scale) or by a heterogeneous soft pattern in those cases with cystic degeneration or necrosis present [2, 9–13]. There are no evidence for a correlation between the tumor stiffness and the tumor grading [34, 38]. In some studies, different elastography image color pattern classification to do differential diagnosis between malignant masses and benign lesions were used, but this approach has also been contradicted by other authors [10, 34, 39, 40]. Giovannini et al. [12, 39] used in two studies a five-score classification system for endoscopic ultrasound elastography, as reported in Table 3.1.

Giovannini et al. reported in the first study [39] this five-score classification based on different color patterns with a sensitivity of 100 % and a specificity of 67 % in differentiating benign from malignant lesions. Then the same group in the second study [12], basing on the same scoring system, proved that the accuracy was 89.2 % for the differential diagnosis, with both sensitivity and positive predictive value (PPV) over 90 % [34]. A second group, Iglesias-Garcia et al. [13], used a four-score classification (Table 3.2), and they prove that EUS elastography has diagnostic sensitivity, specificity, and overall accuracy of 100 %, 85.5 %, and 94 %, respectively, in diagnosing malignancy [34].

Itokawa et al. [11] showed in their study that at qualitative EUS elastography all pancreatic ductal adenocarcinomas had intense blue pattern (hardest color in their color map), whereas inflammatory masses had mixed colorations (green, yellow, and low-intensity blue). Again there are at least two studies that give disappointing results about qualitative endoscopic ultrasound elastography [9, 10, 34]. Hirche et al.

Table 3.1 Five-score classification system for endoscopic ultrasound elastography according to Giovannini studies [12, 34, 39]

Score	Color pattern	Stiffness	Histology
1	Green	Homogeneous soft	Normal pancreatic tissue
2	Green, yellow, and red	Soft heterogeneity	Fibrosis
3	Mostly blue with minimal heterogeneity	Hard	Early pancreatic adenocarcinoma
4	Central green hypoechoic region and blue tissue outer layer	Hard	Neuroendocrine tumor, metastasis
5	Blue lesions with heterogeneity due to necrosis	Hard	Advanced pancreatic adenocarcinoma

Table 3.2 Four-score classification system for endoscopic ultrasound elastography according to Iglesias-Garcia study [13, 34]

Score	Color pattern	Stiffness	Histology
1	Homogeneous green	Soft	Normal pancreas
2	Heterogeneous, green predominant	Soft	Inflammatory pancreatic masses
3	Heterogeneous, blue predominant	Hard	Pancreatic malignant tumors
4	Homogeneous blue	Hard	Pancreatic neuroendocrine malignant lesions

[10] found in their study very low values in predicting the nature of pancreatic lesions, such as diagnostic sensitivity, specificity, and accuracy just 41 %, 53 %, and 45 %, respectively. Janssen et al. [9] instead conclude that it is not possible to distinguish chronic pancreatitis from hard malignant tumors with elastography, probably due to their similar fibrous structure. These different values of diagnostic accuracy in qualitative EUS elastography among different studies can be explained probably because of the subjective interpretation of the elastographic pattern [14, 34, 41]. By the way due to the desmoplasia of ductal adenocarcinoma, it is possible to exclude malignancy with high accuracy when in the ROI is seen a predominantly green pattern, so this examination have a negative predictive value usually higher than 90 % [10, 12, 31, 42–44]. With EUS elastography strain ratio (SR) that gives a relative quantitative value, Iglesias-Garcia et al. [40] proved that in differential diagnosis of pancreatic solid lesions quantitative EUS elastography with SR has an accuracy (97.7 %) and a specificity (92.9 %) higher than qualitative analysis and these data could be explained with comparing two regions of interest (ROI), one inside the lesion and one inside adjacent pancreatic parenchyma. They said that a lesion with a SR higher than 6.04 or a mass elasticity lower than 0.05 % has 100 % sensitivity to be classified as a malignant tumor [34, 40]. Furthermore, the specificity can reach 100 % value with a SR higher than 15.41 or a mass elasticity value below 0.03 %. So EUS elastography with SR could be an important tool in the differential diagnosis among pancreatic masses and could differentiate pancreatic cancers from inflammatory masses, with a sensitivity of 100 % and a specificity of 96 %, and pancreatic adenocarcinoma from neuroendocrine tumors, with 100 % sensitivity and 88 % specificity [34, 40]. Another study confirms different values with EUS quantitative techniques with a mean SR of 39.08 (±20.54) for pancreatic ductal adenocarcinoma and a mean SR of 23.66 (±12.65) for inflammatory masses [11, 34]. At the acoustic radiation force impulse (ARFI), being a rigid mass, stiffer than the adjacent pancreatic parenchyma for the pathological features previously described, pancreatic ductal adenocarcinoma is characterized by higher wave velocity values than normal parenchyma with predominately hard pattern at Virtual Touch Tissue Imaging (VTI) and at Virtual Touch Tissue Quantification (VTQ); shear wave velocities are usually >3 m/s, higher than ones measured in the adjacent parenchyma [2, 16, 29, 45]. Park et al. [30] concluded in their study that ARFI elastography identified relative stiffness values between the lesion and background pancreatic parenchyma using VTI and VTQ, which could be helpful in differentiating malignant tumors from benign inflammatory lesions, although there was a considerable degree of overlap between the ARFI values of the benign and malignant lesions. In D'Onofrio et al. experience, a wide range of wave velocity values results from ARFI analysis on pancreatic adenocarcinoma, but in any case a differential diagnosis with chronic pancreatitis is really difficult, and still now no cutoff values exist [2]. Pancreatic ductal adenocarcinoma usually presents at elastography, both qualitative and quantitative, as a harder mass than normal pancreatic adjacent parenchyma; it is also usually harder than benign lesions, but this last feature is not very simple to appreciate at elastographic study, and of course it is harder in relation to the adjacent parenchyma than benign lesions.

3.2.3.2 Other Solid Neoplasms

Neuroendocrine tumors are the second most common pancreatic solid neoplasms, accounting for about 1–2 % of all pancreatic neoplasms. They are epithelial tumors with neuroendocrine differentiation. Most neuroendocrine tumors present as a solitary, solid, well-circumscribed mass with sharp, rounded, or multi-lobulated borders, with an expansive growth pattern compared to the infiltrative one of ductal adenocarcinoma. At pathology neuroendocrine neoplasms typically have an organoid growth pattern, characterized by solid nests. They are tumors with very rich vascularization, responsible of the hypervascular radiological appearance [32, 46–48]. According to studies of Janssen, Hirche, Itokawa, and Giovannini, pancreatic neuroendocrine tumors can appear with a predominantly blue (the hardest color in the map) honeycomb pattern [9–12]; according to Hirche and Iglesias-Garcia, they can appear as homogeneous blue pattern [10, 13]; or according to Itokawa and Giovannini, they can appear as a green central area surrounded by blue tissue [11, 12]. Furthermore, Itokawa and Giovannini [11, 12] demonstrated also a homogeneous green pattern for pancreatic neuroendocrine neoplasms [2]. Iglesias-Garcia et al. [40] proved that endocrine tumors presented the highest strain ratio (mean 52.34) among pancreas focal lesions, leading EUS elastography to be helpful for differentiating pancreatic adenocarcinoma from neuroendocrine tumors with a sensitivity of 100 % and a specificity close to 88 %.

Other solid tumors of the pancreas can be metastases, although pancreatic metastases are very uncommon entities. In Giovannini and Iglesias-Garcia studies, metastases appear with a heterogeneously blue pattern [2, 12, 13].

3.2.4 Pancreatic Cystic Neoplasms

In pancreatic cystic lesions study, elastography can have a role, both with strain elastography and with share wave elastography, in particular with ARFI. In literature, there are few studies on cystic lesions and elastography, more about ARFI imaging. The application of ARFI quantification in fluids analysis is absolutely innovative. The basic concept is that different fluids are present into cystic lesions. Even though mechanical waves can propagate through both solid and liquid tissues, instead shear waves are more and highly attenuated in liquids, where only longitudinal waves or the shear wave reflection at the solid–fluid interface can be measured. The large range tissues with different fluid content in vivo, due to different viscosities and the presence of suspended particles, may generate different responses on ARFI imaging [49–51]. Experimental studies on fluid models that showed non-numerical values of share waves velocity at ARFI imaging (XXXX or 0 or X.XX on the monitor) in simple non-viscous fluids such as water have been made [49, 52–54]. The X.XX value can also be registered in solid lesions for several reasons, such as incorrect measurements or technical impairments. On the other hand, the possible result in ARFI fluid analysis is the achievement of a numerical value that can be considered related to the presence of viscous fluid [49–52]. In fluid contents, the obtained values with ARFI are related to the molecular motion inside the region of interest. In simple fluids, such as water, the excessive motion probably determines a too great variation of the individual velocity estimates between tracking beams with the obtaining of an unreliable measurement. In viscous fluids instead the molecular motion is reduced owing to the complex content, with the obtaining of a greater mechanical wave speed [20].

ARFI with the Virtual Touch tissue quantification seems to be able to do a not invasive study of fluid content of pancreatic cystic lesions, potentially improving the lesion characterization, that is nowadays still based on their morphology and architecture at imaging study with an invasive analysis of the fluid content still necessary to make a definitive diagnosis in all doubtful cases [51, 52].

3.2.4.1 Serous Neoplasms

The most common serous neoplasm is the serous cystadenoma, a neoplasm that tends to have a benign behavior. Its typical aspect is characterized by a cluster of microcysts (maximum 2 cm) separated by thin enhancing septa, sometimes forming a central scar, without connection with pancreatic duct. They could also have microcystic, macrocystic, and oligocystic aspects, and, in small percentage, about 5 % of cases, they could resemble a solid lesion due to enhancing septa and absence of visualization of the tiny cysts [20, 55, 56]. As specified by their name, serous cystadenomas are full of simple fluid that could be associated to water as intrinsic features. The value mainly measured in these pancreatic cystic lesions at ARFI quantification imaging is XXXX/0 m/s, as previously explained [20, 49, 52].

In literature microcystic serous cystadenoma aspect at endoscopic elastography was described by Janssen et al. affirming that it appears as a honeycomb predominantly blue pattern [9] and by Hirche et al. reporting that it appears as a homogeneously blue pattern or as a green area surrounded by blue tissue [10].

3.2.4.2 Mucinous Producing Neoplasms

Cystic pancreatic neoplasms producing mucinous are principally mucinous cystadenoma and intraductal papillary mucinous tumor. All these kinds of tumors produce mucus and, as a consequence, are filled by mucina that in this case can be considered a complex fluid. For these reasons, at ARFI quantitative imaging, it is reasonable to expect number values of share waves [49, 52].

3.2.4.3 Differential Diagnosis of Pancreatic Cystic Lesions

Pseudocyst is a complication of acute or chronic pancreatitis. To make diagnosis of pseudocyst of course is very important to know the patient medical history. This kind of pancreatic cyst has a fibrotic wall and is filled by fluid that can be different for hemorrhage or necrosis presence. For these reasons, at ARFI quantification imaging, it is possible to obtain different values of share waves depending on fluid contents, from serous type to very complex one [49, 52].

3.3 Clinical Indications and Guidelines

Transabdominal and endoscopic elastography can sufficiently and reproducibly distinguish between normal pancreatic parenchyma and most pancreatic tumors dominated by stiff (blue) areas. In pancreatic focal solid masses' characterization, a green predominant pattern is reported to exclude malignancy with high accuracy, whereas a hard or harder than normal pancreatic parenchyma pattern has been reported for tumors [2, 9, 13].

The clinical role of elastographic technique in pancreatic diseases differential diagnosis is however limited, as also showed by Hirche et al. [2, 10]. As a consequence of course, elastography examination cannot substitute the pathologic examination given by FNA or biopsy, so it cannot give a certain pathological diagnosis, but it can be a very useful tool in setting suspicious diagnosis and in guiding diagnostic and treatment management. An important role, giving information about tissue stiffness, can be found for the decision-making process, in particular in those patients with negative or inconclusive FNA in case of very strong clinical suspicious of malignancy. Regarding pancreatic ductal adenocarcinoma, other future applications of elastography could be the tumor stratification based on tissue stiffness predicting differentiation and response to therapy. Moreover a potential pancreatic surgical application of elastography before tumor resection can be the study of pancreatic parenchyma adjacent to the tumor in predicting the risk of postoperative fistula [2, 34].

In the 2013 EFSUMB guidelines about clinical use of ultrasound elastography [57], the role of predominately endoscopic ultrasound elastography is described also, and the recommendations for this study are:

- EUS elastography is useful as a complementary tool for the characterization of focal pancreatic lesions.
- When there is strong clinical suspicion of pancreatic cancer, but the biopsy is inconclusive or negative, a hard focal lesion on elastography and/or suggestive endoscopic contrast enhancement ultrasound (hypovascular lesion) [58] should guide clinical management by indicating repeat EUS-FNA or direct referral to surgery.
- EUS elastography cannot be currently recommended for differentiating advanced chronic pancreatitis from pancreatic carcinoma due to their similar tissue stiffness in a large proportion of cases.

3.4 Image Gallery

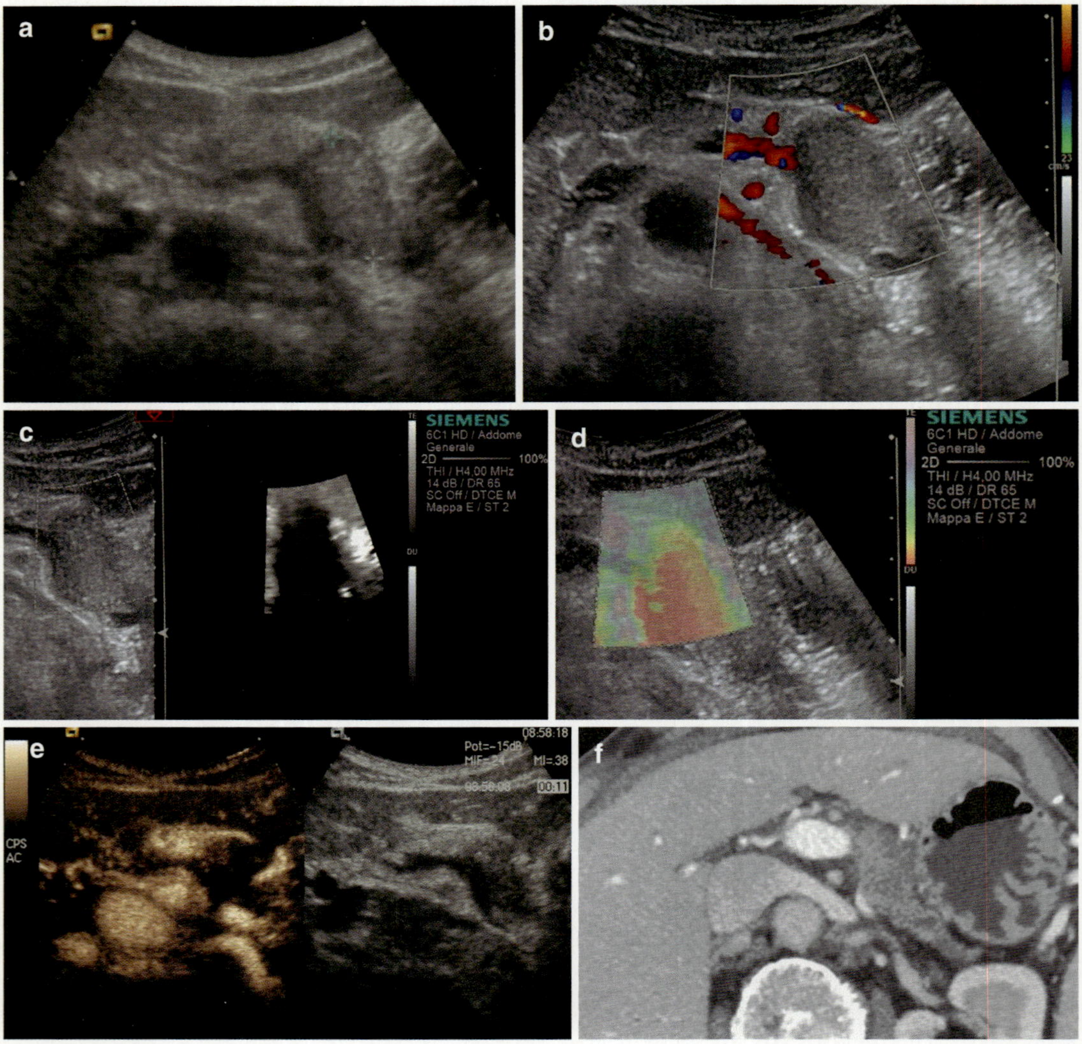

Fig. 3.1 Ductal adenocarcinoma. (**a**–**e**) Complete US study: round-shaped hypoechoic mass (*calipers* in **a**) located in the pancreatic body with no visible Doppler signals according to the very low vascular density of the neoplastic tissue at color Doppler analysis (**b**) and resulting stiff (*black* in **c**, *red* in **d**) due to the rich desmoplastic stroma in the elastogram. At CEUS the lesion typically shows markedly hypovascular pattern (**e**). (**f**) Dynamic CT: hypovascular hypodense mass with upstream dilated Wirsung duct

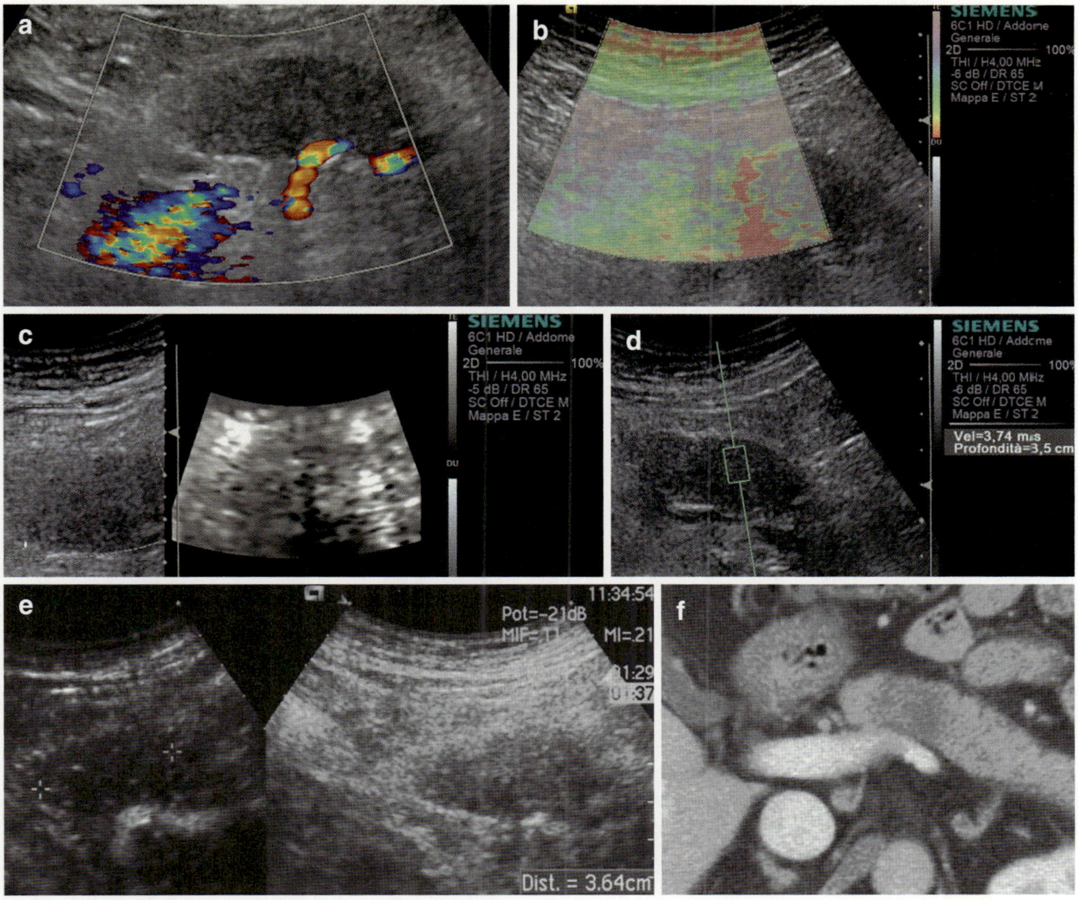

Fig. 3.2 Ductal adenocarcinoma. (**a**–**e**) Complete US study: round-shaped hypoechoic mass (**a**) located in the pancreatic body resulting stiff (marginally *red* in **b**, inhomogeneously *black* in **c**) due to the rich desmoplastic stroma in the elastogram. At the quantitative ARFI elastography, a velocity value of 3.74 m/s is detected (**d**). At color Doppler analysis (**a**), no Doppler signal is visible within the lesion according to the very low vascular density of the neoplastic tissue. At CEUS the lesion typically shows markedly hypovascular pattern (*calipers* in **e**). (**f**) CT study: typical appearance of a pancreatic ductal adenocarcinoma, presenting as a hypovascular lesion (**f**) in comparison to the adjacent pancreatic parenchyma at venous phase

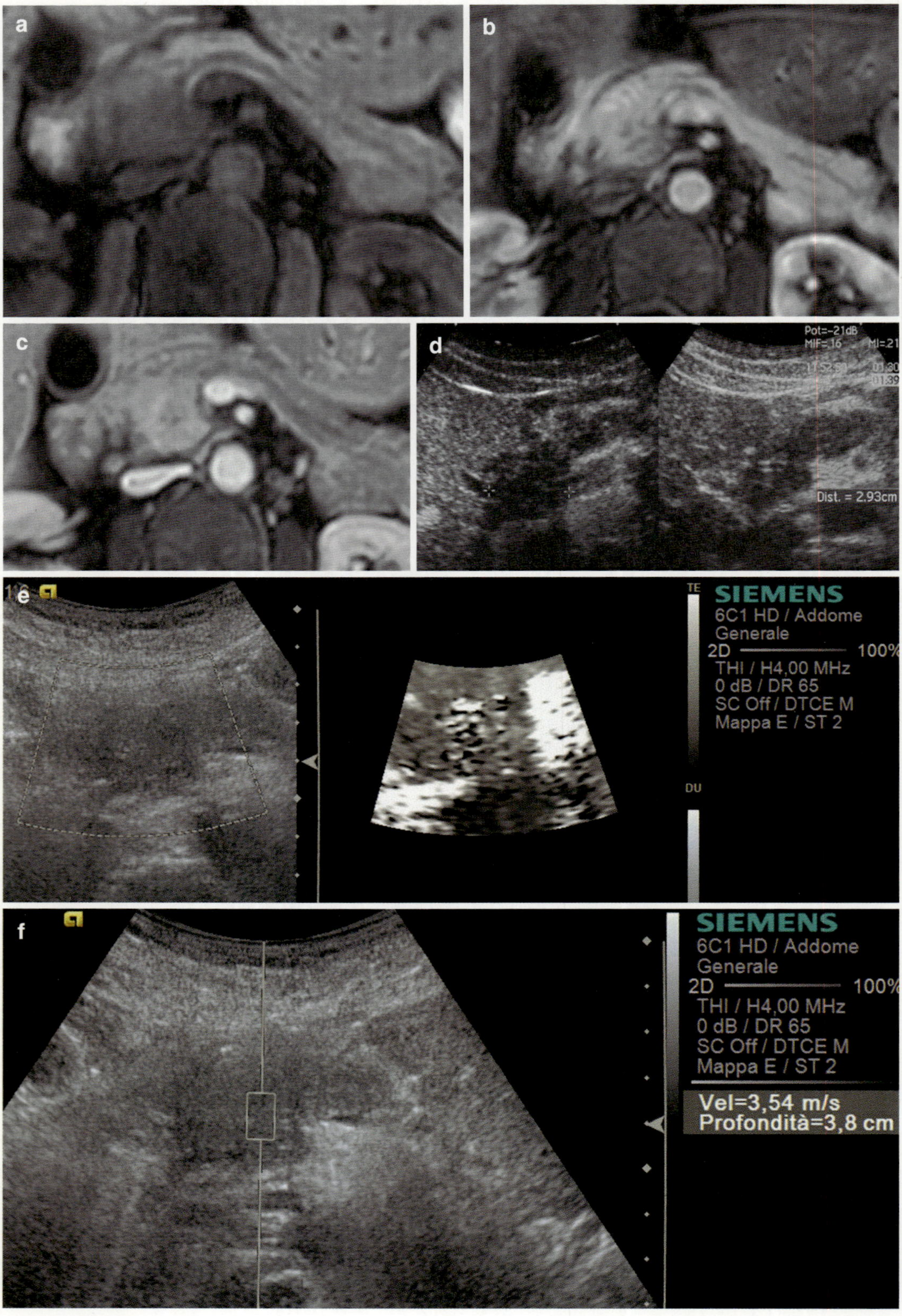
a
b
c
d
Pot=-21dB
MIF=16
Dist. = 2.93cm
e
TE
DU
SIEMENS
6C1 HD / Addome Generale
2D 100%
THI / H4,00 MHz
0 dB / DR 65
SC Off / DTCE M
Mappa E / ST 2
f
SIEMENS
6C1 HD / Addome Generale
2D 100%
THI / H4,00 MHz
0 dB / DR 65
SC Off / DTCE M
Mappa E / ST 2
Vel=3,54 m/s
Profondità=3,8 cm

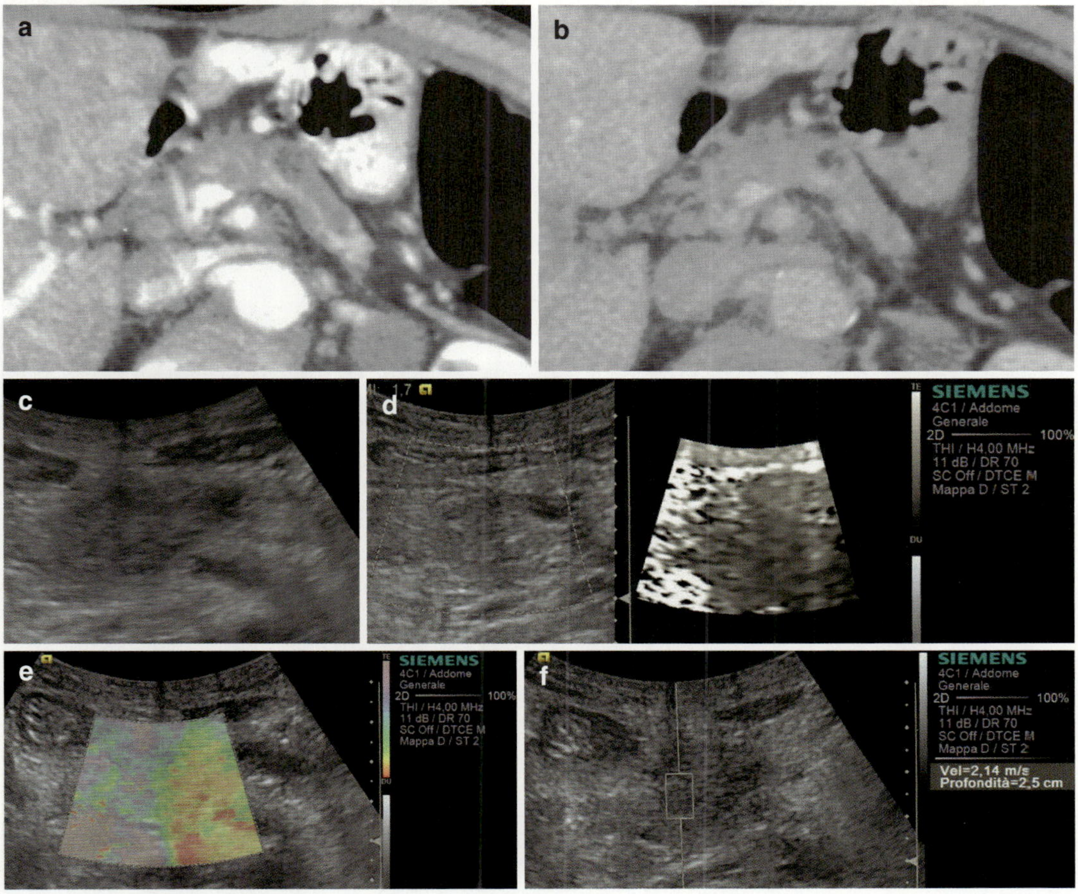

Fig. 3.4 Ductal adenocarcinoma. (**a–b**) CT study: slightly hypovascular mass in the pancreatic isthmus at pancreatic (**a**) and venous (**b**) dynamic phases, causing upstream dilation of the Wirsung duct. (**c–f**) US study: round-shaped hypoechoic mass (**c**) located in the pancreas resulting stiff (*black* in **d**, *red* in **e**) due to the rich desmoplastic stroma in the elastogram. At the quantitative ARFI elastography, a velocity value of 2.14 m/s is detected (**f**)

Fig. 3.3 Pancreatic adenocarcinoma. (**a–c**) MRI study: pancreatic mass hypointense on T1-weighted fat-saturated (**a**) image. In the pancreatic dynamic phase, the mass is hypovascular (**b**) with progressive contrast medium retention in the following phases (**c**). The Wirsung duct is upstream dilated. (**d–f**) US study: round-shaped hypoechoic mass located in the pancreatic head resulting stiff (slightly *black* in **e**) in the elastogram due to the rich desmoplastic stroma. At the quantitative ARFI elastography, a velocity value of 3.54 m/s is detected (**f**). At CEUS the lesion typically shows markedly hypovascular pattern (*calipers* in **d**)

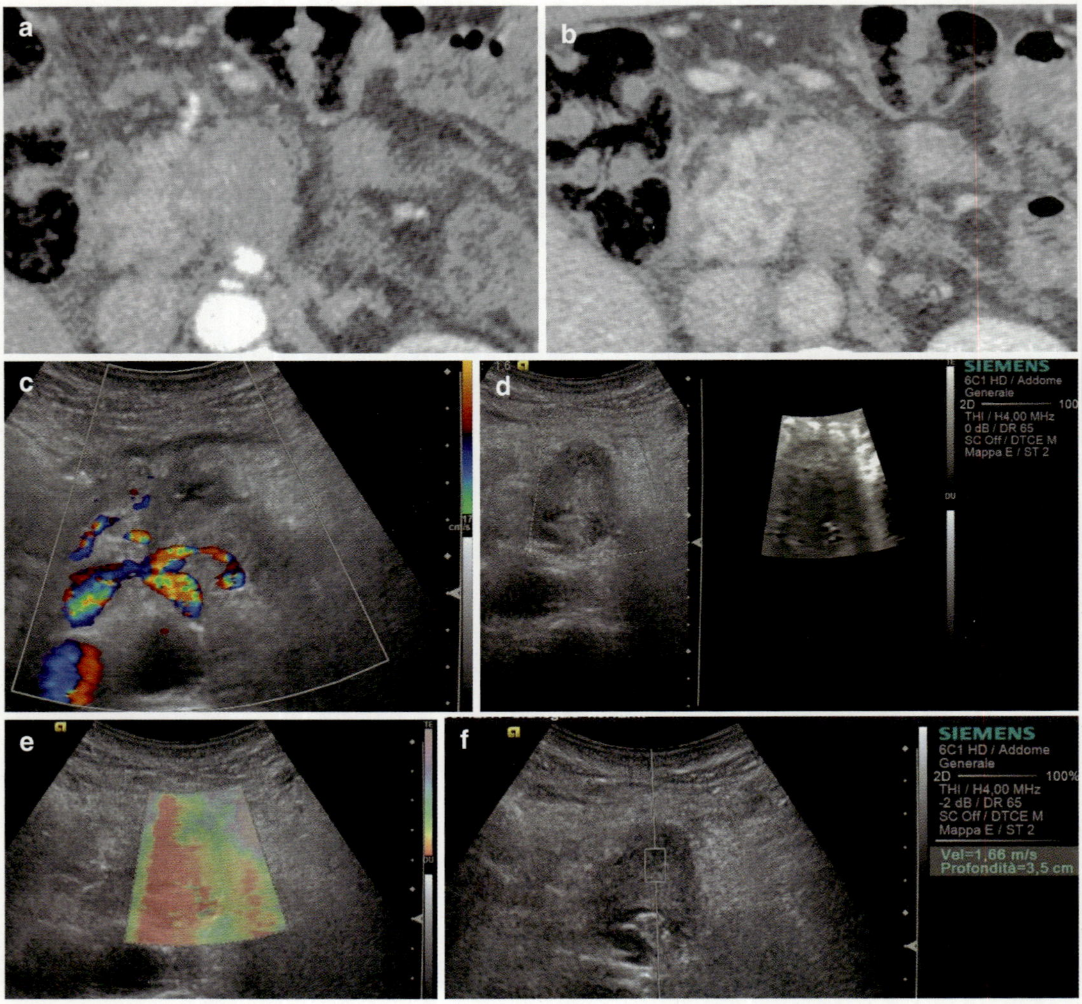

Fig. 3.5 Ductal adenocarcinoma. (**a–b**) CT study: typical appearance of a pancreatic ductal adenocarcinoma, presenting hypovascular in comparison to the adjacent pancreatic parenchyma at pancreatic (**a**) and venous (**b**) dynamic phases. (**c–f**) US study: round-shaped hypoechoic mass (**c**) located in the pancreas resulting stiff (*black* in **d**, *red* in **e**) due to the rich desmoplastic stroma in the elastogram. At color Doppler analysis (**c**), no Doppler signal is visible within the lesion according to the very low vascular density of the neoplastic tissue. At the quantitative ARFI elastography, a velocity value of 1.66 m/s is detected (**f**)

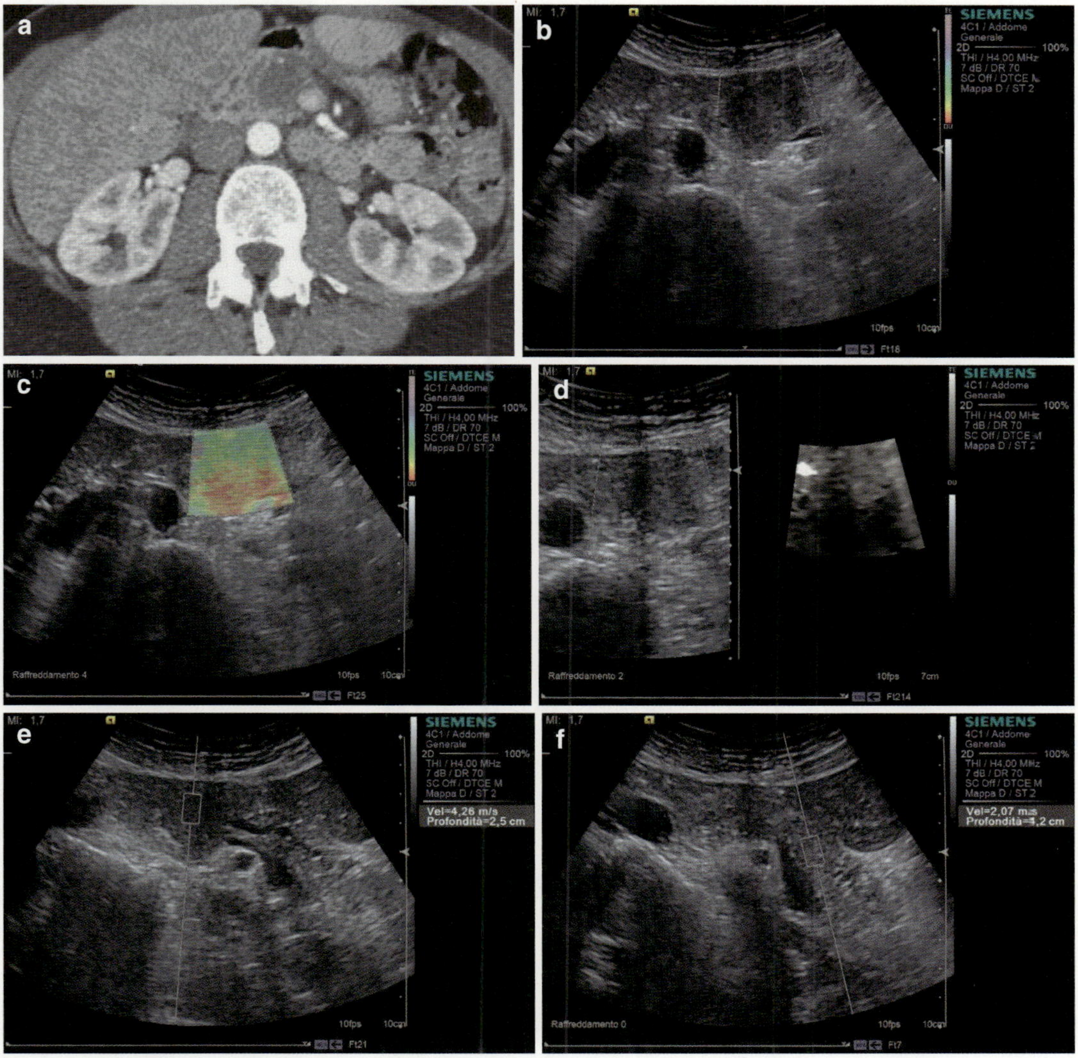

Fig. 3.6 Ductal adenocarcinoma. (**a**) CT study: study demonstrates a round-shaped lesion hypovascular on pancreatic (**a**) phase located in the pancreatic head. (**b–f**) Conventional US study: round-shaped hypoechoic mass (**b**) located in the pancreatic head resulting stiff (*red* in **c**, *black* in **d**) due to the rich desmoplastic stroma in the elastogram. At the quantitative ARFI elastography, high velocity value (4,26 m/s in **e**) is confirmed within the lesion in respect to the pancreatic body parenchyma (2,07 m/s in **f**)

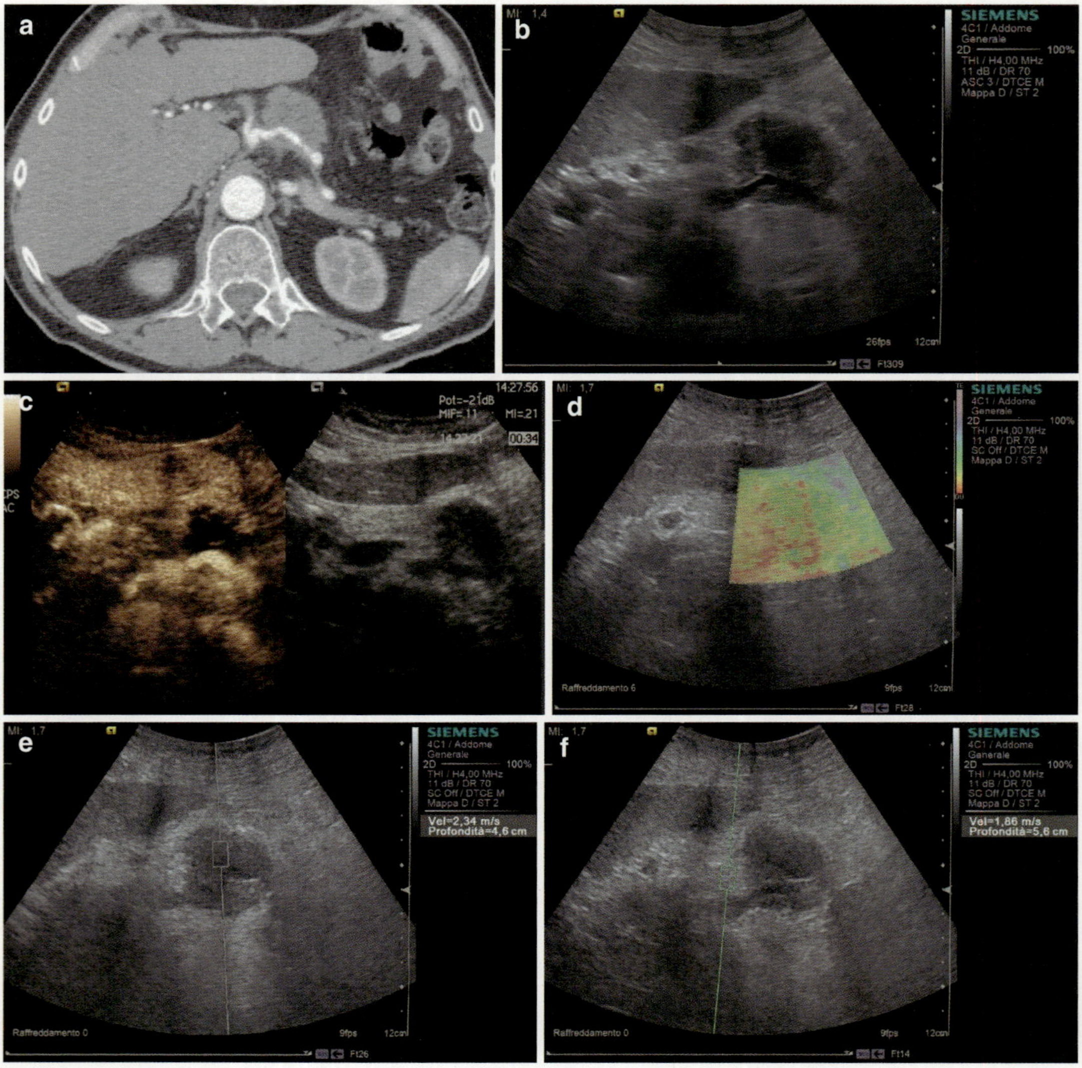

Fig. 3.7 Ductal adenocarcinoma. (**a**) CT study: study demonstrates a round-shaped lesion hypovascular hypodense on pancreatic (**a**) phase located in the pancreatic body. (**b–f**) Complete US study: round-shaped hypoechoic mass (**b**) located in the pancreatic body. At CEUS the lesion typically shows markedly hypovascular pattern (**c**). The lesion results stiff (*red*) due to the rich desmoplastic stroma at the previously performed elastographic study (**d**), and at the quantitative ARFI elastography, high velocity value (2.34 m/s in **e**) is confirmed in respect to the pancreatic body parenchyma (1.86 m/s in **f**)

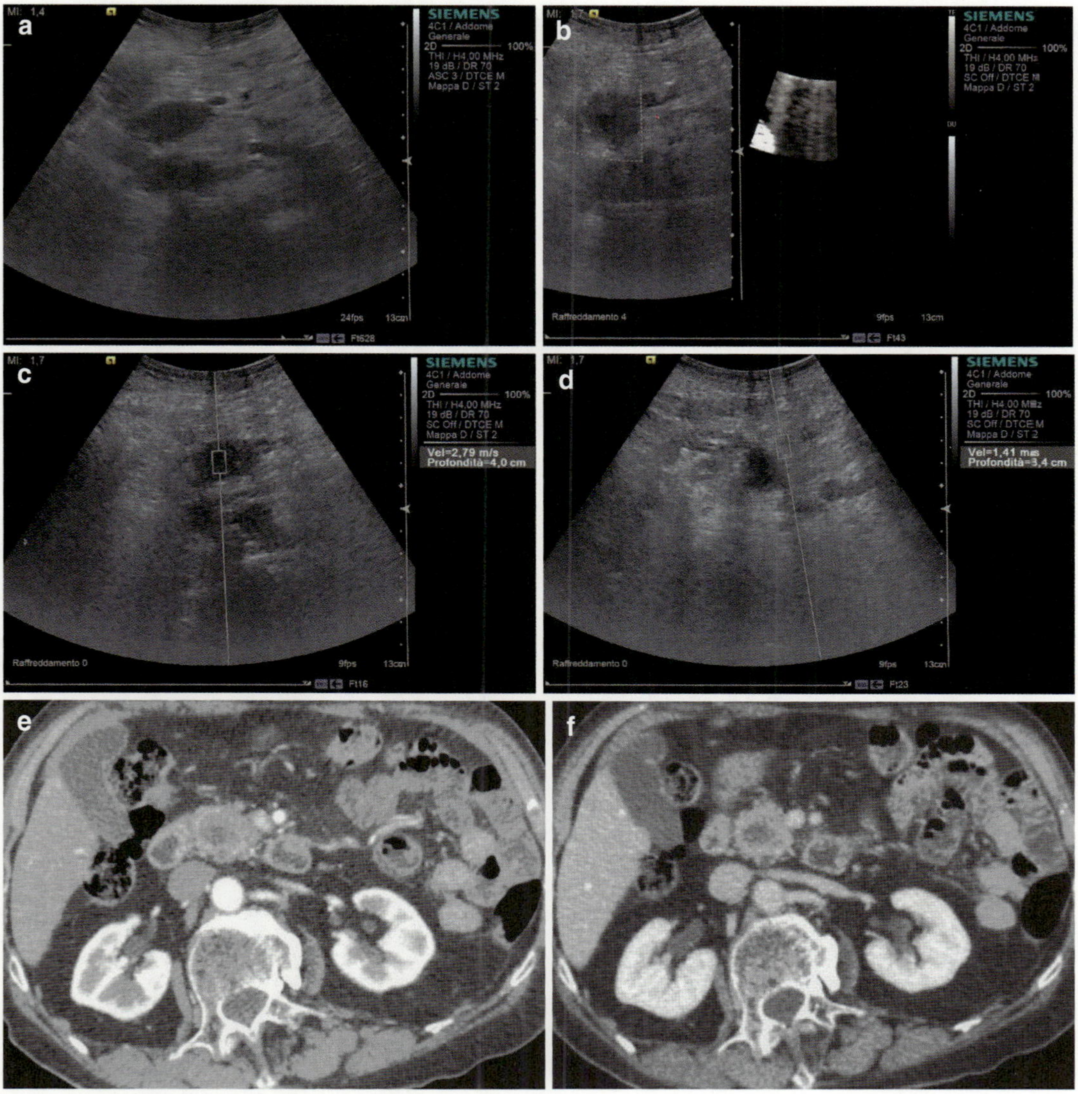

Fig. 3.8 Ductal adenocarcinoma. (**a–d**) US study: round-shaped hypoechoic mass (**a**) located in the pancreatic head resulting stiff (*black*) due to the rich desmoplastic stroma in the elastogram (**b**). At the quantitative ARFI elastography, high velocity value (2.79 m/s in **c**) is confirmed in respect to the pancreatic body parenchyma (1.41 m/s in **d**). (**e–f**) Dynamic CT: study demonstrates a round-shaped lesion hypovascular hypodense on pancreatic phase (**a**) located in the pancreatic head that is in strict contact with superior mesenteric vein, better visible in venous phase (**f**)

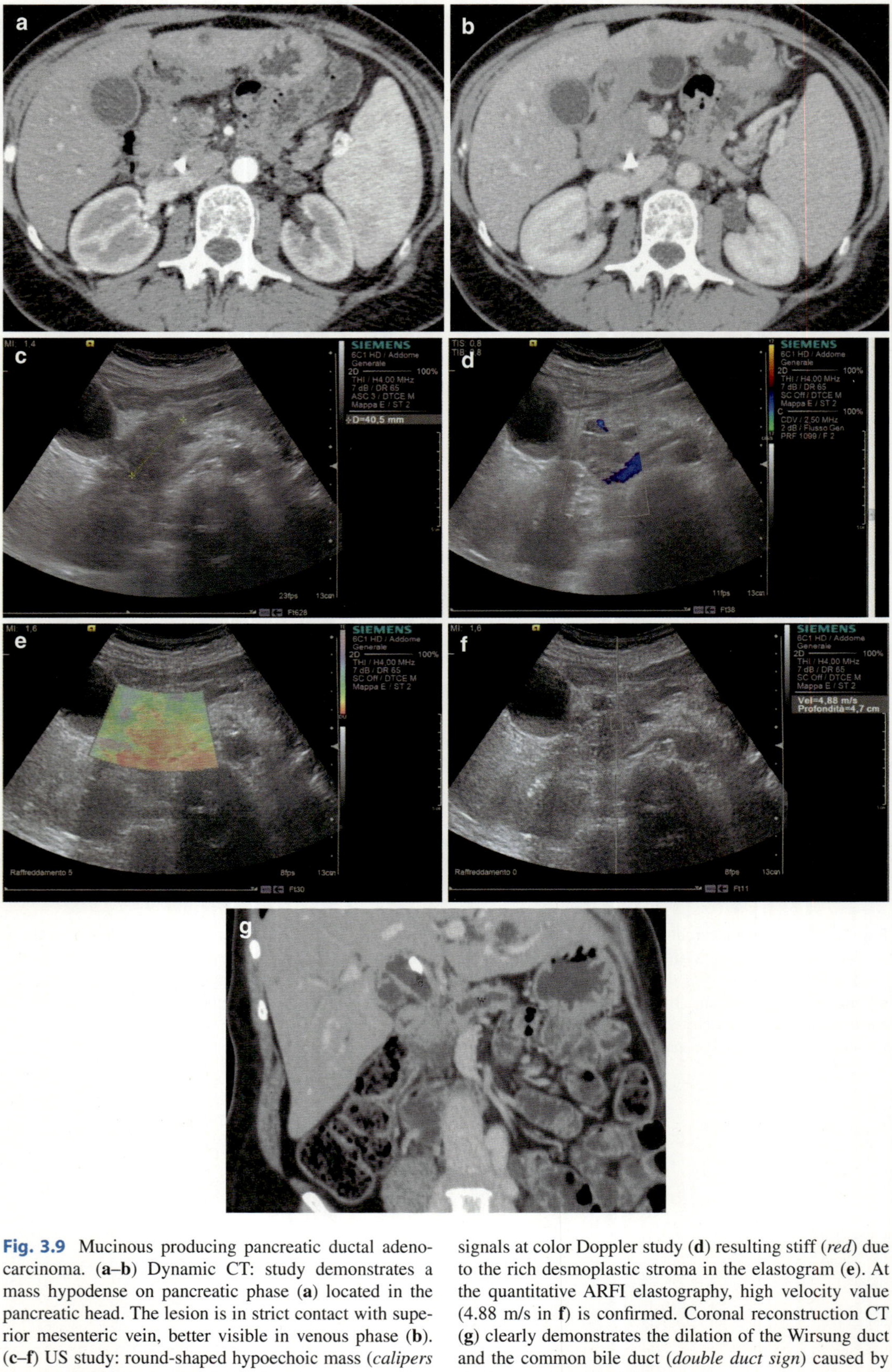

Fig. 3.9 Mucinous producing pancreatic ductal adenocarcinoma. (**a–b**) Dynamic CT: study demonstrates a mass hypodense on pancreatic phase (**a**) located in the pancreatic head. The lesion is in strict contact with superior mesenteric vein, better visible in venous phase (**b**). (**c–f**) US study: round-shaped hypoechoic mass (*calipers* in **c**) located in the pancreatic head with no vascular flow signals at color Doppler study (**d**) resulting stiff (*red*) due to the rich desmoplastic stroma in the elastogram (**e**). At the quantitative ARFI elastography, high velocity value (4.88 m/s in **f**) is confirmed. Coronal reconstruction CT (**g**) clearly demonstrates the dilation of the Wirsung duct and the common bile duct (*double duct sign*) caused by the tumor in pancreatic head

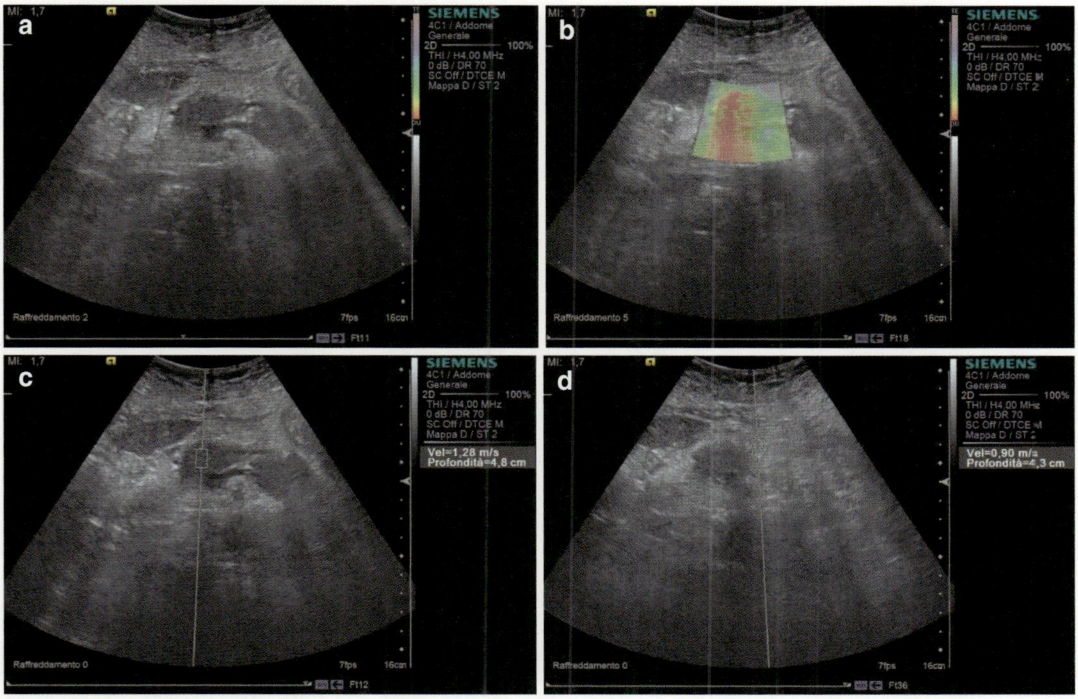

Fig. 3.10 Ductal adenocarcinoma. (**a–d**) US study: hypoechoic round-shaped lesion (**a**) with blurred margins located in the pancreatic neck resulting stiff (*red*) due to the rich desmoplastic stroma in the elastogram (**b**). At the quantitative ARFI elastography, high velocity value (1,28 m/s in **c**) is confirmed in respect to the pancreatic body parenchyma (0,90 m/s in **d**)

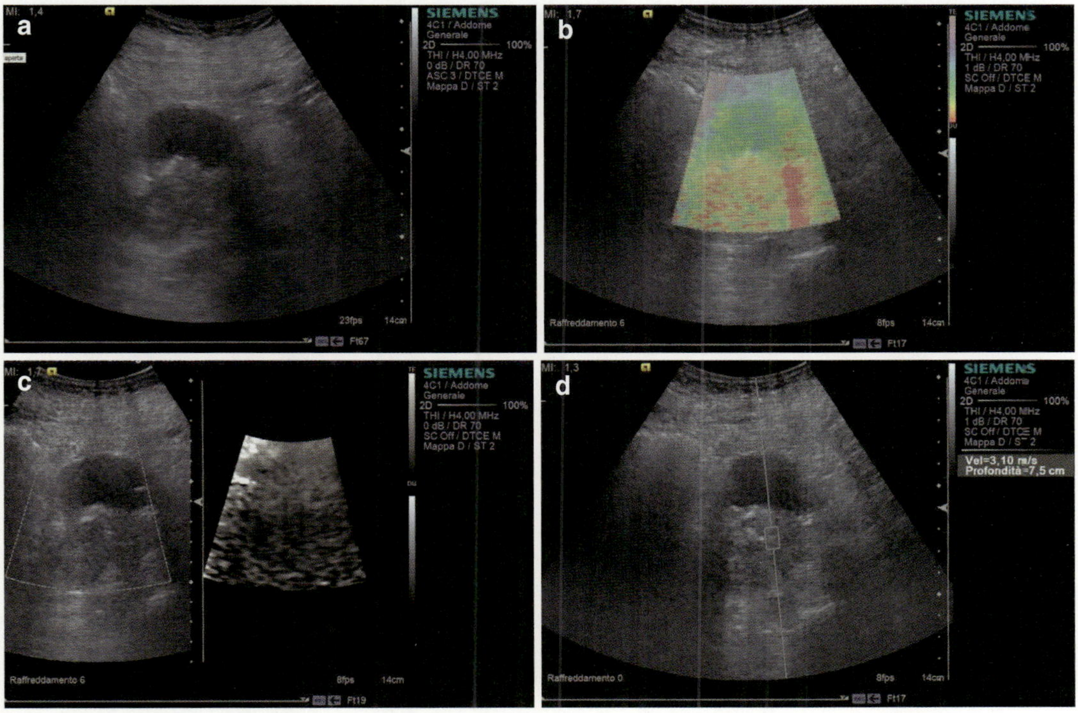

Fig. 3.11 Pancreatic ductal adenocarcinoma with cystic cavity. (**a–d**) US study: complex solid and cystic mass (**a**) in the pancreatic head. Solid component results stiff (*red* in **b** and *black* in **c**) due to the rich desmoplastic stroma in the elastogram. At the quantitative ARFI elastography, high velocity value (3,10 m/s in **b**) is confirmed within the solid lesion portion

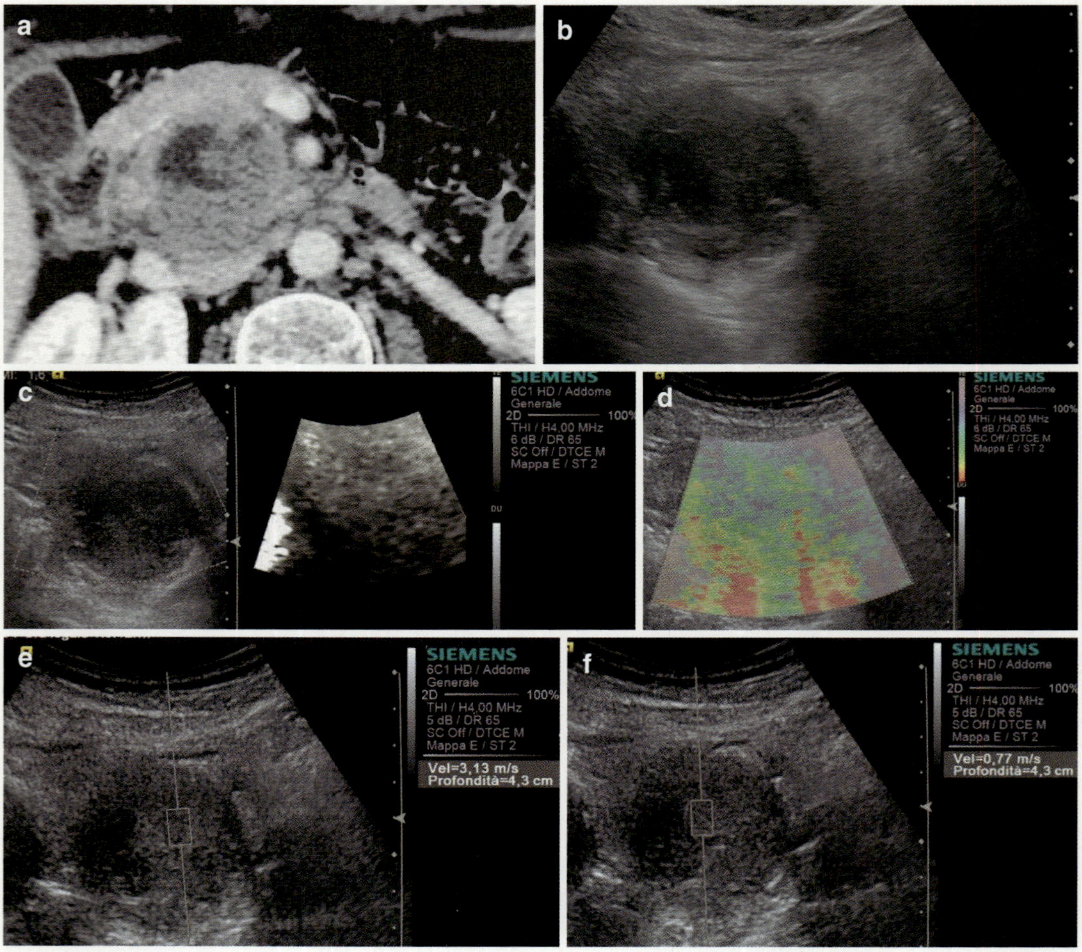

Fig. 3.12 Anaplastic carcinoma. (**a**) CT study: pancreatic mass appearing hypovascular hypodense on pancreatic (**a**) phase with central evident avascular necrotic area. (**b–f**) Ultrasound study: in the pancreas an round-shaped mass markedly hypoechoic (**b**) on conventional ultrasound is visible. It results moderately soft (slightly *black* in **c** and *blue-green* in **d**) due to the central necrotic area in the elastogram. At the quantitative ARFI elastography, a velocity value of 3.13 m/s is detected in the solid viable part of the lesion (**e**), whereas a velocity value of 0.77 m/s is detected in the necrotic component of the lesion (**f**)

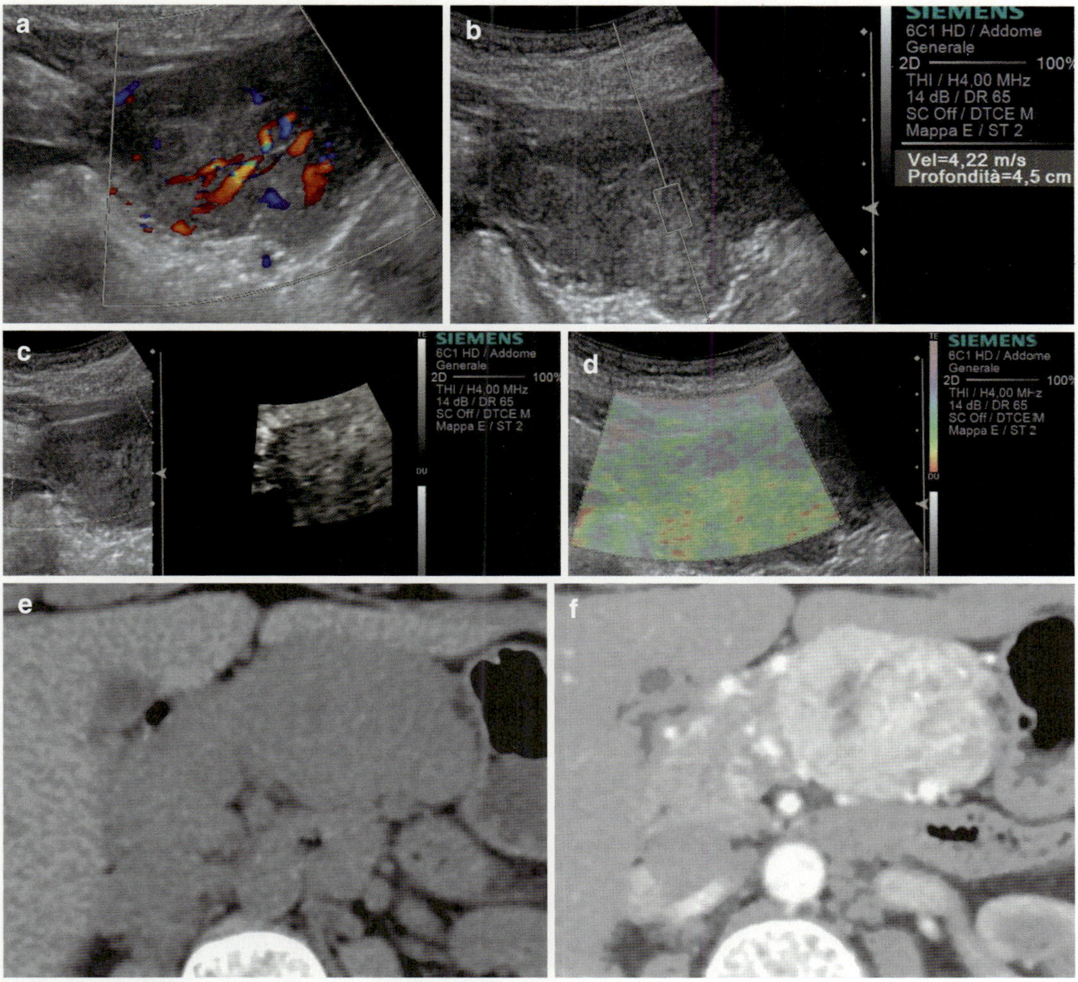

Fig. 3.13 Neuroendocrine pancreatic tumor. (**a–d**) US study: typical US presentation of neuroendocrine pancreatic tumor (NET) as a well-demarked homogeneous hypoechoic mass (**a**) located in the pancreatic body resulting stiff (*black* in **c**, *yellow-green* in **d**) in the elastogram. At the color Doppler examination, the lesion shows a pronounced "spot" pattern (**a**). At the quantitative ARFI elastography, a velocity value of 4.22 m/s is detected (**b**). (**e–f**) CT study: solid mass of the pancreas isodense (**e**) in the baseline study and hypervascularized on pancreatic (**f**) phase in comparison to the adjacent pancreatic parenchyma

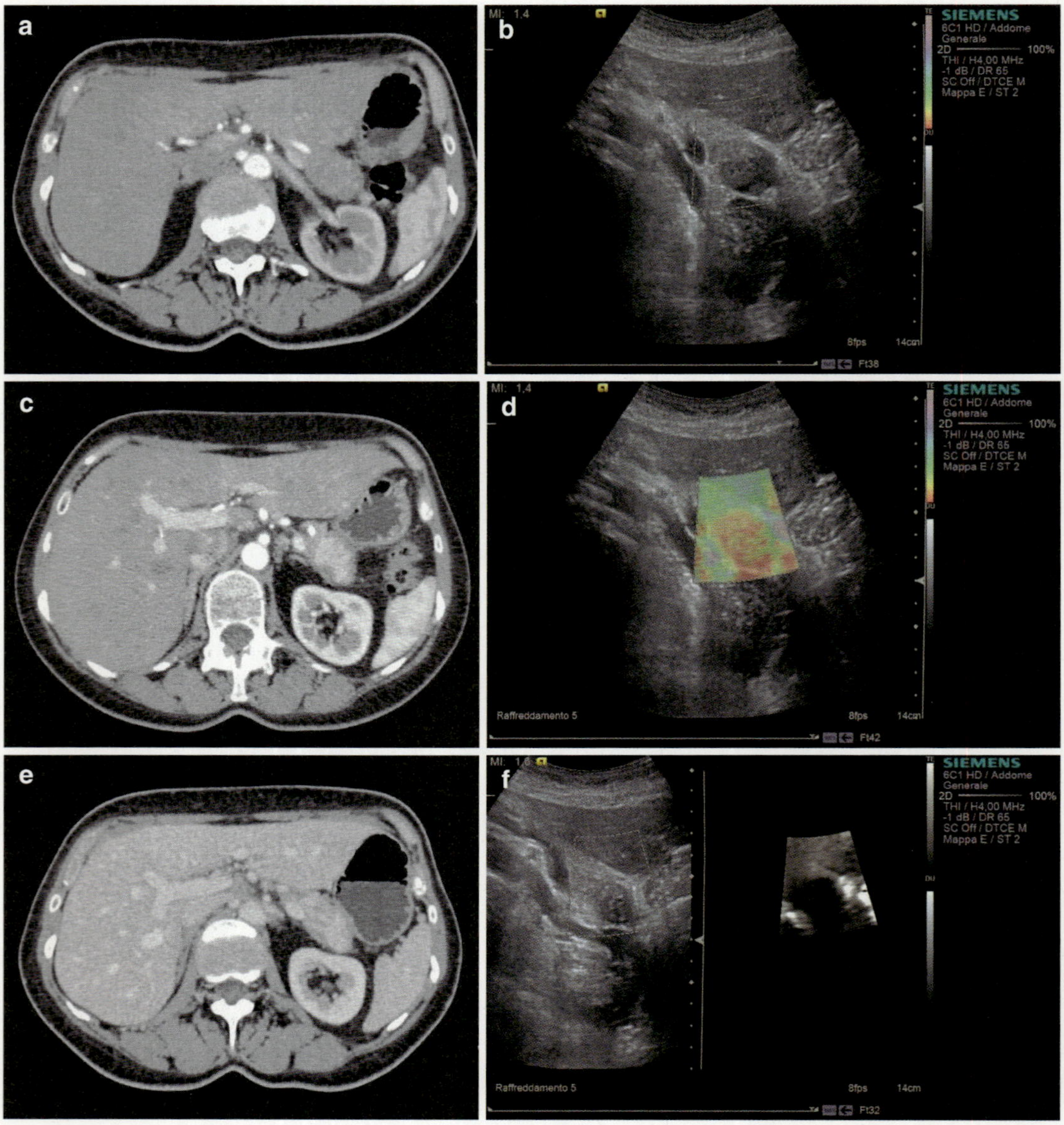

Fig. 3.14 Neuroendocrine pancreatic tumor. (**a**, **c**, **e**) CT study: solid mass of the pancreatic body slightly hyperdense in the arterial phase (**a**) and hyperdense on pancreatic (**c**) phase in comparison to the adjacent pancreatic parenchyma. During the venous phase, the lesion appears slightly hyperdense (**e**). (**b**, **d**, **f**) US study: typical US presentation of neuroendocrine pancreatic tumor (NET) as a well-demarked homogeneous hypoechoic mass (**b**) resulting stiff due to the rich desmoplastic stroma in the elastogram (*red* in **d** and *black* in **f**)

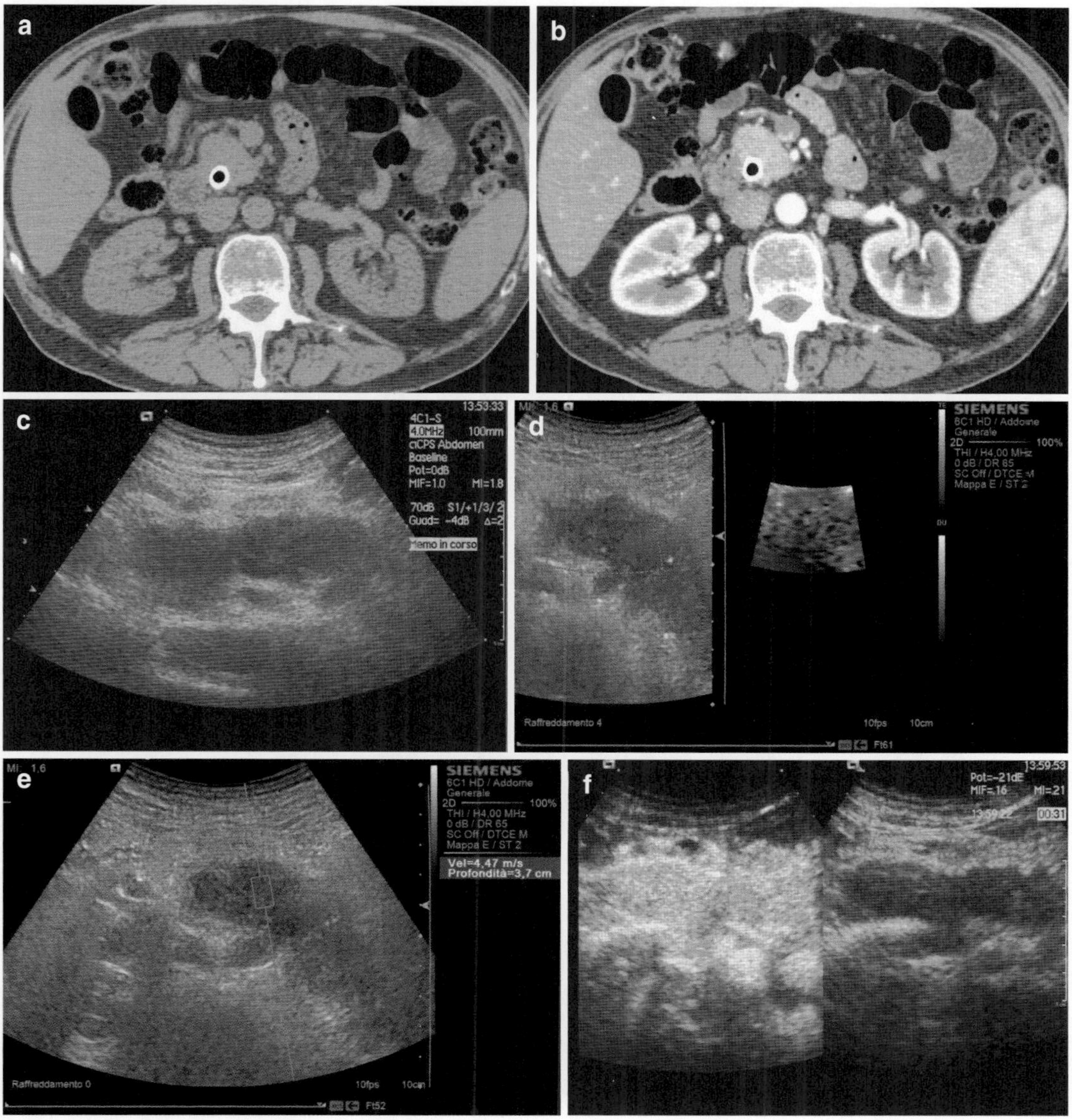

Fig. 3.15 Autoimmune pancreatitis. (**a**–**b**) CT study: diffuse form with slightly enlargement of pancreatic head isodense on basal (**a**) and pancreatic (**b**) phases. Presence of biliary endoprothesis but no dilation of main pancreatic duct. (**c**–**f**) Complete US study: diffuse form of autoimmune pancreatitis appearing as diffuse enlargement with typical "sausage" shape of pancreatic gland slightly hypoechoic on conventional ultrasound (**c**). The gland resulting stiff (slightly *black*) in the elastogram (**d**). At the quantitative ARFI elastography, high velocity value (4.47 m/s in **e**) is confirmed (**e**). At CEUS all part of gland result isovascular (**f**)

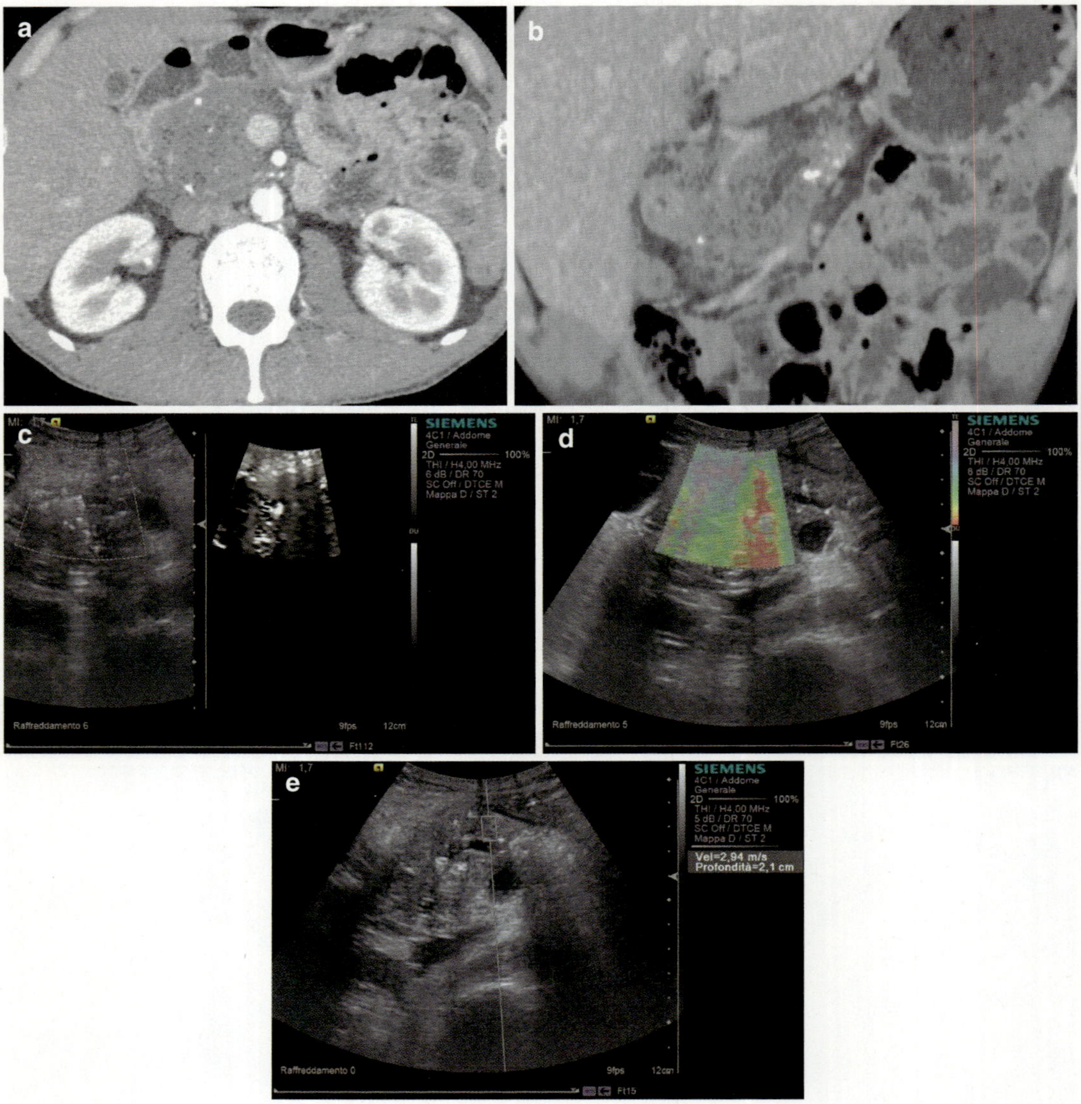

Fig. 3.16 Paraduodenal (groove) pancreatitis. (**a**–**b**) CT study: study demonstrates an enlargement of pancreatic head resulting hypovascular and hypodense due to chronic inflammation on pancreatic phase (**a**) with some calcifications and small cysts within the mass. In addition, there is a thickening of duodenal wall. Coronal reconstruction on venous phase shows a mass causing dilation of Wirsung duct. (**c**–**e**) US study: hypoechoic and heterogeneous mass located in the pancreatic head causes dilation of Wirsung duct and resulting stiff (*black* in **c** and *red* in **d**) in the elastogram due to the rich fibrotic tissue. At the quantitative ARFI elastography, high velocity value (2,94 m/s in **e**) is confirmed

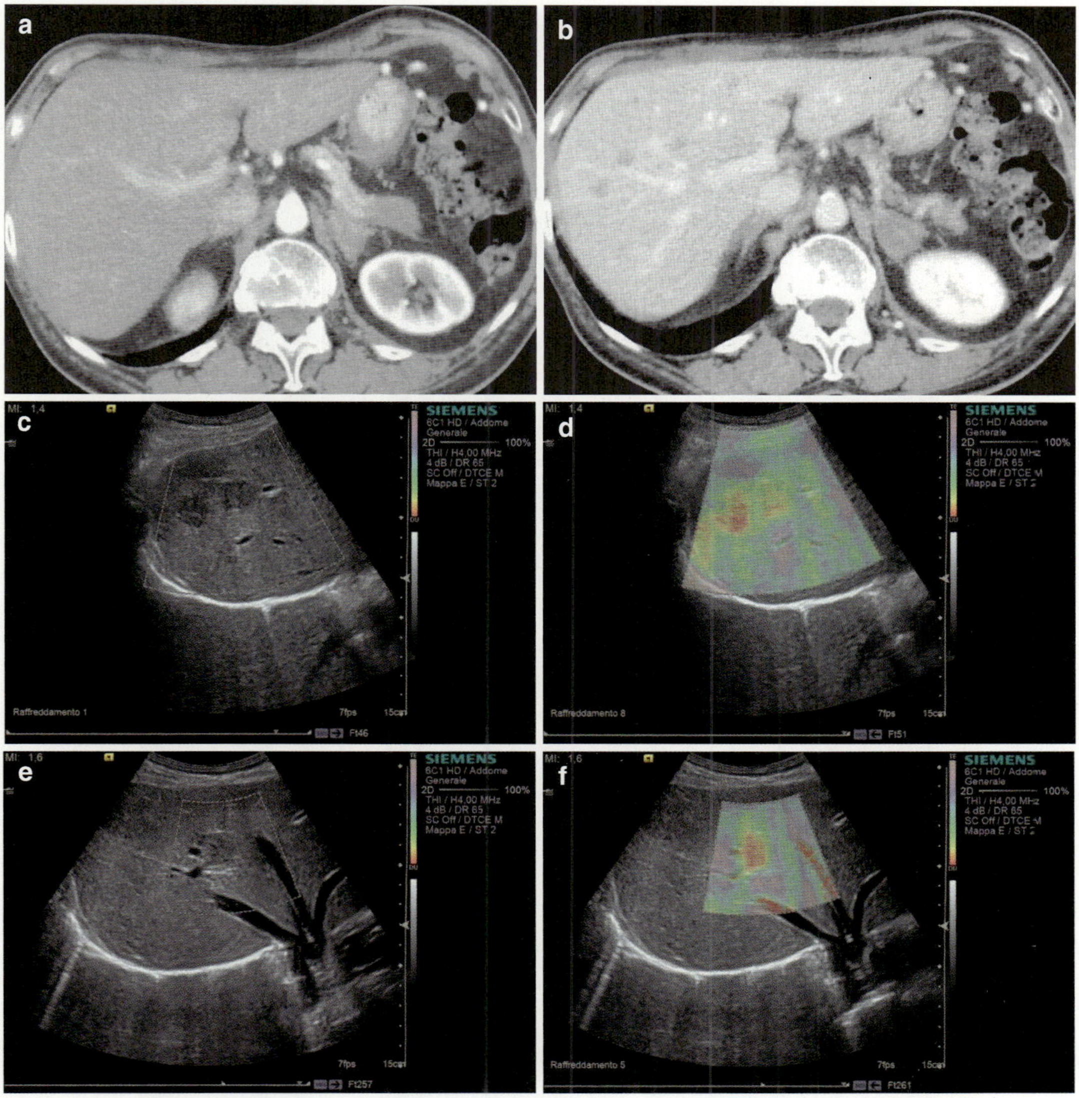

Fig. 3.17 Pancreatic adenocarcinoma with metastatic spread. (**a–b**) CT study: hypodense mass in the pancreatic (**a**) phase located in the tail of the pancreas. Liver metastases are visible as hypodense lesions in the venous (**b**) phase. (**c–f**) US study: round-shaped hypoechoic nodules (**c**, **e**) located in the right lobe of the liver resulting stiff (*red*) in the elastogram (**d**, **f**)

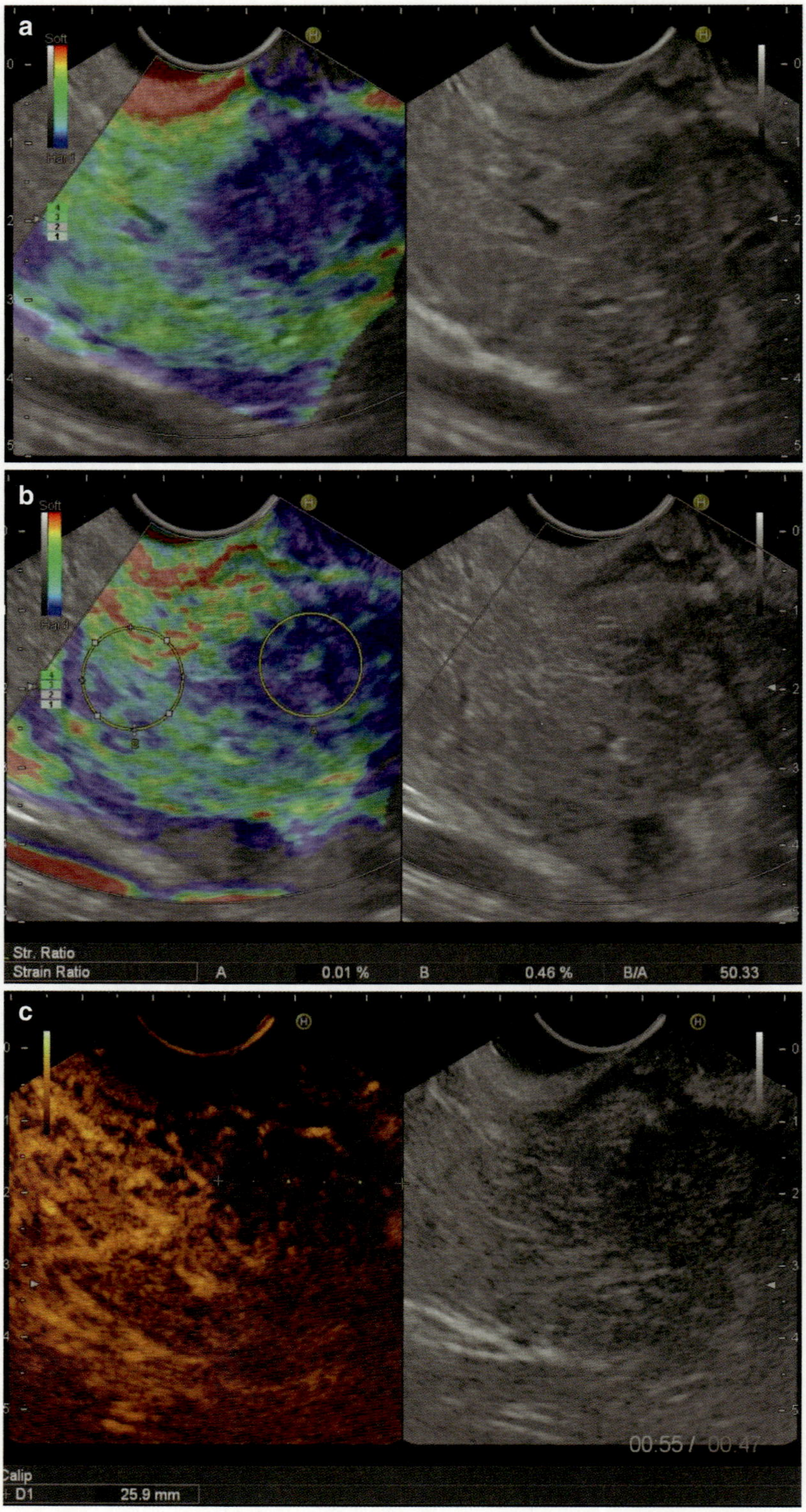

Fig. 3.18 Ductal adenocarcinoma (**a**, **b**). EUS elastosonographic study shows a hypoechoic lesion in the head of the pancreas with a homogeneous *blue pattern* surrounded by normal *green* parenchyma (**a**), a mass elasticity of 0.46% with strain ratio of 50 at semiquantitative study (**b**). (**c**) E-CEUS study. After infusion of echographic contrast, the lesion appears hypovascularized (**c**)

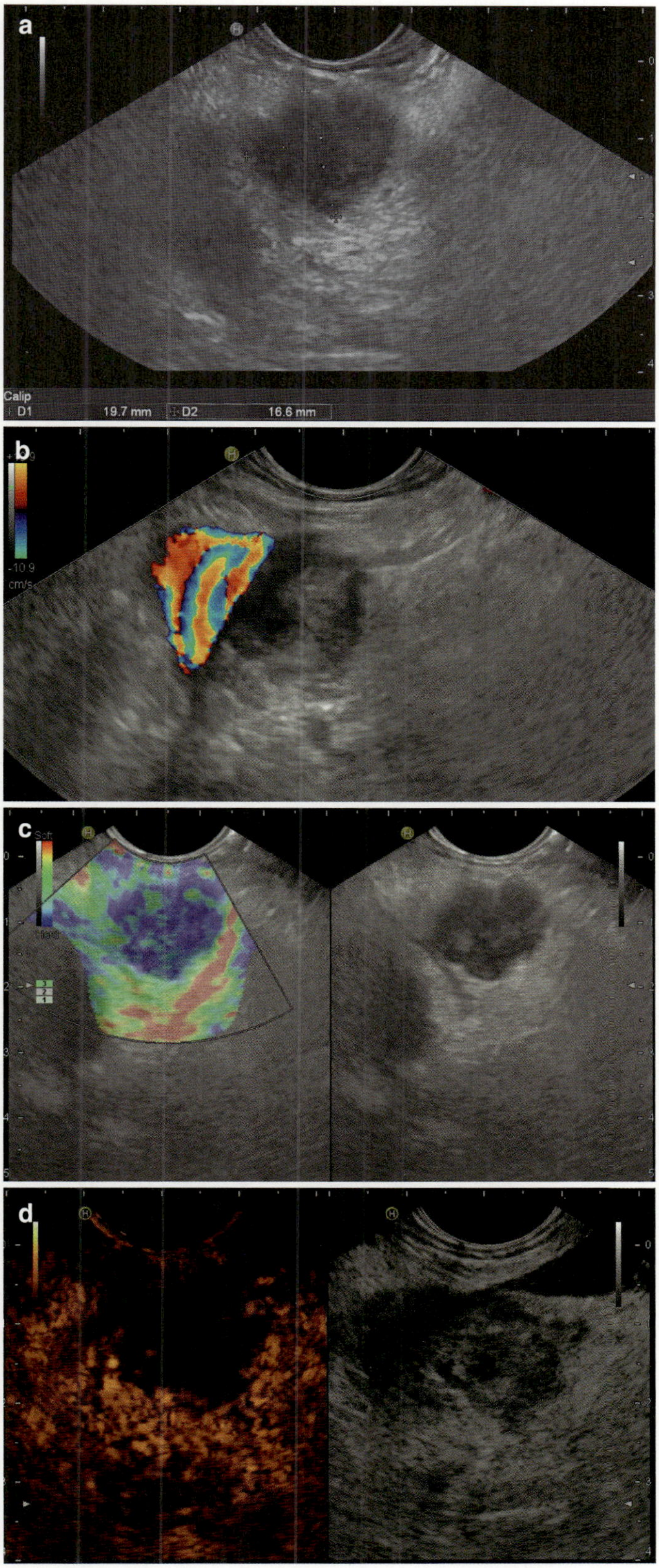

Fig. 3.19 Ductal adenocarcinoma. (**a–d**) EUS study. Hypoechoic pancreatic mass with irregular margins in B-mode EUS imaging (**a**) infiltrating splenomesenteric venous confluence with Doppler signal (**b**). With qualitative EUS, elastosonography adenocarcinoma shows a homogeneous *blue pattern* (**c**) and appears hypovascular after injection of contrast (**d**)

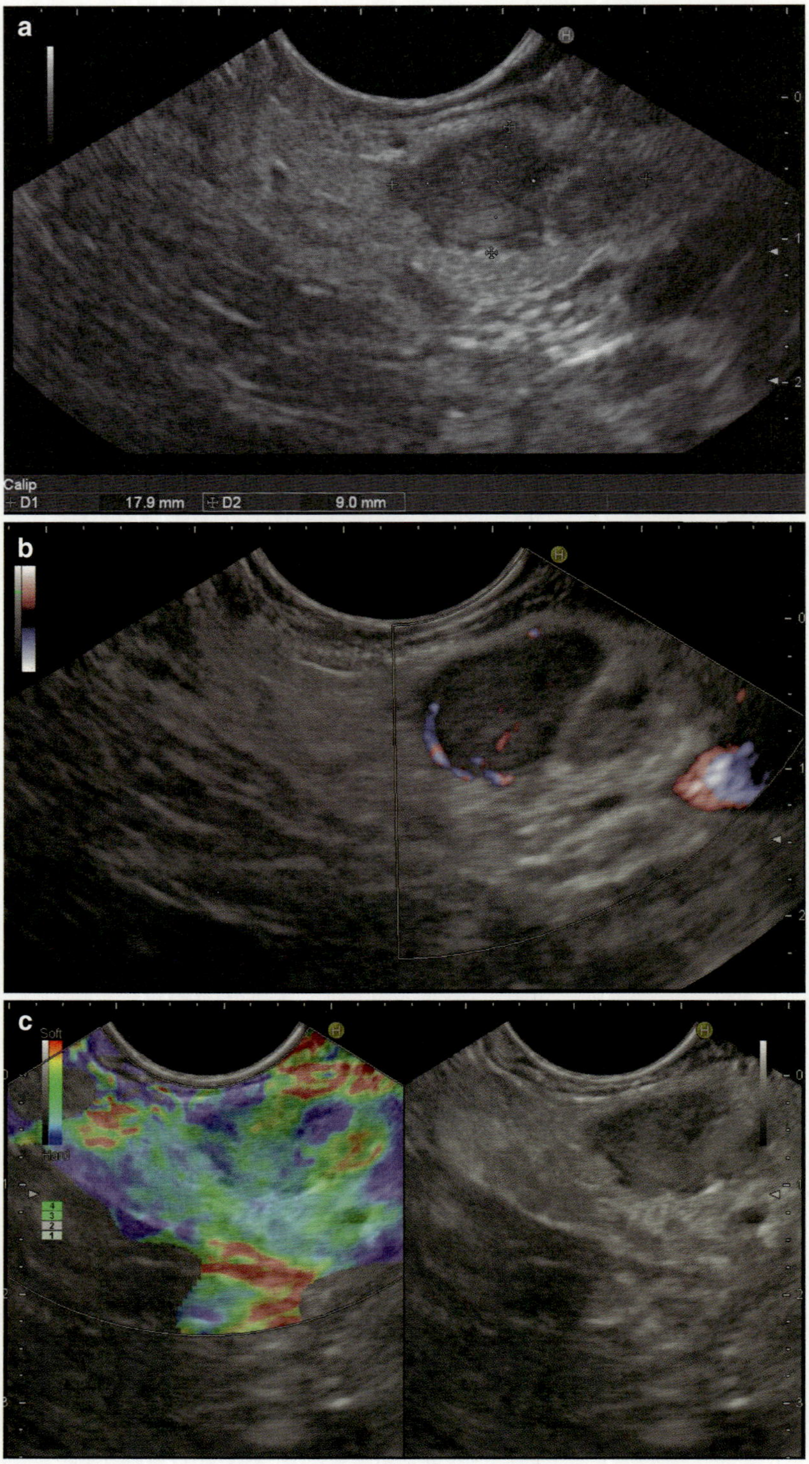

Fig. 3.20 Neuroendocrine tumor. (**a–f**) EUS study. B-mode image shows a small incidentally hypoechoic solid mass (**a**) with a peripheral vascularization at the fine flow Doppler signal (**b**). Qualitative elastosonographic study shows a mixed *blue-green pattern* (**c**) with a strain ratio and a mass elasticity of 0.45 and 0.12 %, respectively (**d**). The typical rapid intense enhancement in early phase after injection of contrast (**e**) and adequate fine needle aspiration (**f**) is definitively diagnostic

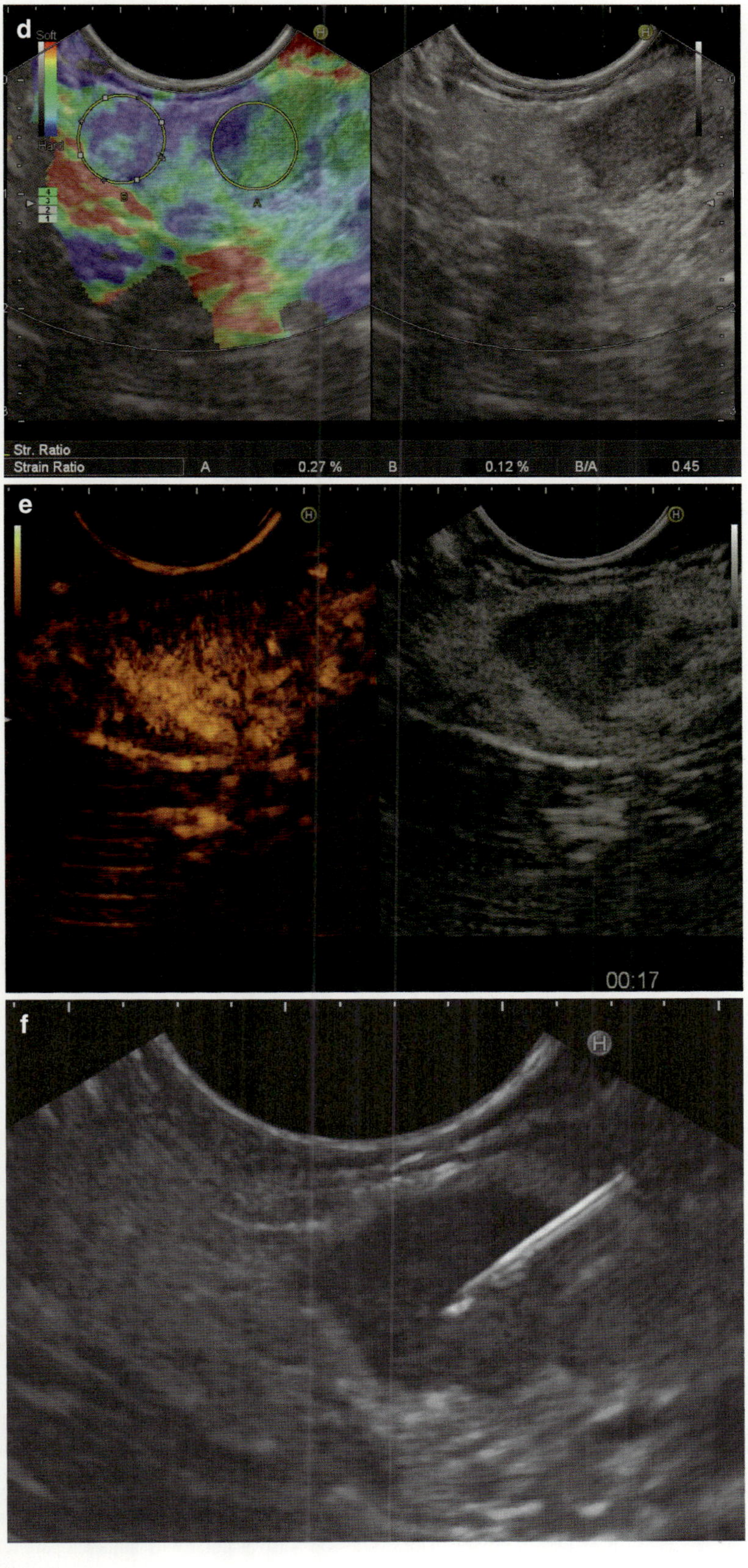

Fig. 3.20 (continued)

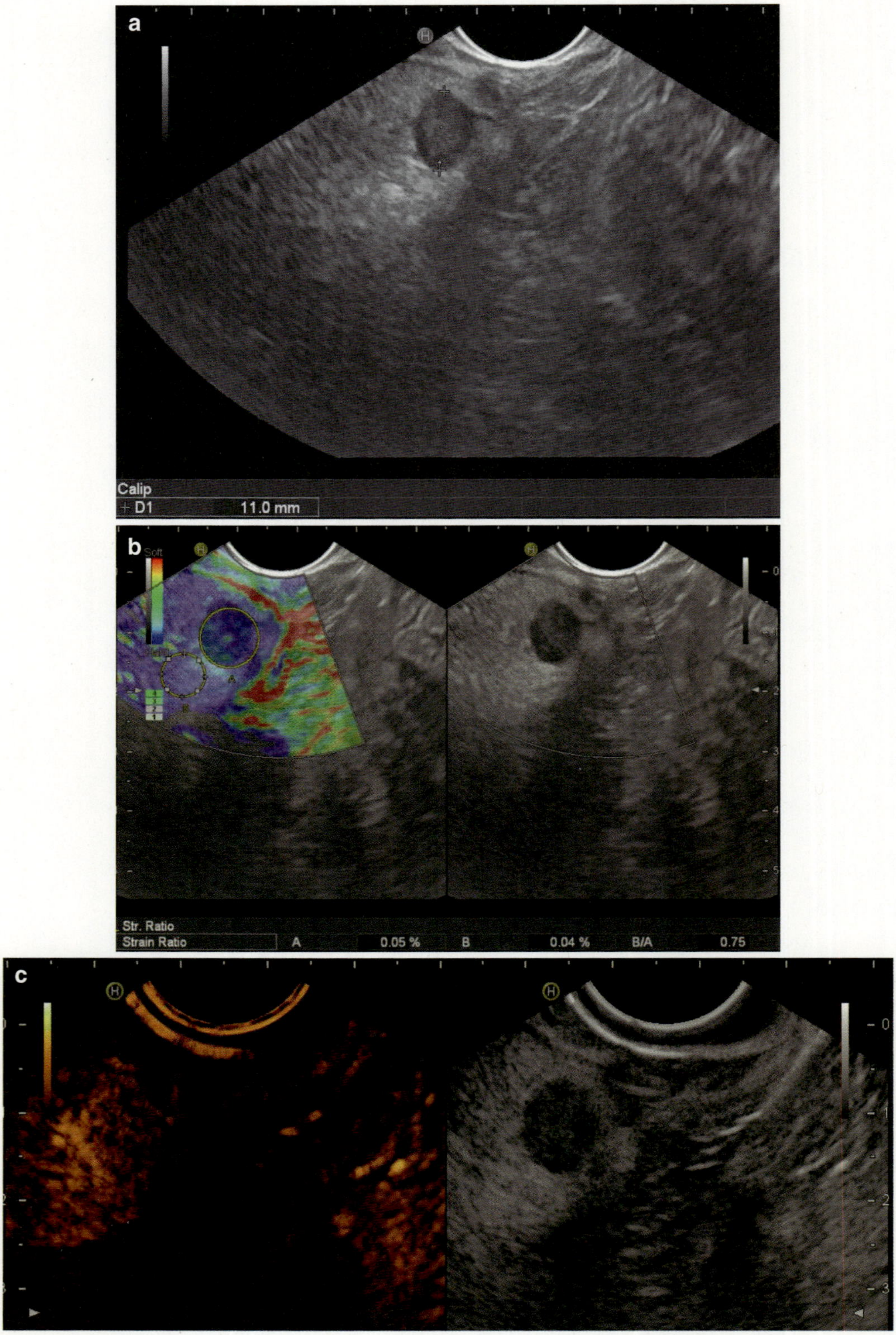

Fig. 3.21 Neuroendocrine tumor. (**a–c**) EUS study. A little hypoechoic mass in uncinate process inside the pancreatic parenchyma (*calipers* in **a**) with a homogeneous *blue pattern* at qualitative EUS elastography and a strain ratio of 0.75 at semiquantitative study (**b**). At E-CEUS, lesion is isovascular with adjacent parenchyma (**c**)

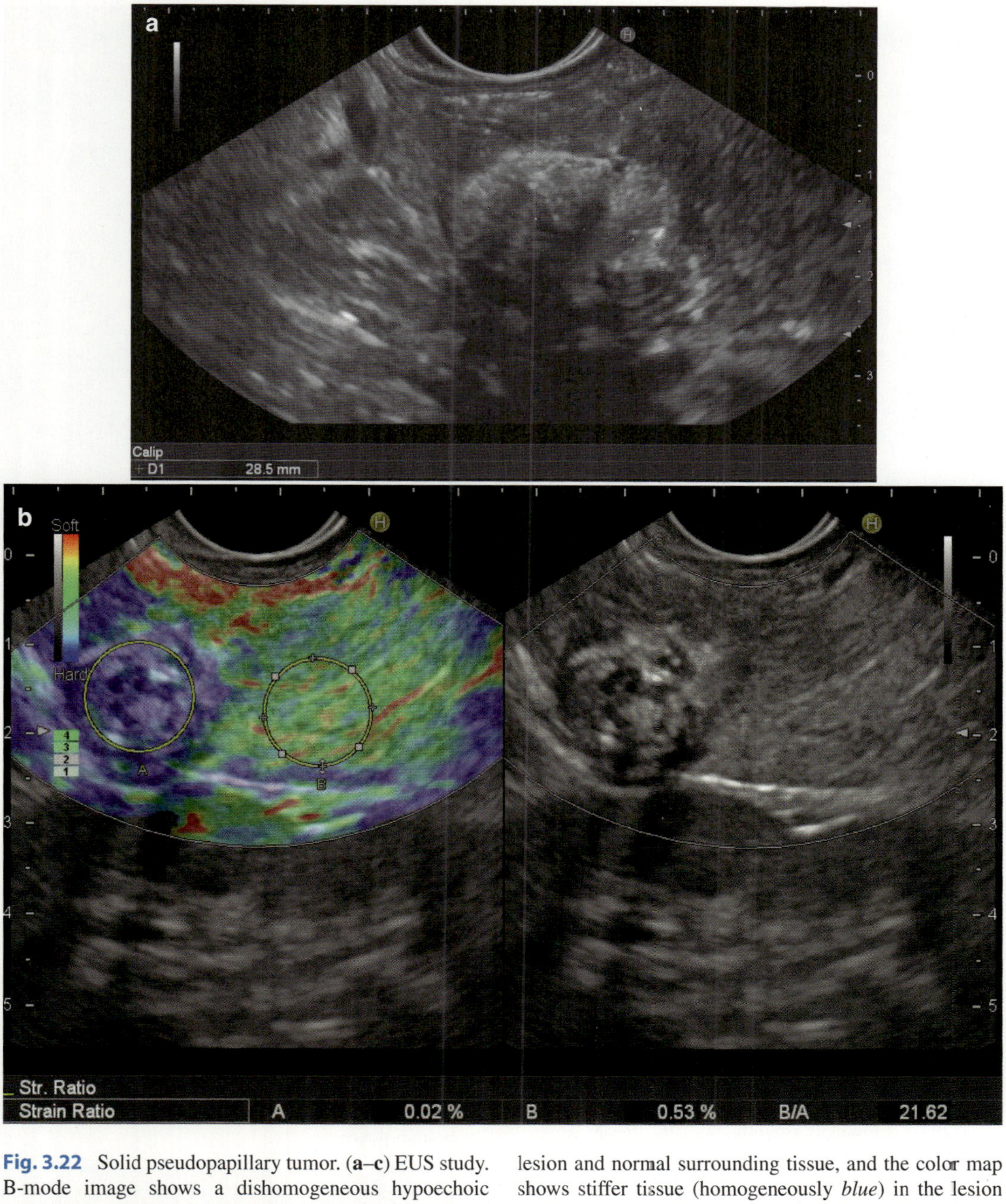

Fig. 3.22 Solid pseudopapillary tumor. (**a–c**) EUS study. B-mode image shows a dishomogeneous hypoechoic solid lesion of pancreatic gland (**a**). The ROI (region of interest) of elastosonographic study includes both the lesion and normal surrounding tissue, and the color map shows stiffer tissue (homogeneously *blue*) in the lesion (**b**). The dynamic study shows an inhomogeneous vascularization (**c**)

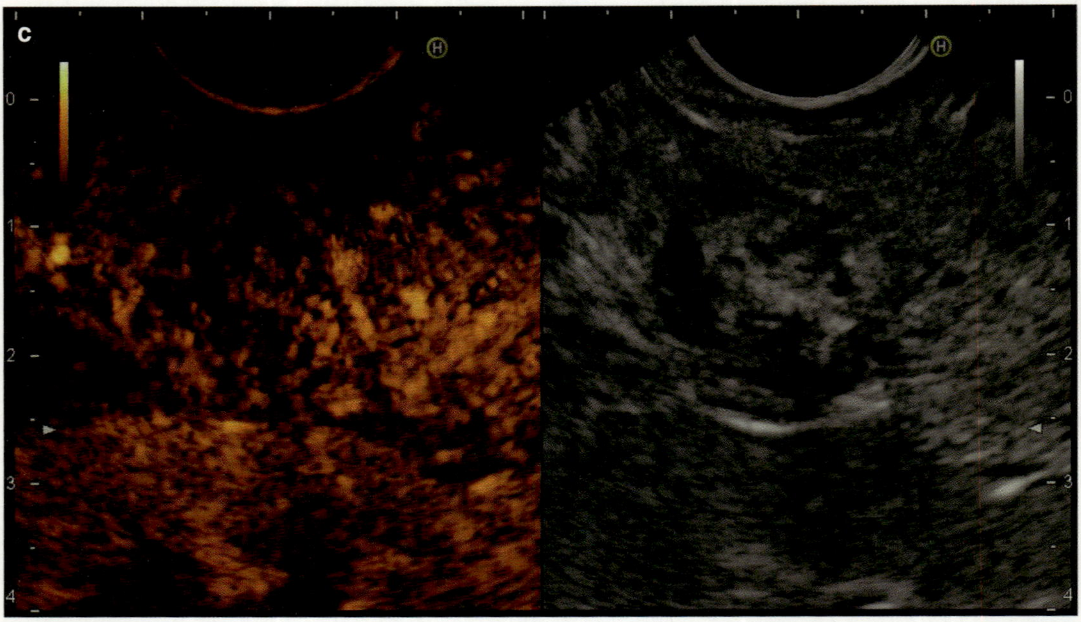

Fig. 3.22 (continued)

References

1. D'Onofrio M, editor. Ultrasonography of the pancreas. Imaging and pathological correlations. Italia: Springer; 2012.
2. D'Onofrio CS, De Robertis R, et al. Elastography of the pancreas. Eur J Radiol. 2014;83:415–9.
3. Ophir J, Cespedes I, Ponnekanti H, et al. Elastography: a quantitative method for imaging the elasticity of biological tissues. Ultrason Imaging. 1991;13: 111–34.
4. Itoh A, Ueno E, Tohno E, et al. Breast disease: clinical application of US elastography for diagnosis. Radiology. 2006;239:341–50.
5. Shiina T, Nitta N, Ueno E, et al. Real time tissue elasticity imaging using the combined autocorrelation method. J Med Ultrasound. 2002;29:119–28.
6. Evans A, Whelehan P, Thomson K, et al. Quantitative shear wave ultrasound elastography: initial experience in solid breast masses. Breast Cancer Res. 2010;12(6):R104.
7. Nightingale K, Soo MS, Nightingale R, et al. Acoustic radiation force impulse imaging: in vivo demonstration of clinical feasibility. Ultrasound Med Biol. 2002;28:227–35.
8. Nightingale K, McAleavey S, Trahey G. Shear-wave generation using acoustic radiation force: in vivo and ex vivo results. Ultrasound Med Biol. 2003;29:1715–23.
9. Janssen J, Schlorer E, Greiner L. EUS elastography of the pancreas: feasibility and pattern description of the normal pancreas, chronic pancreatitis, and focal pancreatic lesions. Gastrointest Endosc. 2007;65:971–8.
10. Hirche TO, Ignee A, Barreiros A, et al. Indications and limitations of endoscopic ultrasound elastography for evaluation of focal pancreatic lesions. Endoscopy. 2008;40:910–7.
11. Itokawa F, Itoi T, Sofuni A, et al. EUS elastography combined with the strain ratio of tissue elasticity for diagnosis of solid pancreatic masses. J Gastroenterol. 2011;46:843–53.
12. Giovannini M, Botelberge T, Bories E, et al. Endoscopic ultrasound elastography for evaluation of lymph nodes and pancreatic masses: a multicenter study. World J Gastroenterol. 2009;15:1587–93.
13. Iglesias-Garcia J, Larino-Noia J, Abdulkader I, et al. JEEUS. Elastography for the characterization of solid pancreatic masses. Gastrointest Endosc. 2009;70:1101–8.
14. Lee TH, Cha SW, Cho YD. EUS Elastography: advances in diagnostic EUS of the pancreas. Korean J Radiol. 2012;13(S1):S12–6.
15. D'Onofrio M, Gallotti A, Pozzi Mucelli R. Imaging techniques in pancreatic tumors. Expert Rev Med Devices. 2010;7:257–73.
16. Gallotti A, D'Onofrio M, Pozzi Mucelli R. Acoustic radiation force impulse (ARFI) technique in ultrasound with virtual touch tissue quantification of the upper abdomen. Radiol Med. 2010;115:889–97.
17. Banks PA, Bollen TL, Dervenic C, et al. Classifications of acute pancreatitis – 2012: revision of the Atlanta classification and definitions by international consensus. Gut. 2013;62(1):102–11.

18. Dietrich CF. Real-time tissue elastography. Multiple clinical applications. Multiple clinical solutions. Endoskopie Heute. 2011;24:177–212.
19. Hiroki U, Yoshiki H, Akihiro I, et al. Feasibility of tissue elastography using transcutaneous ultrasonography for the diagnosis of pancreatic diseases. Pancreas. 2009;38:17–22.
20. D'Onofrio M, Galloti A, Martone E, et al. Solid appearance of pancreatic serous cystadenoma diagnosed as cystic at ultrasound acoustic radiation force impulse imaging. JOP. 2009;10:543–6.
21. Mateen MA, Muheet KA, Mohan RJ, et al. Evaluation of ultrasound based acoustic radiation force impulse (ARFI) and eSie touch sonoelastography for diagnosis of inflammatory pancreatic diseases. JOP. 2012;13:36–44.
22. Goya C, Hamidi C, Hattapoglu S, et al. Use of acoustic radiation force impulse elastography to diagnose acute pancreatitis at hospital admission: comparison with sonography and computed tomography. J Ultrasound Med. 2014;33(8):1453–60.
23. Dimcevski G, Erchinger FG, Havre R, et al. Ultrasonography in diagnosing chronic pancreatitis: new aspects. World J Gastroenterol. 2013;19(42): 7247–57.
24. Mondal U, Henkes N, Patel S, et al. Endoscopic ultrasound elastography. Current clinical use in pancreas. Pancreas. 2016;45:929–33.
25. Wiersema MJ, Hawes RH, Lehman GA, et al. Prospective evaluation of endoscopic ultrasonography and endoscopic retrograde cholangiopancreatography in patients with chronic abdominal pain of suspected pancreatic origin. Endoscopy. 1993;25:555–64.
26. Catalano MF, Sahai A, Levy M, et al. EUS-based criteria for the diagnosis of chronic pancreatitis: the Rosemont classification. Gastrointest Endosc. 2009;69:1251–61.
27. Catalano MF, Lahoti S, Geenen JE, et al. Prospective evaluation of endoscopic ultrasonography, endoscopic retrograde pancreatography, and secretin test in the diagnosis of chronic pancreatitis. Gastrointest Endosc. 1998;48:11–7.
28. Kloppel G, Detlefsen S, Feyerabend B. Fibrosis of the pancreas: the initial tissue damage and the resulting pattern. Virchows Arch Int J Pathol. 2004; 445:1–8.
29. Yashima Y, Sasahira N, Isayama H, et al. Acoustic radiation force impulse elastography for noninvasive assessment of chronic pancreatitis. J Gastroenterol. 2012;47:427–32.
30. Park MK, Jo JH, Cho JH, et al. Usefulness of acoustic radiation force impulse elastography in the differential diagnosis of benign and malignant solid pancreatic lesions. Ultrason. 2014;33(1):26–33.
31. Dietrich CF, Hirche TO, Ott M, et al. Real-time tissue elastography in the diagnosis of autoimmune pancreatitis. Endoscopy. 2009;41:718–20.
32. D'Onofrio M, Capelli P, Pederzoli P, editors. Imaging and pathology of pancreatic neoplasms. A pictorial atlas. Italia: Springer; 2015.
33. Saftoiu A, Vilmann P, Gorunescu F, et al. (2011) European EUS Elastography Multicentric Study Group. Accuracy of endoscopic ultrasound elastography used for differential diagnosis of focal pancreatic masses: a multicenter study. Endoscopy. 43:596–603.
34. Cui XW, Chang JM, Kan QC, et al. Endoscopic ultrasound elastography: current status and future perspectives. World J Gastroenterol. 2015;21(47):13212–24.
35. Hu DM, Gong TT, Zhu Q. Endoscopic ultrasound elastography for differential diagnosis of pancreatic masses: a meta-analysis. Dig Dis Sci. 2013;58:1125–31.
36. Mei M, Ni J, Liu D, et al. EUS elastography for diagnosis of solid pancreatic masses: a meta-analysis. Gastrointest Endosc. 2013;77:578–89.
37. Li X, Xu W, Shi J, et al. Endoscopic ultrasound elastography for differentiating between pancreatic adenocarcinoma and inflammatory masses: a meta-analysis. World J Gastroenterol. 2013;19:6284–91.
38. Schrader H, Wiese M, Ellrichmann M, et al. Diagnostic value of quantitative EUS elastography for malignant pancreatic tumors: relationship with pancreatic fibrosis. Ultraschall Med. 2012;33:E196–201.
39. Giovannini M, Hookey LC, Bories E. Endoscopic ultrasound elastography: the first step towards virtual biopsy? Preliminary results in 49 patients. Endoscopy. 2006;38(4):344–8.
40. Iglesias-Garcia J, Larino-Noia J, Abdulkader I, et al. Quantitative endoscopic ultrasound elastography: an accurate method for the differentiation of solid pancreatic masses. Gastroenterol. 2010;139:1172–80.
41. Gheonea DI, Săftoiu A. Beyond conventional endoscopic ultrasound: elastography, contrast enhancement and hybrid techniques. Curr Opin Gastroenterol. 2011;27:423–9.
42. Dietrich CF, Saftoiu A, Jenssen C. Real time elastography endoscopic ultrasound (RTE-EUS), a comprehensive review. Eur J Radiol. 2014;83:405–14.
43. Saftoiu A, Vilmann P, Gorunescu F, et al. Efficacy of an artificial neural network-based approach to endoscopic ultrasound elastography in diagnosis of focal pancreatic masses. Clin Gastroenterol Hepatol. 2012;10(1):84–90.
44. Giovannini M. The place of endoscopic ultrasound in bilio-pancreatic pathology. Gastroenterol Clin Biol. 2010;34(8–9):436–45.
45. Uchida H, Hirooka Y, Itoh A, et al. Feasibility of tissue elastography using transcutaneous ultrasonography for the diagnosis of pancreatic diseases. Pancreas. 2009;38:17–22.
46. Procacci C, Biasiutti C, Carbognin G, et al. Pancreatic neoplasms and tumor-like conditions. Eur Radiol. 2001;11(S2):S167–92.
47. Hruban RH, Pitman MB, Klimstra DS, American Registry of Pathology, Armed Forces Institute of Pathology (US). Tumors of the pancreas. Washington, DC: Armed Forces Institute of Pathology; 2007.
48. Bosman FT, World Health Organization, International Agency for Research on Cancer. WHO classification of tumours of the digestive system. Lyon: International Agency for Research on Cancer; 2010.

49. D'Onofrio M, Crosara S, Canestrini S, et al. Virtual analysis of pancreatic cystic lesion fluid content by ultrasound acoustic radiation force impulse quantification. J Ultrasound Med. 2013;32:647–51.
50. Hutchins GF, Draganov PV. Cystic neoplasms of the pancreas: a diagnostic challenge. World J Gastroenterol. 2009;15:48–54.
51. Garcea G, Ong SL, Rajesh A, et al. Cystic lesions of the pancreas: a diagnostic and management dilemma. Pancreatology. 2008;8:236–51.
52. D'Onofrio M, Gallotti A, Salvia R, et al. Acoustic radiation force impulse (ARFI) ultrasound imaging of pancreatic cystic lesions. Eur J Radiol. 2011;80:241–4.
53. D'Onofrio M, Gallotti A, Falconi M, et al. Acoustic radiation force impulse imaging of pancreatic cystic lesions: preliminary results. Pancreas. 2010;39:939–40.
54. Barr RG. Shear wave Imaging of the breast: still on the learning curve. J Ultrasound Med. 2012;31:347–50.
55. Lewin M, Hoeffel C. Imaging of incidental cystic lesions of the pancreas. J Radiol. 2008;89:197–207.
56. Gabata T, Terayama N. Solid serous cystadenoma of the pancreas: MR imaging with pathologic correlation. Abdom Imaging. 2005;30:605–9.
57. Cosgrove D, Piscaglia F, Bamber J, et al. EFSUMB Guidelines and recommendations on the clinical use of ultrasound elastography. Part 2: clinical applications. Ultraschall Med. 2013;34:238–53.
58. Piscaglia F, Nolsoe C, Dietrich CF, et al. The EFSUMB guidelines and recommendations on the clinical practice of contrast enhanced ultrasound (CEUS): update 2011 on non-hepatic applications. Ultraschall Med. 2012;33:33–59.

Kidney

4

Costanza Bruno, Alessandra Bucci, Valentina Ciaravino, Giorgia Tedesco, Alessandro Sarno, and Emilio Quaia

4.1 Introduction

Kidney evaluation using elastographic technique has been very challenging from the beginning, giving often conflicting results. A clue to understand this can come from the analysis of the many factors which can influence ARFI measurements. Many of them are shared with other target tissues, while others are peculiar of the kidney, the most important being related to its anatomical organization [1].

The kidney is a highly anisotropic organ, where anisotropy reflects the direction dependence of some properties that some organs demonstrate. Particularly, the medulla (where Henle loops and vasa recta are parallel to each other, all being oriented from the capsule to the papilla) is very different from the cortex, mostly occupied by glomeruli and by convoluted proximal and distal tubules, being approximately spherical in shape. It means that when a US beam is sent parallel to a renal segment, it generates SW traveling perpendicular to the medullary structures, thus encountering multiple interfaces and thus decreasing their speed of propagation; on the contrary when an US beam is sent perpendicularly to Henle loops and vasa recta, it originates SW traveling parallel to these structures and meeting few interfaces; this is reflected by higher SW; in an experimental [2] model obtained using Supersonic Shear Wave Elastography, the mean variation of the apparent shear modulus due to the medullary anisotropy was 31.8 % which is very similar to the 40 % fractional anisotropy demonstrated using diffusion MRI [3]. Besides anisotropy other elements closely related to its physiology can affect kidney evaluation by means of ARFI.

In the same experimental model [2], a linear relationship between the increasing of urinary pressure induced by ligation of the ureter was demonstrated. Changes in the arterial and venous fluxes were also found to induce modifications in the SWV; particularly occlusion of the renal artery caused their decrease and ligation of the renal vein caused their increase.

The same results were found using a different experimental model [4], particularly when considering two different conditions: ureter obstruction and renal vein occlusion. The

C. Bruno (✉)
Department of Radiology, Policlinico GB Rossi, P.le LA Scuro, 37134 Verona, Italy
e-mail: clgbruno@gmail.com; costanza.bruno@ospedaleuniverona.it

A. Bucci
Department of Radiology, GB Rossi University Hospital, University of Verona, Verona, Italy

V. Ciaravino • G. Tedesco • A. Sarno
Department of Radiology, GB Rossi University Hospital, University of Verona, Verona, Italy

E. Quaia
Clinical Research Imaging Centre, Queen's Medical Research Institute, 47 Little France Crescent, Edinburgh EH16 4TJ, UK
e-mail: equaia@ed.ac.uk

D.-A. Clevert et al. (eds.), *Atlas of Elastosonography*, DOI 10.1007/978-3-319-44201-3_4

degree of fibrosis was significantly different when compared with normal kidneys; fibrosis induced by ureter obstruction was lower than fibrosis induced by renal vein occlusion. SWV was positively correlated with this histologic finding.

Besides these elements, strictly correlated to the target, also all the other factors generally influencing the propagation of the SW must be taken into account when evaluating the kidney using ARFI, particularly compression – which is crucial when evaluating the superficial transplanted kidneys [5]. Being so, an accurate and standardized technique must be used, in order to reduce the variability of measurements.

Since urinary stasis induced by bladder repletion can modify the data, the exams should be performed after micturition, with the ROI parallel to the main US beam and completely included in the cortex (which can be difficult to be obtained when the cortical thickness is reduced, since the dimensions of the ROI are fixed) and – to reduce the effects of anisotropy – with the same axis of the pyramids; this can be easily obtained at the middle third in the sagittal scan.

A relationship is described between the frequency of the probe and the SWV [6]. Therefore, attention must be paid in order to use always the same (i.e., high-frequency probe, 6 MHz, when evaluating children, and low-frequency probes – 4 MHz – when evaluating adults) in order to obtain comparable results.

There is no consensus about position, some authors using the prone position [7, 8], some the lateral one [9], and some the supine one [10, 11].

4.2 Healthy Kidney

As a consequence of the many elements affecting ARFI evaluation of the kidneys, the first reports found a vast difference in the SWV of healthy adults [12]. After standardizing the technique, these differences were gradually reduced [9], with a strong agreement between the operators, concluding that ARFI can be considered a useful tool in the evaluation of kidneys.

ARFI values are lower in children and gradually increase with age, most notably in children under 5 years of age [10].

Possible applications of ARFI to the kidneys include evaluation of diffuse and focal disease.

4.3 Diffuse Disease

After the good results obtained in the liver evaluation using ARFI, an extension to the evaluation of the kidney was postulated, on the basis that a hypercellular, high-grade interstitial fibrosis leading to a progressive loss of functioning nephrons is the cause of chronic kidney disease. As already said also experimental models support this approach.

A noninvasive approach to chronic kidney disease was ever more needed because both morphological US parameters (i.e., renal size, cortical thickness, and pelvis diameter) and arterial resistive index evaluated with color Doppler can only approximately quantify the extension and the degree of the damage [13, 14]. This makes renal biopsy often necessary and scintigraphy with dimercaptosuccinic acid labeled with technetium-99m (99mTc-DMSA) (a procedure associated with a certain amount of radiation exposure) recommended by the current guidelines in the evaluation of some pediatric forms [15].

4.3.1 Renal Allografts

The results are very controversial.

In a pilot study, Arndt showed that parenchymal stiffness evaluated using transient elastography was related with interstitial fibrosis [16]; a good correlation of the cortical stiffness with the global histological deterioration was demonstrated using Supersonic Shear Wave Elastography [17, 18].

A significant correlation of SWV values with the estimated glomerular filtration rate with 72 % sensitivity and 86.5 % specificity in the diagnosis of allograft dysfunction was found by He et al. [19]; kidneys with acute allograft rejection showed slightly lower SWV than those with chronic allograft nephropathy; a higher mean SWV value was found in patients with lower eGFR (<50 vs. > −50 ml/min).

On the other hand, Syversveen et al. found that ARFI cannot detect allograft fibrosis [20], with a mean decreasing trend of SWV from lower to higher degrees of fibrosis, and similarly Gao et al. [21] reported higher values of stiffness in patients with <25 % of fibrosis than patients with >26 % of fibrosis.

4.3.2 Chronic Disease

As for the evaluation of chronic allografts also when considering chronic kidney disease, the findings are very controversial, probably reflecting problems in the standardization of the exams.

Wang reported no correlation between the degree of fibrosis and SWV in 45 patients – most of them affected by IgA nephropathy [22]. Other authors [23] found that a progressive reduction of the SWV was associated with an increase of the CKD stages and with a decrease of the GFR; this can be explained by a progressive reduction of the renal blood flow due to nephroangiosclerosis which could affect the SWV more than tissue fibrosis does. The same results were found when considering patients with chronic kidney disease related to diabetes mellitus. ARFI was found able to distinguish between the different diabetic nephropathy stages, except for stages [5]; also in this subgroup, an inverse relationship between ARFI values and GFR was found [24].

This finding is consistent with Gennisson's experimental findings demonstrating a SWV reduction after ligation of the renal artery.

4.4 Pediatric Evaluation

Evaluating pediatric kidney is particularly challenging, due to the need and the difficulty of breath holding in children. The main applications are in the workout of chronic disease and in the managing of renal damage in hydronephrosis.

In children under 2 years of age with pelvis dilation, SWV was found higher in kidneys with high-grade hydronephrosis compared with normal kidneys [25] although ARFI was not able to distinguish between obstructive hydronephrosis and nonobstructive hydronephrosis [26].

Nevertheless a relationship between the type of obstruction and SWV was found; children with chronic kidney disease related to obstructive uropathy had higher ARFI values than children with chronic kidney disease due to nonobstructive uropathy. In children with monolateral disease, the contralateral seeming healthy kidney was characterized by higher SWV than healthy controls [27].

4.5 Focal Disease

Preliminary studies were published about ARFI evaluation of renal masses and particularly the differentiation between benign and malignant ones.

After the first attempts to evaluate renal tumors in order to obtain additional informations about the nature of the lesions [28], more standardized studies were performed.

As demonstrated in other organs, cysts are characterized by low SWV.

In a large cohort of patients [29], a statistically significant difference was found between renal cell carcinomas and angiomyolipomas; with a cutoff point of 1.87 m/s, the sensitivity and specificity were 47.5 % and 33.2 %. Oncocytomas – which often can create problems in the differential diagnosis with RCCs, being hypervascular too – are characterized by lower SWV.

When considering the different subtypes of RCCs, the SWV of the clear cell renal cell carcinomas was significantly higher than the SWV of the papillary renal cell carcinomas, chromophobe renal cell carcinomas, and angiomyolipomas [30].

Given the fixed dimensions of the ROI (1 cm × 0.5 cm), a correct evaluation of an inhomogeneous mass or of a cystic lesion is particularly difficult because it is necessary to avoid the necrotic/cystic areas in order to obtain reproducible results.

4.6 Image Gallery

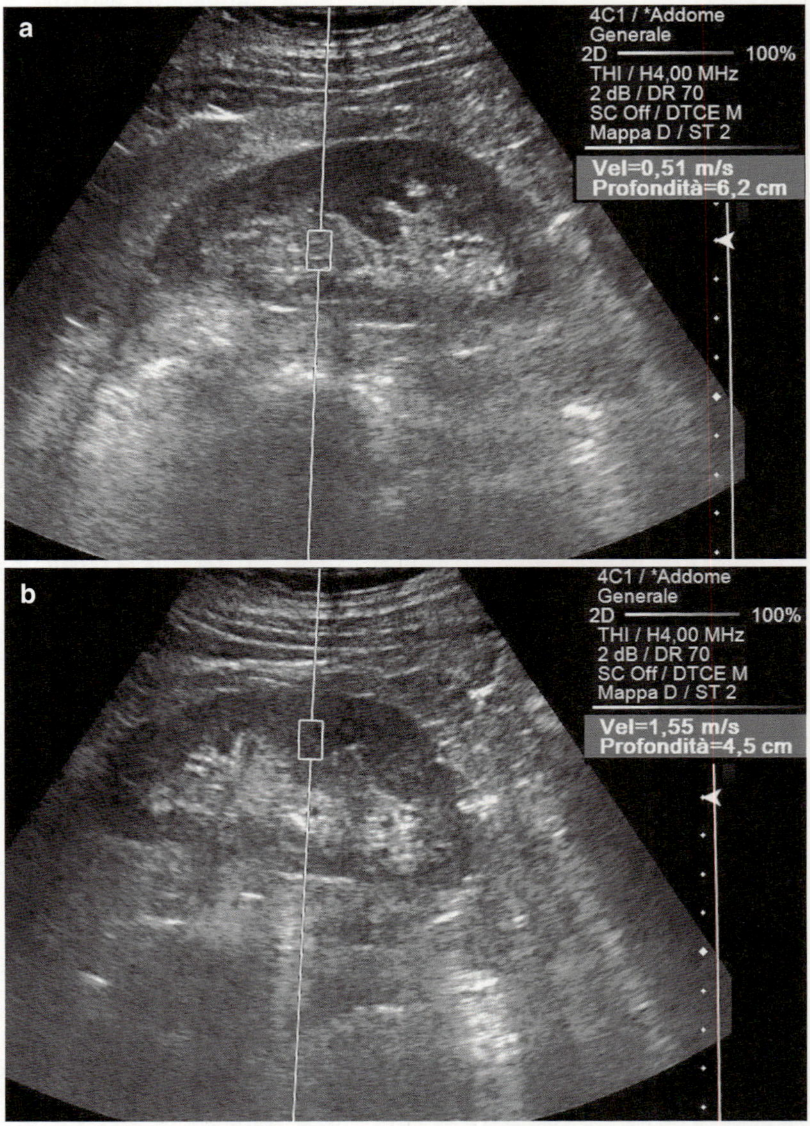

Fig. 4.1 ARFI values in kidneys are deeply affected by many elements. One of them is the anatomical architecture. In fact they are lower in the renal sinus (**a**) where the vascular elements are predominant and where the SW meet more interfaces and higher in the cortex (**b**) where anisotropy plays a major role

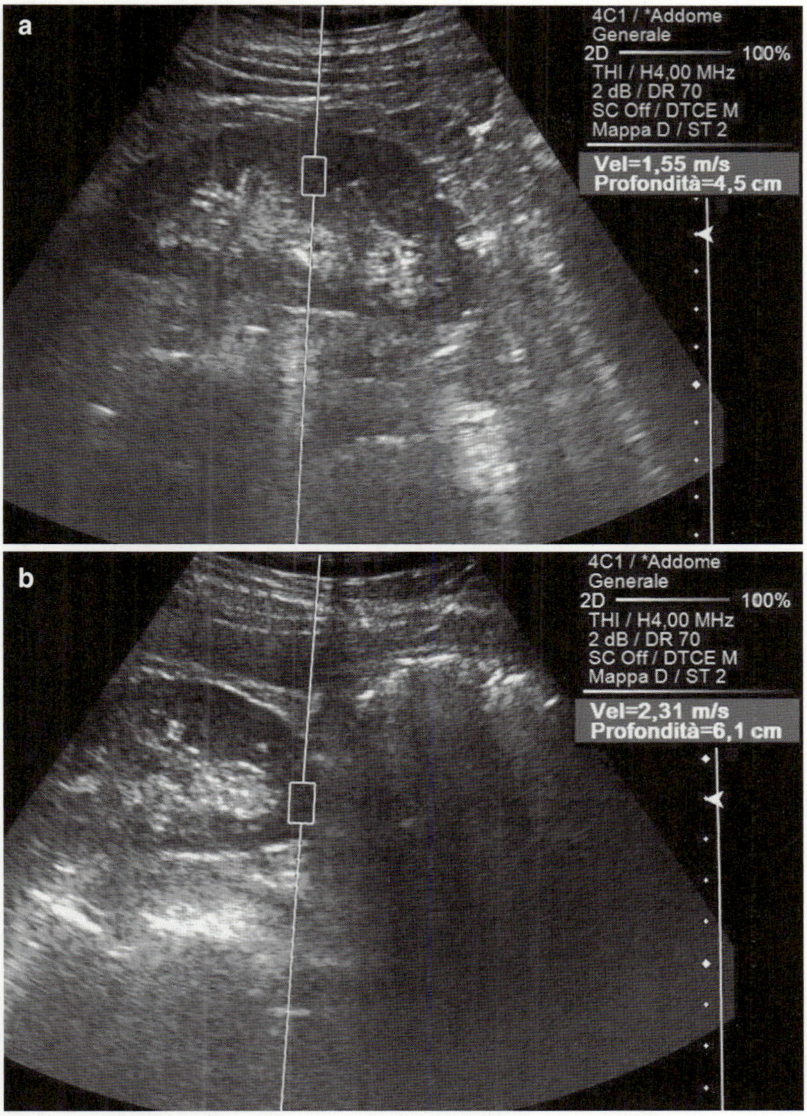

Fig. 4.2 The most important element which influences the SWV in the kidneys is anisotropy. In fact the SWV is lower when the US beam is parallel to the pyramids (**a**) because the SW travel perpendicularly to the Henle loops, thus meeting many interfaces. The SWV is higher when the US beam is perpendicular (**b**) to the pyramids because the SW are parallel to the Henle loops

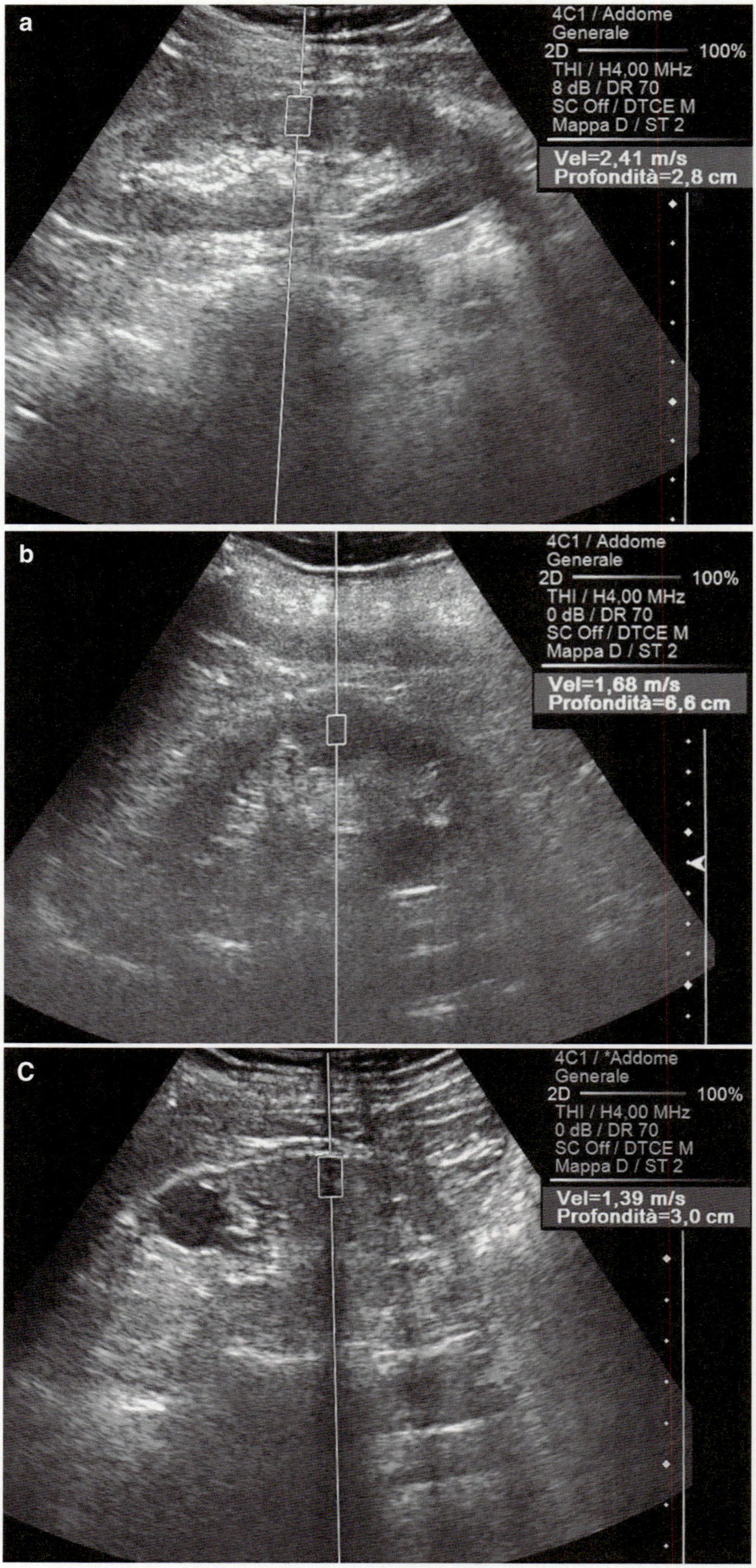

Fig. 4.3 According to many reports, SW is high in the first stages of CKD (**a**) and gradually decreases (**b**, **c**) probably because of the progressive degeneration of the parenchyma

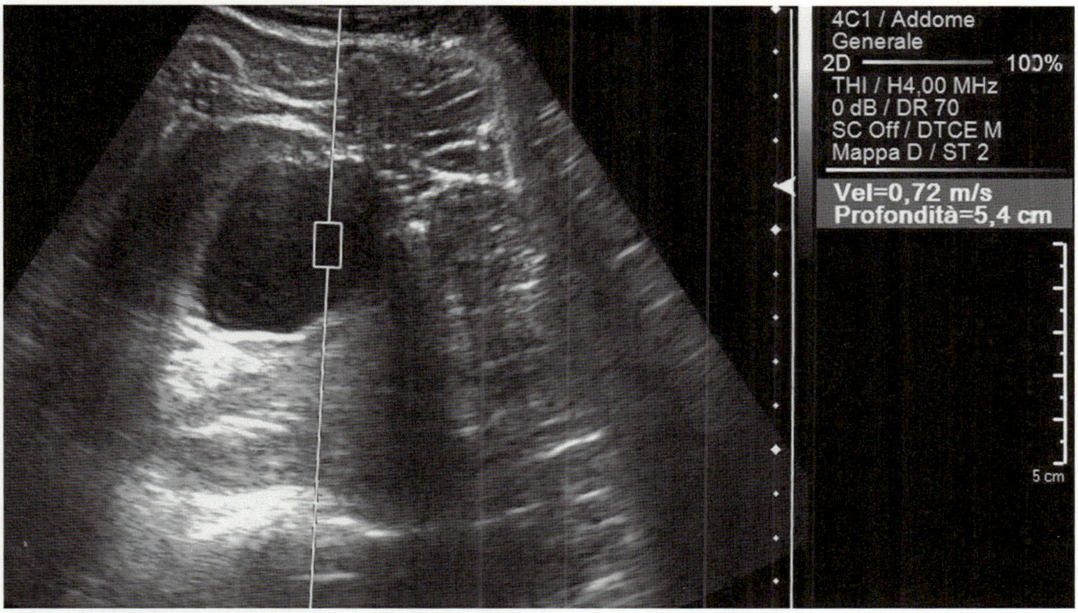

Fig. 4.4 Posttraumatic cyst communicating with calices and characterized by low SWV. Pure fluids are characterized by XXX values

Fig. 4.5 Angiomyolipoma is a lesion composed by smooth muscles, fat elements, and vessels. CEUS can depict the architecture of the large and convoluted vessels (**a**), while ARFI can show the low values characteristic of fat (**b**)

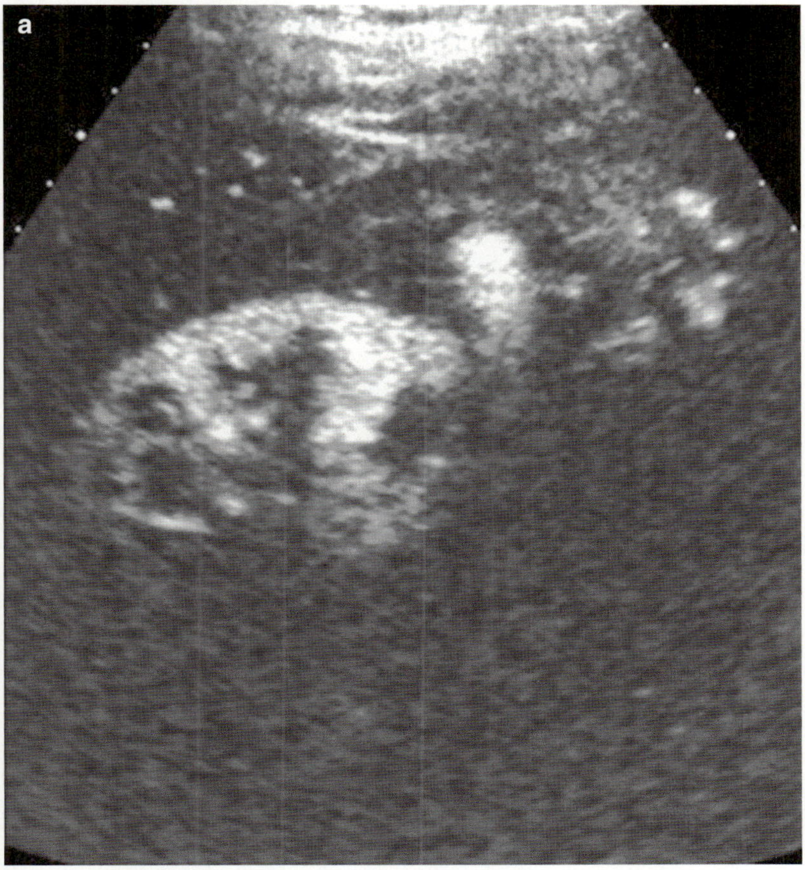

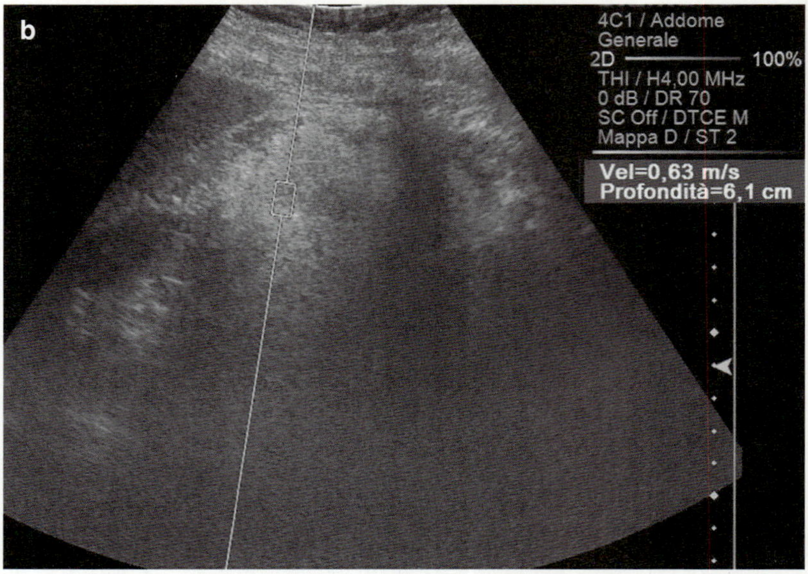

Fig. 4.5 (continued)

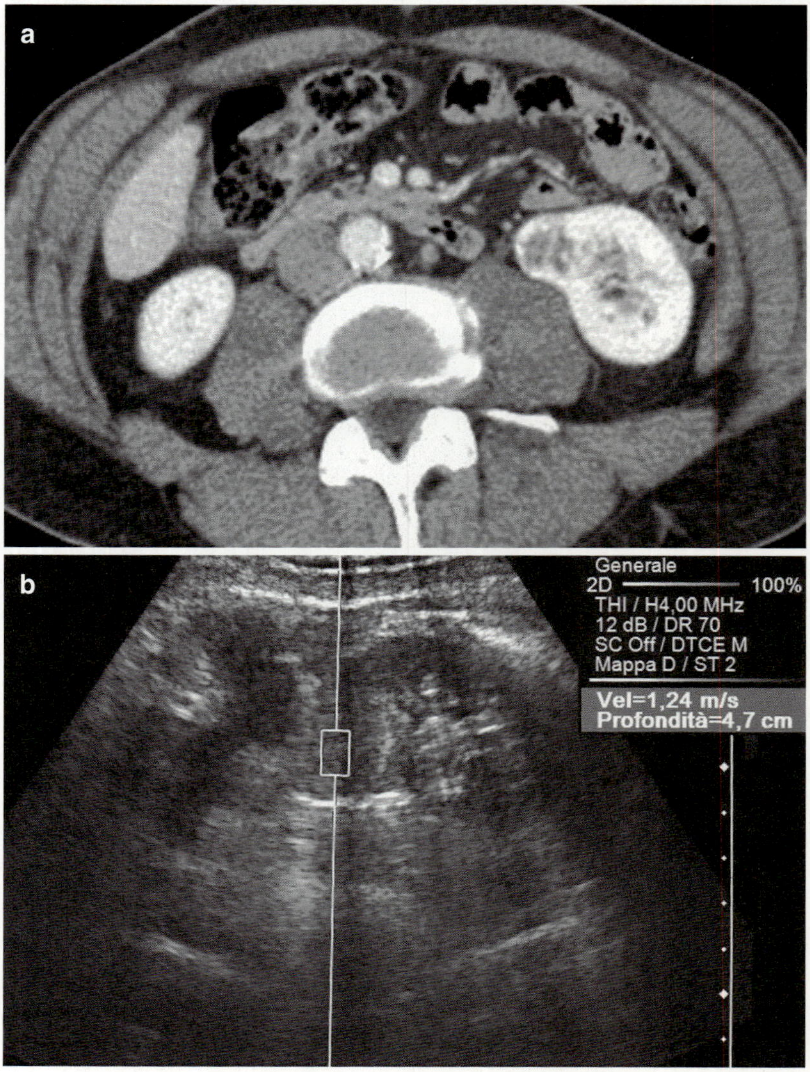

Fig. 4.6 Oncocytomas are highly vascularized too, with a central scar (**a**) which can be misunderstood for necrosis. ARFI can help in the differential diagnosis because the SWV are lower (**b**)

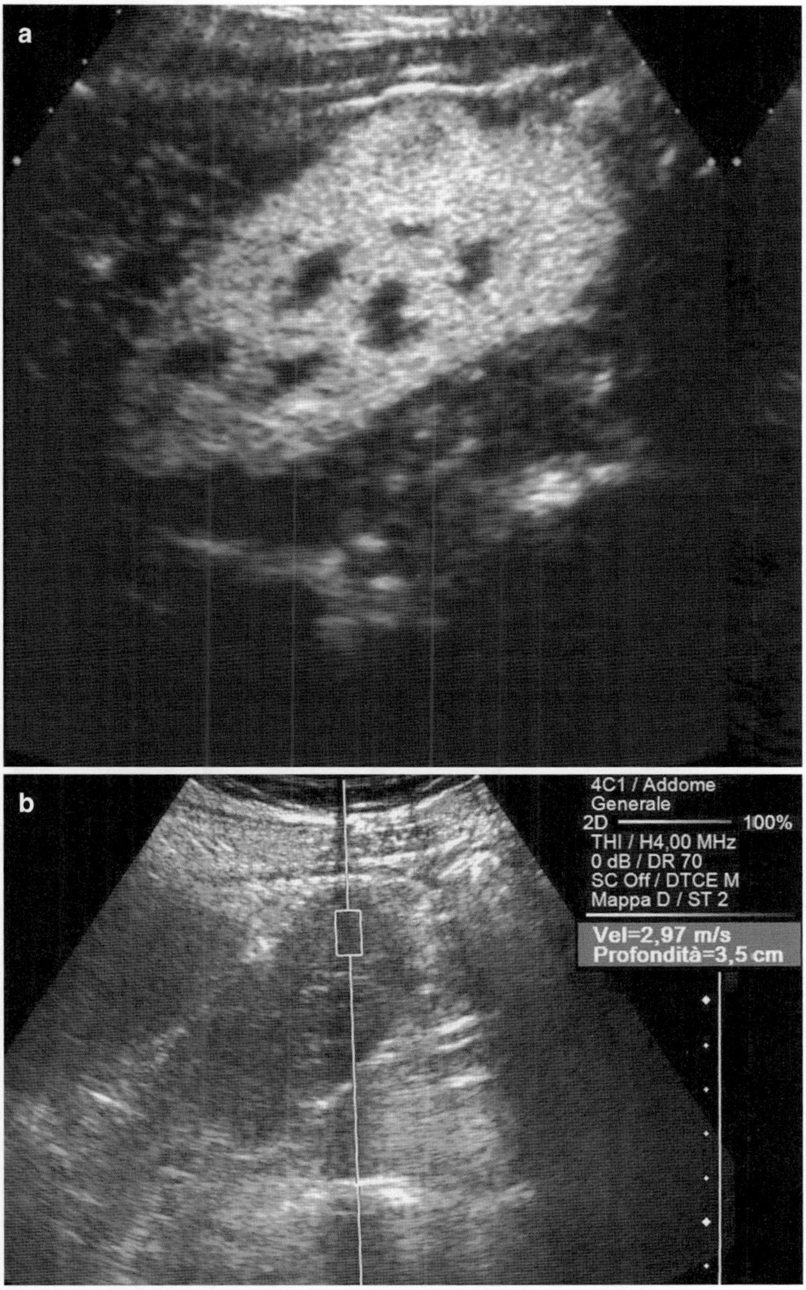

Fig. 4.7 Clear cell renal cell carcinomas are characterized by a highly vascular pattern (**a**) which can be easily depicted by CEUS; in many cases they exhibit an ARFI pattern characterized by high SWV (**b**)

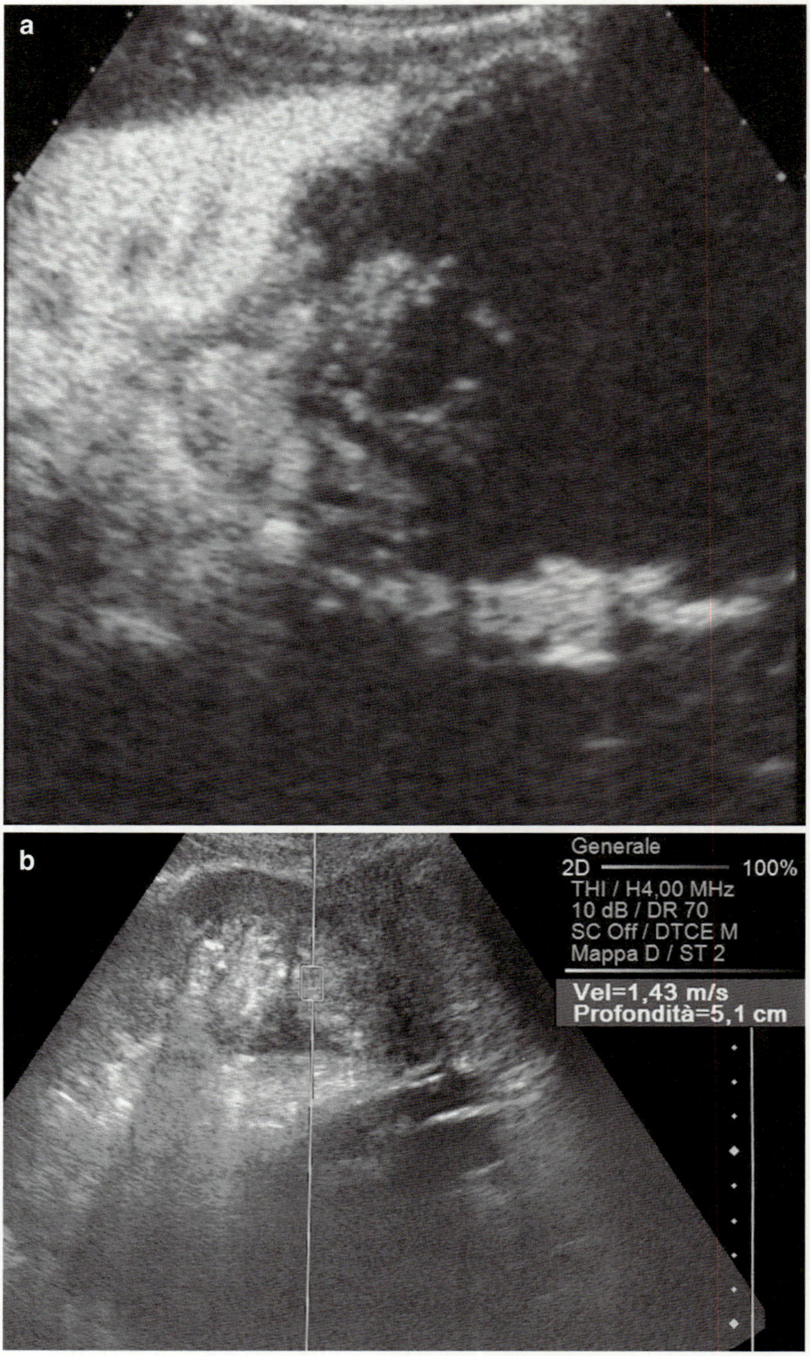

Fig. 4.8 (**a**) The evaluation of a complex cyst is very difficult because the dimensions of the ROI are fixed, and it must be completely included in the lesion in order to obtain correct measurements. In this example the ROI is placed in the solid portion of a cystic papillary RCC and the SWV are far different (**b**) from the values obtained in clear cell renal cell carcinomas and in oncocytomas

References

1. Goertz RS, Amann K, Heide R, et al. An abdominal and thyroid status with acoustic radiation force impulse elastometry – a feasibility study: acoustic radiation force impulse elastometry of human organs. Eur J Radiol. 2011;80:e226–30.
2. Gennisson JL, Grenier N, Combe C, Tanter M. Supersonic shear wave elastography of in vivo pig kidney: influence of blood pressure, urinary pressure and tissue anisotropy. Ultrasound Med Biol. 2012;38:1559–67.
3. Ries M, Jones RA, Basseau F, et al. Diffusion tensor MRI of the human kidney. J Magn Reson Imaging. 2001;14:42–9.
4. Moon SK, Kim SY, Cho JY, Kim SH. Quantification of kidney fibrosis using ultrasonic shear wave elastography. Experimental study with a rabbit model. J Ultrasound Med. 2015;34:869–77.
5. Syversveen T, Midtvedt K, Berstad AE, et al. Tissue elasticity estimated by acoustic radiation force impulse quantification depends on the applied transducer force: an experimental study in kidney transplant patients. Eur Radiol. 2012;22:2130–7.
6. Chang S, Kim MJ, Kim J, Lee MJ. Variability of shear wave velocity using different frequencies in acoustic radiation force impulse (ARFI) elastography: a phantom and normal liver study. Ultraschall Med. 2013;34:260–5.
7. Guo LH, Xu HX, Fu HJ, Peng A, Zhang YF, Liu NH. Acoustic radiation force impulse imaging for noninvasive evaluation of renal parenchyma elasticity: preliminary findings. PLoS One. 2013;8(7), e68925.
8. Zheng XZ, Yang B, Fu NH. Preliminary study on the kidney elasticity quantification in patients with chronic kidney disease using virtual touch tissue quantification. Iran J Radiol. 2015;12(1):e1206.
9. Bob F, Bota S, Sporea I, Şirli R, Petrica L, Schiller A. Kidney shear wave speed values in subjects with and without renal pathology and inter-operator reproducibility of acoustic radiation force impulse elastography (ARFI) – preliminary results. PLoS One. 2014;9(11):e113761.
10. Lee MJ, Kim MJ, Han KH, Yoon CS. Age related changes in liver, kidney and spleen stiffness in healthy children measured with acoustic radiation force impulse imaging. Eur J Radiol. 2013;82(6):e290–4.
11. Zaffanello M, Piacentini G, Bruno C, Brugnara M, Fanos V. Renal elasticity quantification by acoustic radiation force impulse applied to the evaluation of kidney disease: a review. J Investig Med. 2015;63(4):605–12.
12. Gallotti A, D'Onofrio M, Pozzi MR. Acoustic radiation force impulse technique in ultrasound with virtual touch tissue quantification of the upper abdomen. Radiol Med. 2010;1115:889–97.
13. Stock KF, Klein BS, Cong MT, et al. ARFI-based tissue elasticity quantification and kidney graft dysfunction: first clinical experiences. Clin Hemorheol Microcirc. 2011;49(1–4):527–35.
14. Brader P, Riccabona M, Schwarz T, Seebacher U, Ring E. Value of comprehensive renal ultrasound in children with acute urinary tract infection for assessment of renal involvement: comparison with DMSA scintigraphy and final diagnosis. Eur Radiol. 2008;18(12):2981–9.
15. Riccabona M, Avni FE, Blickman JG, et al. Imaging recommendations in paediatric uroradiology: minutes of the ESPR uroradiology task force session on childhood obstructive uropathy, high-grade fetal hydronephrosis, childhood hematuria, and urolithiasis in childhood. ESPR Annual Congress, Edinburgh, UK, June 2008. Pediatr Radiol. 2009;39(8):891–8.
16. Arndt R, Schmidt S, Loddenkemper C, et al. Noninvasive evaluation of renal allograft fibrosis by transient elastography – a pilot study. Transpl Int. 2010;23(9):871–7.
17. Grenier N, Gennisson JL, Cornelis F, et al. Renal ultrasound elastography. Diagn Interv Imaging. 2013;94:545–50.
18. Grenier N, Poulain S, Lepreux S, et al. Quantitative elastography of renal transplants using supersonic shear imaging: a pilot study. Eur Radiol. 2012; 22(10):2138–46.
19. He WY, Jin YJ, Wang WP, Li CL, Ji ZB, Yang C. Tissue elasticity quantification by acoustic radiation force impulse for the assesment of renal allograft function. Ultrasound Med Biol. 2014;40:(2):322–9.
20. Syversveen T, Brabrand K, Midtvedt K, et al. Assessment of renal allograft fibrosis by acoustic radiation force impulse quantification – a pilot study. Transpl Int. 2011;24(1):100–5.
21. Gao J, Min R, Hamilton J. Corticomedullary strain ratio: a quantitative marker for assessment of renal allograft fibrosis. J Ultrasound Med. 2013;32:1769–75.
22. Wang L, Xia P, Lv K, et al. Assessment of renal tissue elasticity by acoustic radiation force impulse quantification with histopathological correlation: preliminary experience in chronic kidney disease. Eur Radiol. 2014;24(7):1694–9.
23. Asano K, Ogata A, Tanaka K, et al. Acoustic radiation force impulse elastography of the kidneys: is shear wave velocity affected by tissue fibrosis or renal blood flow? J Ultrasound Med. 2014;33(5):793–801.
24. Goya C, Kilinc F, Hamidi F, Yavuz A, Yildirim Y, Cetincakmac M, Hattapoglu S. Acoustic radiation force impulse imaging for evaluation of renal parenchymal elasticity in diabetic nephropathy. AJR Am J Roentgenol. 2015;204:324–9.
25. Sohn B, Kim MJ, Han SW, Im YJ, Lee MJ. Shear wave velocity measurements using acoustic radiation force impulse in young children with normal kidneys versus hydronephrotic kidneys. Ultrasonography. 2014;33(2):116–21.
26. Dillman JR, Smith EA, Davenport MS, DiPietro MA, Sanchez R, Kraft KH, Brown RK, Rubin JM. Can shear wave elastography be used to discriminate obstructive hydronephrosis from nonobstructive hydronephrosis in children? Radiology. 2015;277(1):259–67.

27. Bruno C, Caliari G, Zaffanello M, et al. Acoustic radiation force impulse (ARFI) in the evaluation of the renal parenchymal stiffness in paediatric patients with vesicoureteral reflux: preliminary results. Eur Radiol. 2013;23:3477–84.
28. Clevert DA, Stock K, Klein B, Slotta Huspenina J, Pranti L, Heemann U, Reiser M. Evaluation of acoustic radiation force impulse (ARFI) imaging and contrast enhanced ultrasound in renal tumors of unknown etiology in comparison to histological findings. Clin Hemorheol Microcirc. 2009;43(1–2):95–107.
29. Lu Q, Wen JX, Huang BJ, Wang WP. Virtual touch tissue quantification using acoustic force impulse (ARFI) technology for the evaluation of focal solid renal lesions: preliminary findings. Clin Radiol. 2015;70(12):1376–81.
30. Goya C, Daggulli M, Hamid C, Yavuz A, Hattapoglu S, Cetincakmak MG, Teke M. The role of quantitative measurement by acoustic radiation force impulse imaging in differentiating benign lesions from malignant renal tumours. Radiol Med. 2015;120(3):296–303.

5 Elastography of the Breast

Dirk-André Clevert

The use of ultrasound in addition to mammography in breast screening has been shown to increase the detection rate of breast cancer, especially in women with dense breast parenchyma, to 4.2 cancers per 1000 women screened. However, its low specificity and low positive predictive value (PPV) remain an unavoidable limitation of this method [1, 2]. Besides interpretive criteria that take into account factors like mass margins, shape, orientation and effects on the surrounding, colour Doppler sonography and strain elastography, also known as strain elastography, have been introduced to further characterize masses of the breast. Colour Doppler sonography has shown a sensitivity of 68.0–91.2 % and a specificity of 92.7–95.0 % in differentiating malignant breast masses from benign lesions by visualizing the presence and morphology of blood vessels [3–7]. Strain elastography, which is an imaging modality that measures tissue stiffness, shows better specificity in distinguishing benign from malignant solid breast lesions (41.0–98.5 %) than B-mode sonography alone and has become a routine tool during the last years. Three different modes of elastography are currently available. Free-hand ultrasound elastography, also known as strain elastography, which is based on comparison of signals acquired before and after tissue displacement due to manual compression, is the most common method to date, whereas more recent elastography techniques such as acoustic radiation force imaging (ARFI) and shear wave elastography (SWE) offer the possibility of an objective and operator-independent quantitative measurement of tissue elasticity. Additionally, the possibility of differentiation between solid masses and cystic lesions has been shown in several studies [7–14].

D.-A. Clevert
Department of Clinical Radiology,
Interdisciplinary Ultrasound-Center,
University of Munich-Grosshadern Campus,
Marchioninistr. 15, 81377 Munich, Germany
e-mail: Dirk.Clevert@med.uni-muenchen.de

D.-A. Clevert et al. (eds.), *Atlas of Elastosonography*, DOI 10.1007/978-3-319-44201-3_5

5.1 Image Gallery

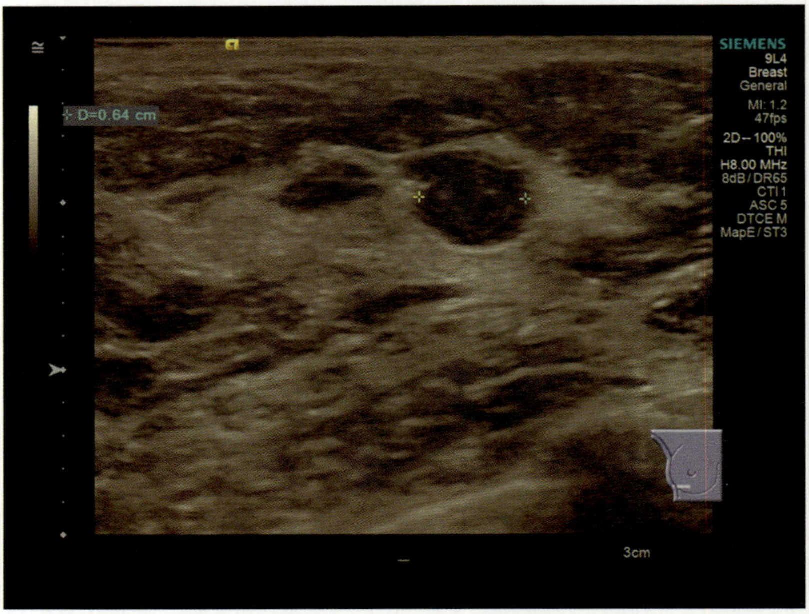

Fig. 5.1 Ultrasound images of a 57-year-old woman. B-mode sonography indicates an ovoid to round hypoechoic lesion with a maximum diameter of 0.6 cm. The diagnosis was a focal fatty tissue area of the breast

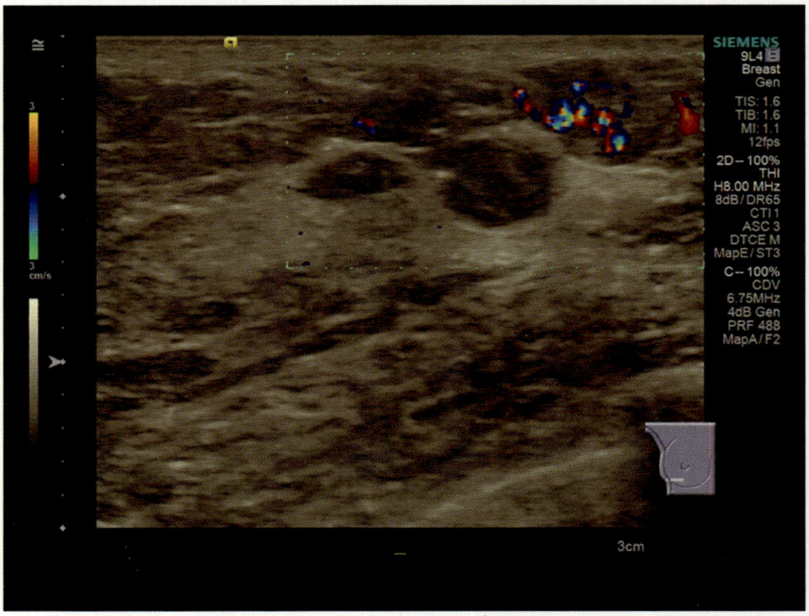

Fig. 5.2 Colour Doppler sonography does not indicate an increased vascularity of the lesion

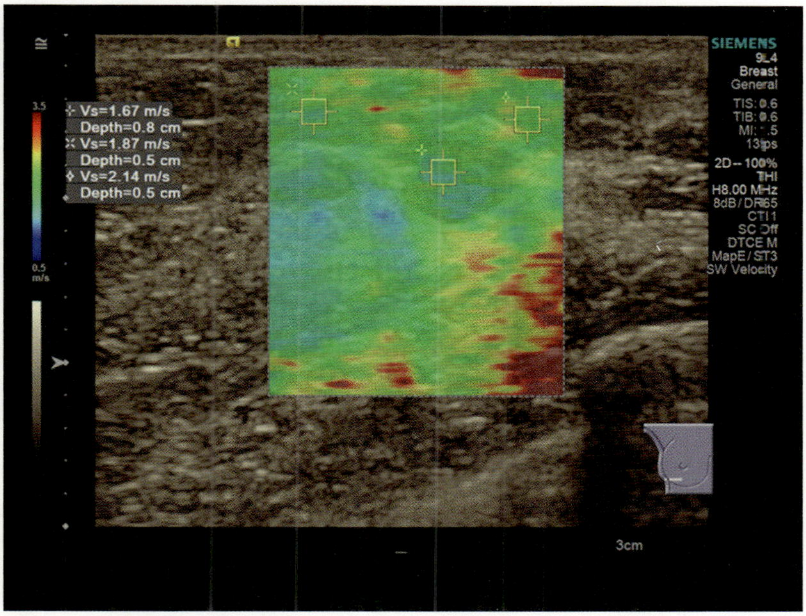

Fig. 5.3 VTIQ velocity colour overlay displayed relative shear wave velocities according to the adjacent colour spectrum, *red areas* corresponding to higher values and *blue areas* corresponding to lower values. Increased shear wave speed relates to increased tissue stiffness. Shear wave velocity was measured in the lesion $v = 1.67$ m/s and in the surrounding tissue level between $v = 1.87–2.14$ m/s

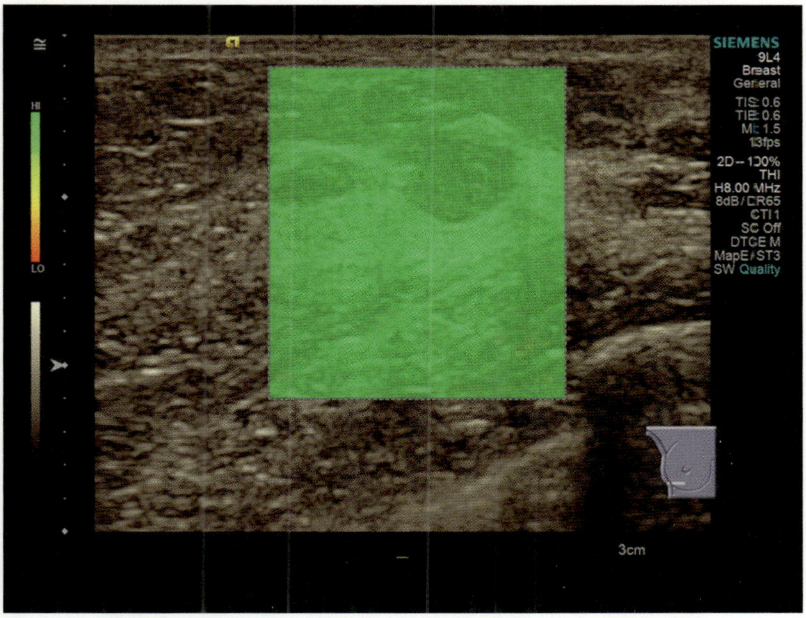

Fig. 5.4 Same lesion as Fig. 5.3. The VTIQ quality map is used to confirm that shear wave formation was adequate and to identify regions where shear wave velocity measurements may be artificially low due to poor shear wave signal quality. Here the VTIQ quality map shows all of the breast tissue and the lesion coloured *green*, an indicator of reliable shear wave velocity measurement

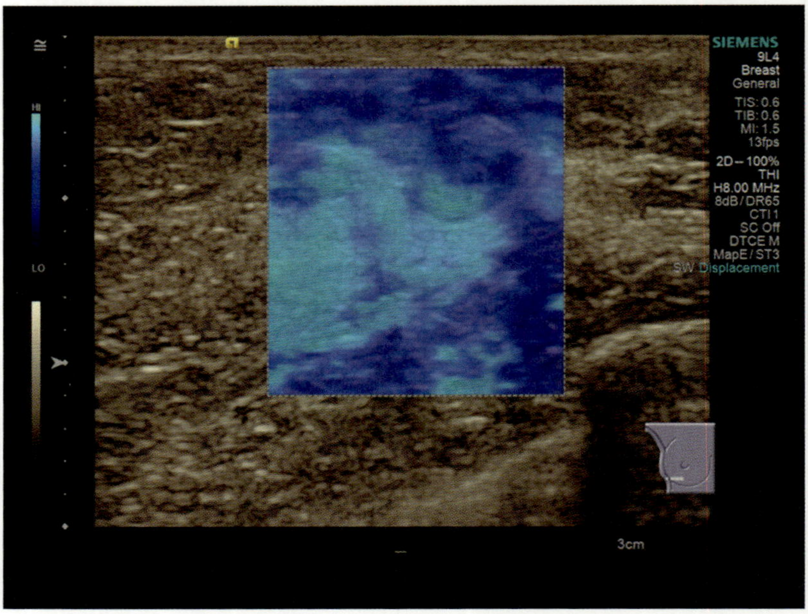

Fig. 5.5 Same lesion as Figs. 5.3 and 5.4. VTIQ displacement mode showed areas of poor lesion deformation displayed as *dark blue* in comparison to good displacement displayed in *bright blue*

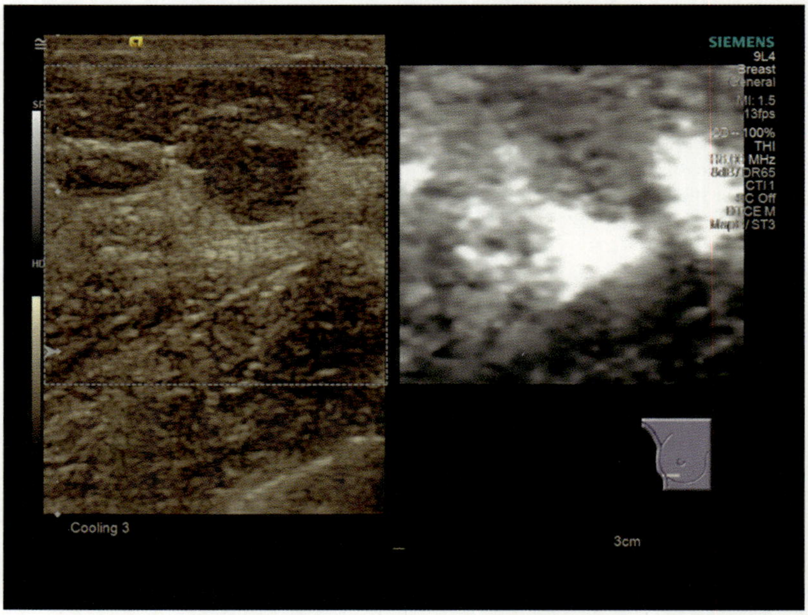

Fig. 5.6 In VTI elastography mode, the lesion appears *grey*, indicating an intermediate stiffness of the lesion

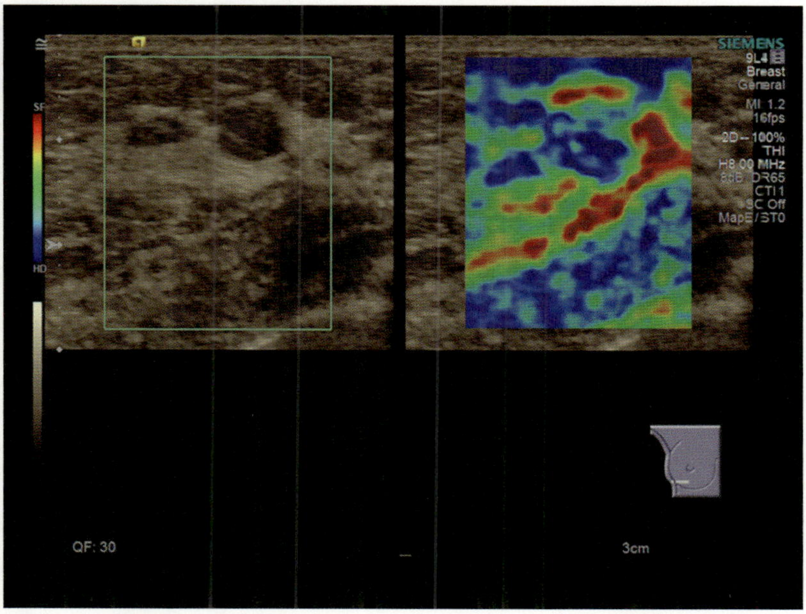

Fig. 5.7 Strain elastography shows a mixture of *green* and *blue*, indicating a lesion of intermediate stiffness in comparison with the surrounding tissue

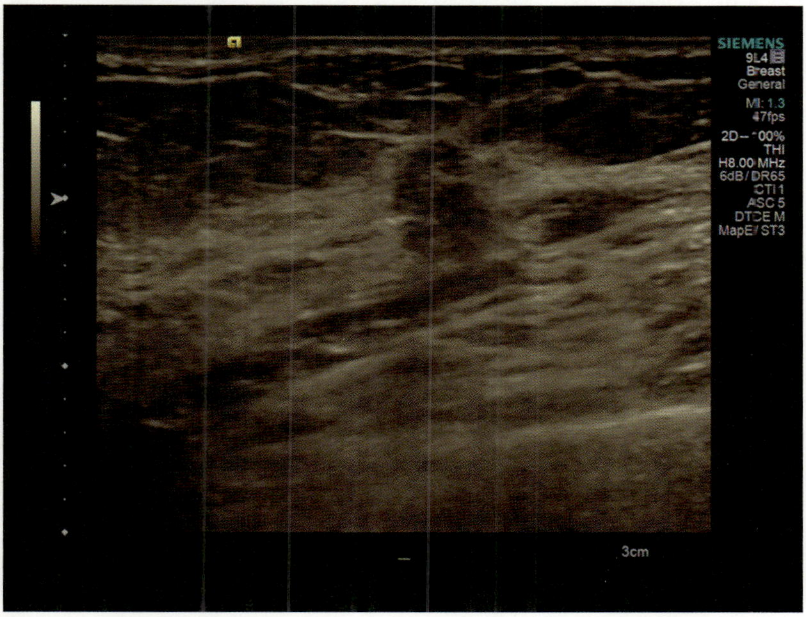

Fig. 5.8 Ultrasound images of a 43-year-old woman. B-mode sonography indicates a hypoechoic mass with angular margins. The histological diagnosis proven by core needle biopsy was of an invasive ductal carcinoma

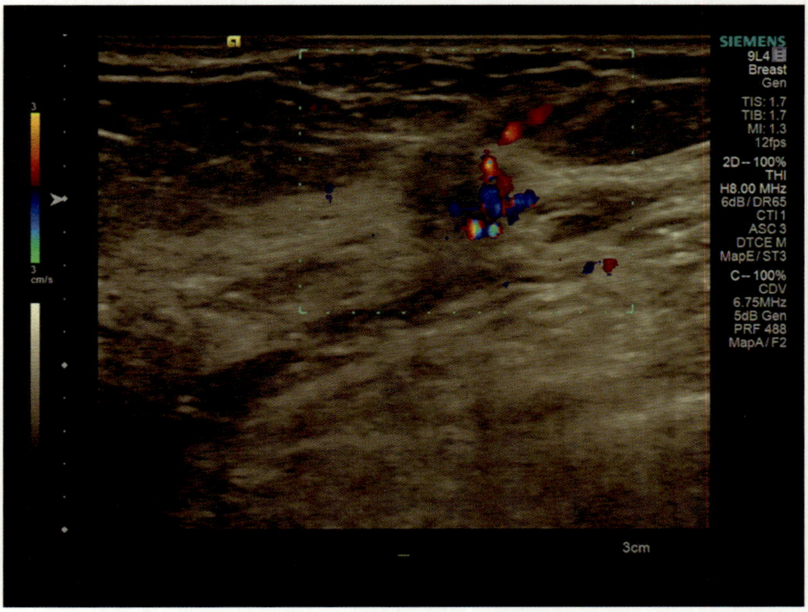

Fig. 5.9 Colour Doppler sonography indicates an increased vascularity of the lesion

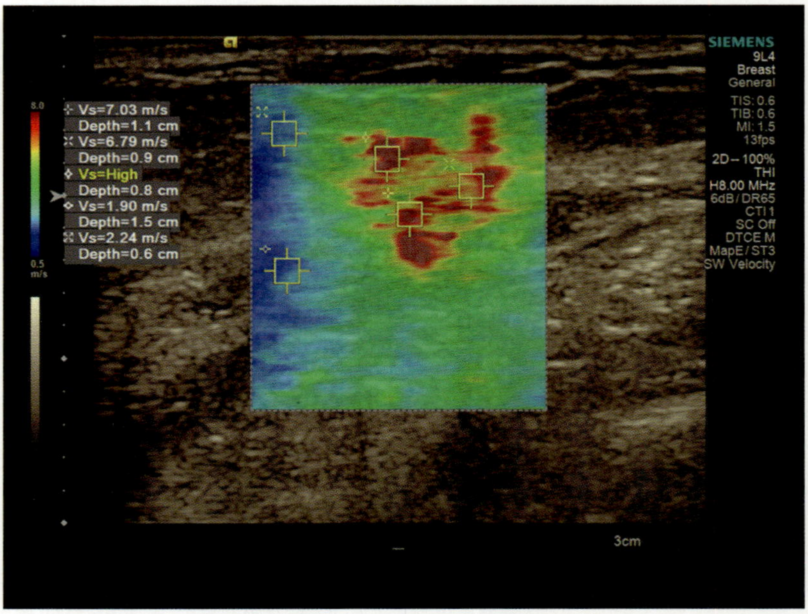

Fig. 5.10 VTIQ velocity colour overlay displayed relative shear wave velocities according to the adjacent colour spectrum, *red areas* corresponding to higher values and *blue areas* corresponding to lower values. Shear wave velocity was measured in the lesion $v = 6.79$–7.03 m/s and in the surrounding tissue level between $v = 1.90$–2.24 m/s

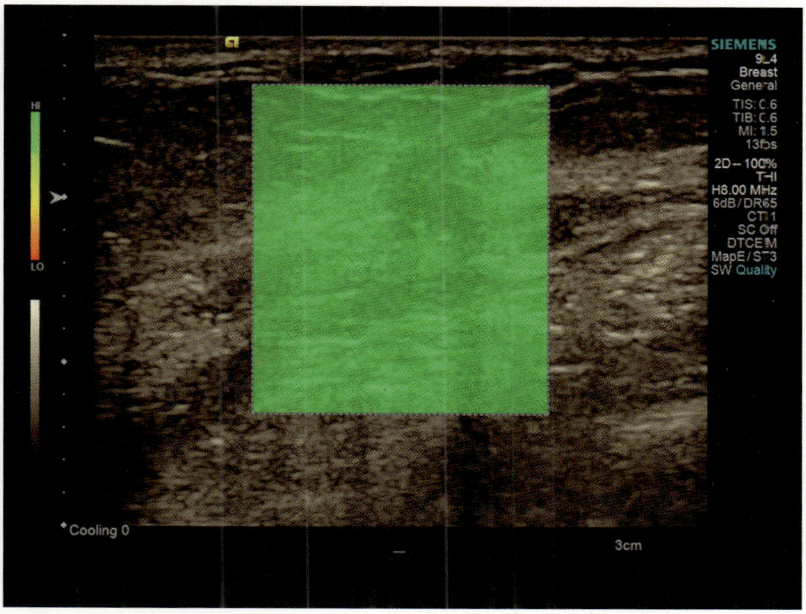

Fig. 5.11 Same lesion as Fig. 5.10. Using the VTIQ quality map, all of the breast tissue and the lesion are coloured in *green*, indicating the high quality of generated shear wave velocity measurements

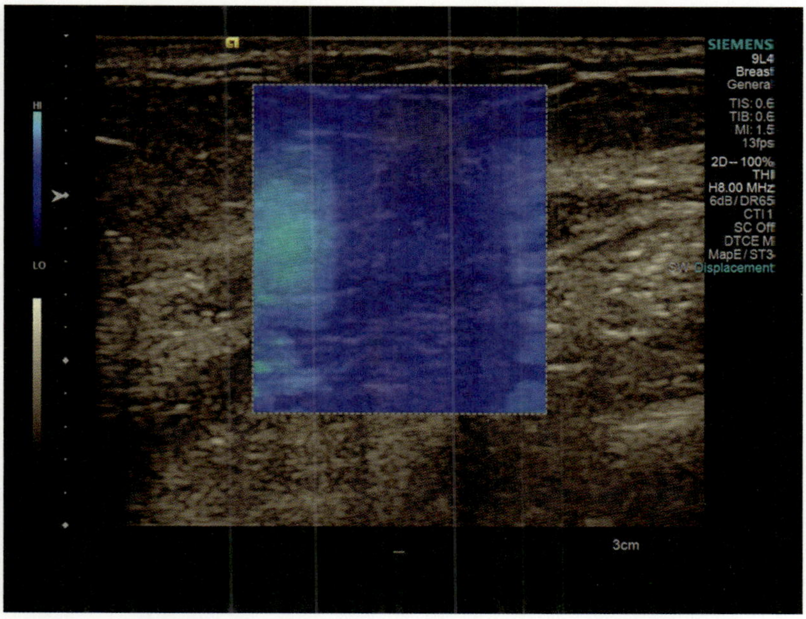

Fig. 5.12 Same lesion as Figs. 5.10 and 5.11. VTIQ displacement mode showed a low deformation of the lesion displayed as *dark blue* in comparison to good displacement of the surrounding tissue as displayed in *bright blue*

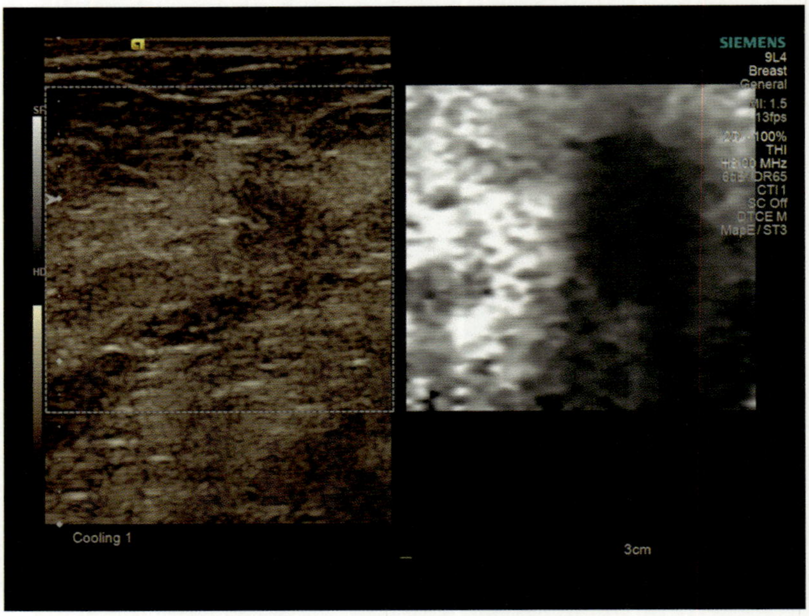

Fig. 5.13 In VTI elastography mode, the lesion appears *black* and is much larger in comparison to the lesion size seen on B-mode, indicative of a very stiff lesion

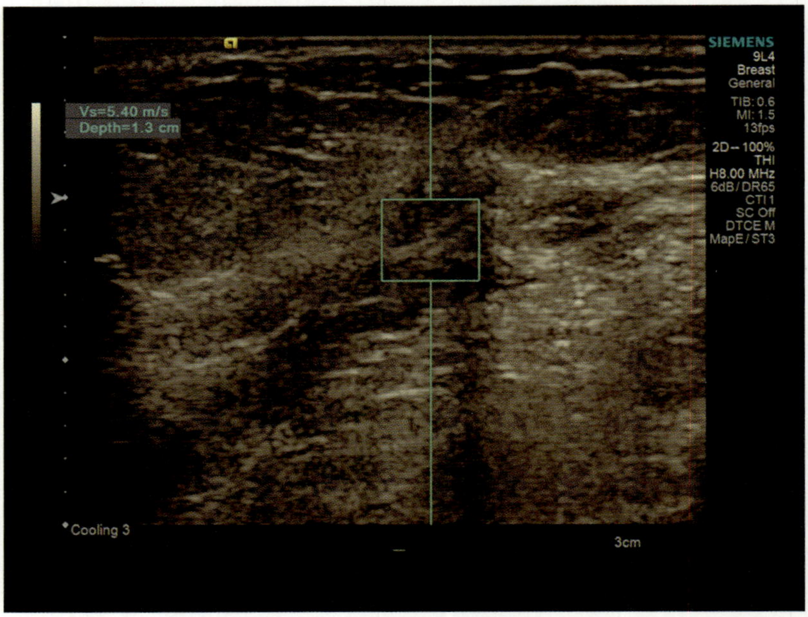

Fig. 5.14 In VTQ mode, the shear wave speed velocity was measured in the lesion with a velocity of $v = 5.40$ m/s

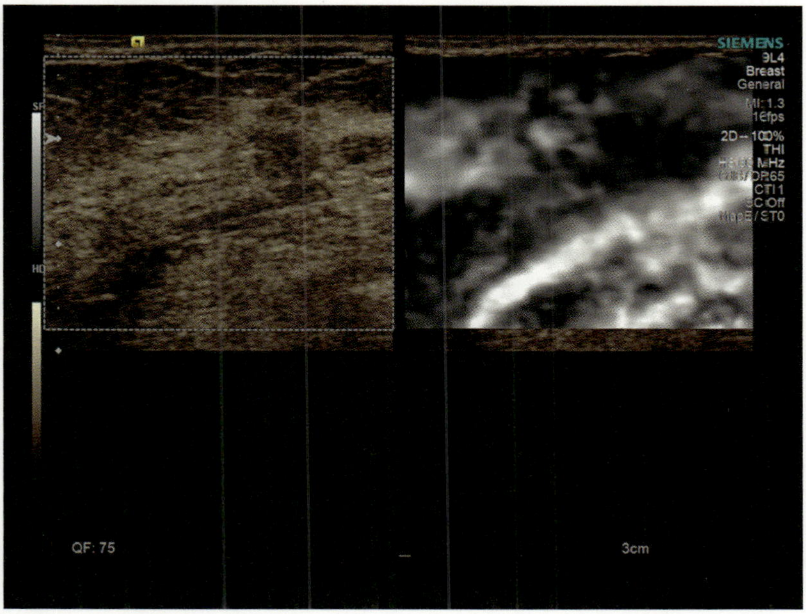

Fig. 5.15 In strain elastography, the lesion appears *black* and is larger in comparison to the B-mode, indicative of a very stiff lesion

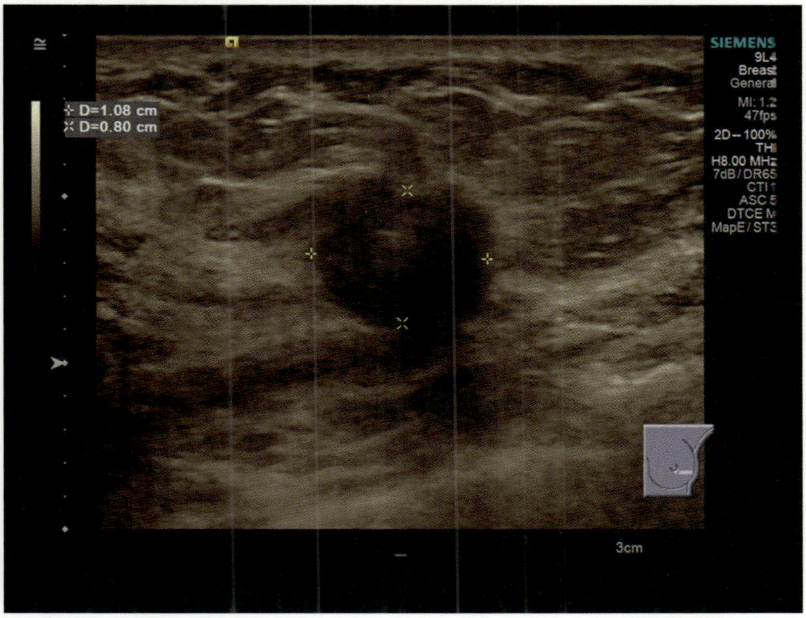

Fig. 5.16 Ultrasound images of a 65-year-old woman. B-mode sonography shows a round hypoechoic lesion with a maximum diameter of 1.1 cm. The histological diagnosis proven by core needle biopsy was of ductal carcinoma in situ (DCIS)

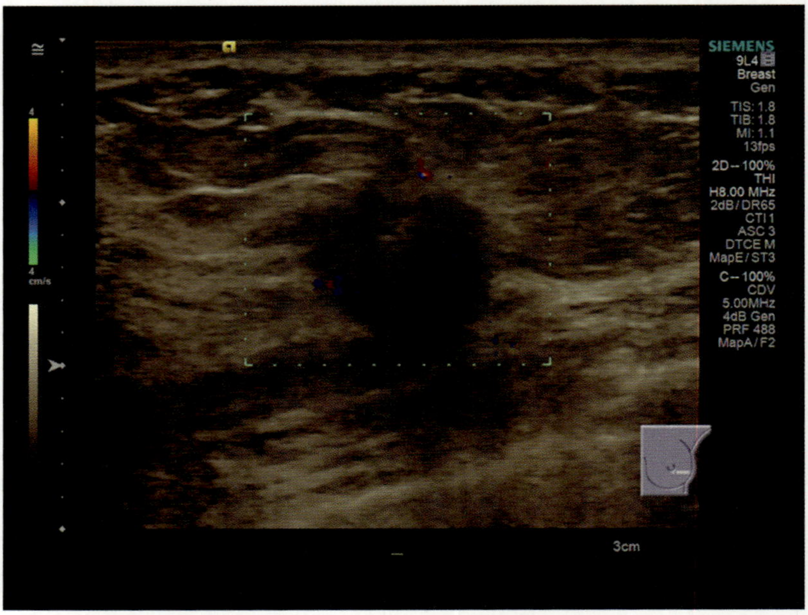

Fig. 5.17 Colour Doppler sonography indicates moderate vascularity of the lesion

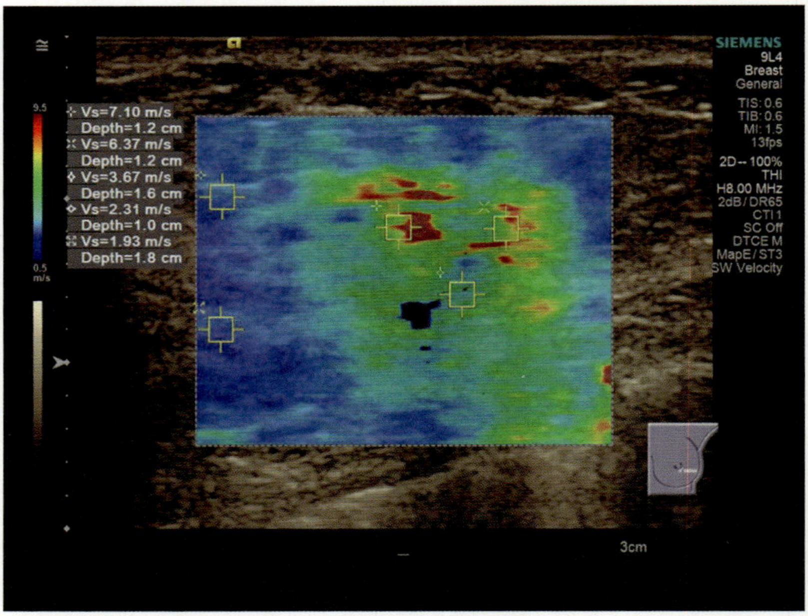

Fig. 5.18 VTIQ velocity colour overlay displayed relative shear wave velocities according to the adjacent colour spectrum, *red areas* corresponding to higher values and *blue areas* corresponding to lower values. Shear wave velocity was measured in the lesion $v=3.67–7.10$ m/s and in the surrounding tissue level between $v=1.93–2.31$ m/s

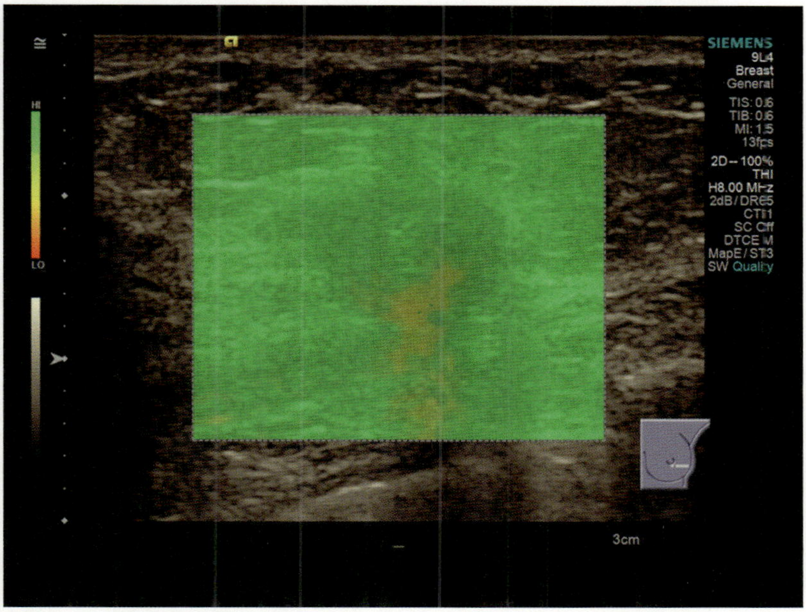

Fig. 5.19 Same lesion as Fig. 5.18. Using the VTIQ quality map, most of the breast tissue and the lesion are coloured *green* with some parts of the lesion coloured *yellow*, indicating a good quality of generated shear waves

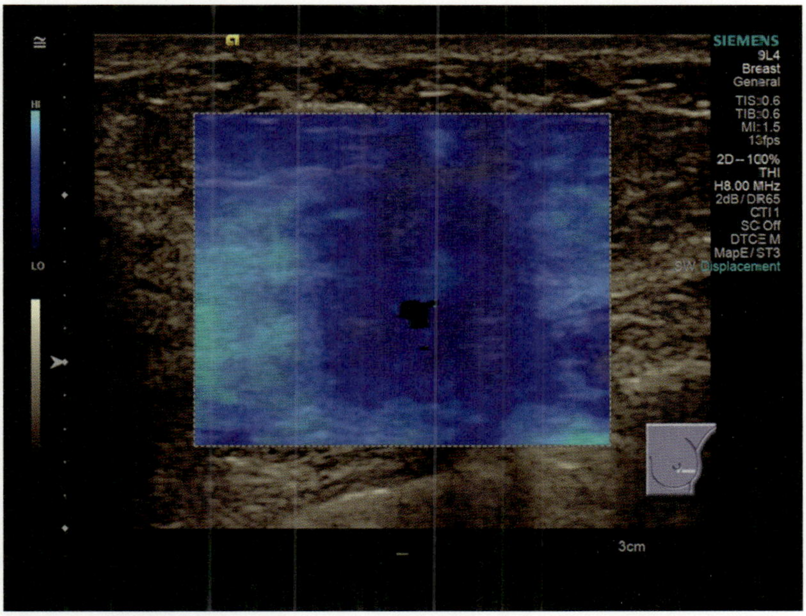

Fig. 5.20 Same lesion as Figs. 5.18 and 5.19. VTIQ displacement mode showed a low deformation of the lesion displayed as *dark blue* in comparison to good displacement of the surrounding tissue displayed in *bright blue*

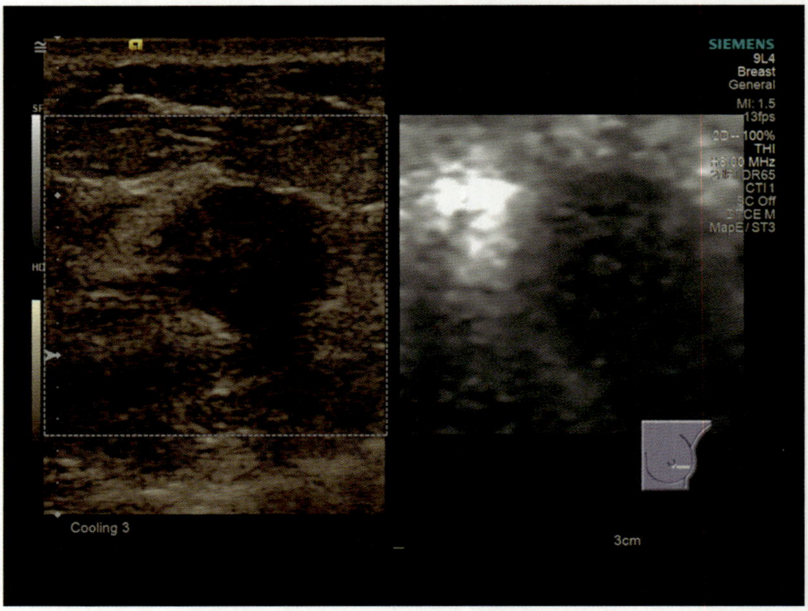

Fig. 5.21 In VTI elastography mode, the lesion appears as *black* and is much larger in VTI-mode in comparison to the B-mode, indicative of a very stiff lesion

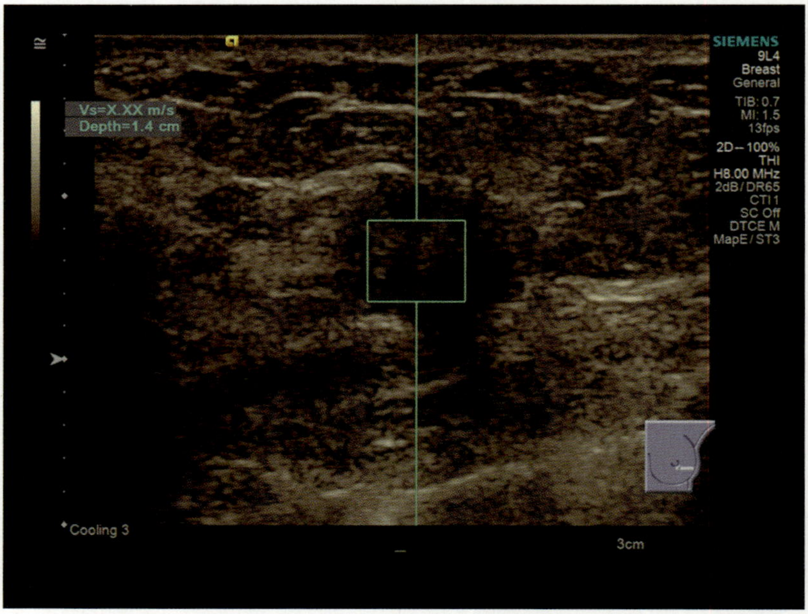

Fig. 5.22 In VTQ mode, the shear wave measurement in the centre of the lesion is displayed as X.XX m/s. This result is likely caused by the heterogeneity of the lesion (as indicated in Fig. 5.18), making a large single point measurement unobtainable. VTIQ is recommended in these cases where a measurement cannot reliably be made with VTQ

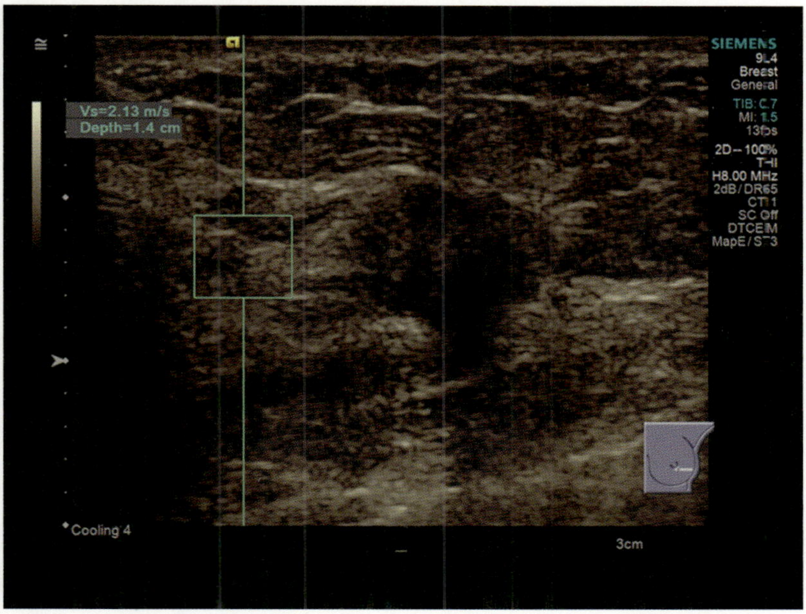

Fig. 5.23 In VTQ mode, the shear wave speed was measured in the surrounding tissue with a velocity of $v = 2.13$ m/s

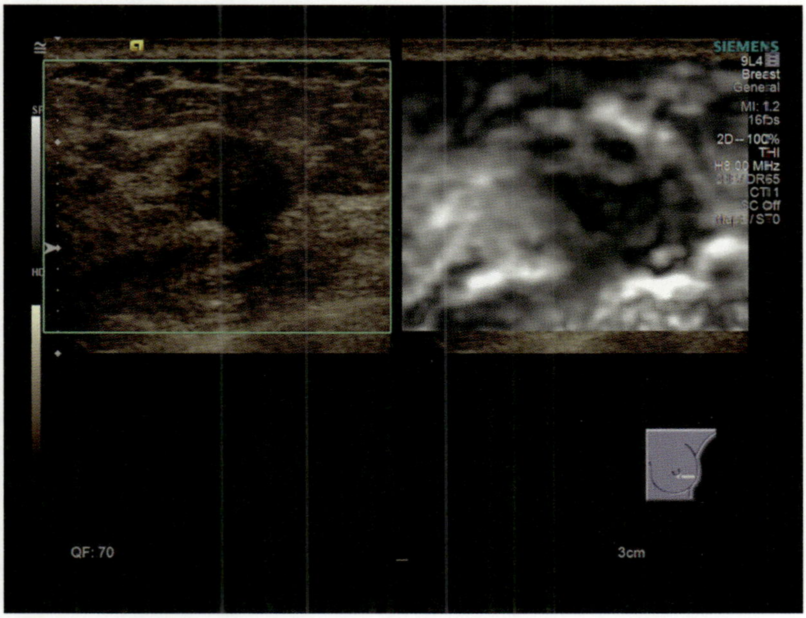

Fig. 5.24 In the strain elastogram, the lesion appears *black* and is larger in comparison to the B-mode, indicative of a very stiff lesion

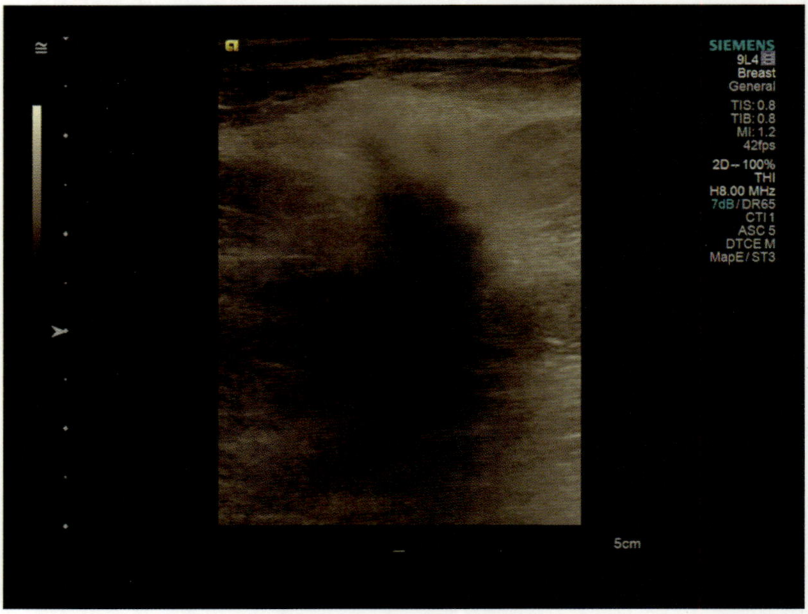

Fig. 5.25 Ultrasound images of a 55-year-old woman. B-mode sonography indicates a hypoechoic lesion with angular margins and significant posterior shadowing measuring a maximum diameter of 2.1 cm. The histological diagnosis proven by core needle biopsy was invasive ductal carcinoma

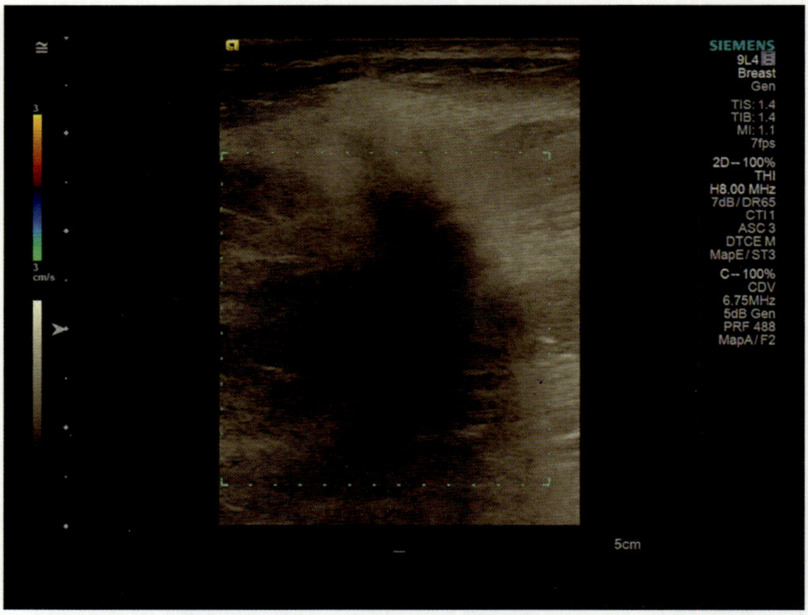

Fig. 5.26 Colour Doppler sonography does not display increased vascularity of the lesion

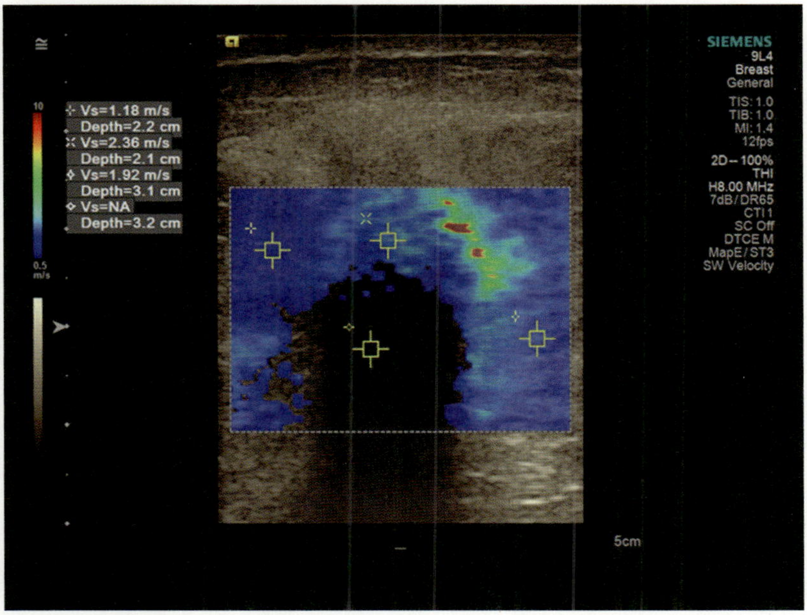

Fig. 5.27 VTIQ velocity colour overlay displayed relative shear wave velocities according to the adjacent colour spectrum, *red areas* corresponding to higher values and *blue areas* corresponding to lower values. Shear wave velocity was measured in the surrounding tissue $v = 1.18$–2.36 m/s. This is a classic example of the "red ring" appearance of cancer VTIQ colour map shown as *black* in the centre of the lesion with no obtainable shear wave velocity. This corresponds to the significant absorption seen in the B-mode image (Fig. 5.25) and is where the VTIQ information has dropped out due to the shear wave signal-to-noise ratio (SNR) being too low for a measurement to be made. Also see quality map in Fig. 5.28

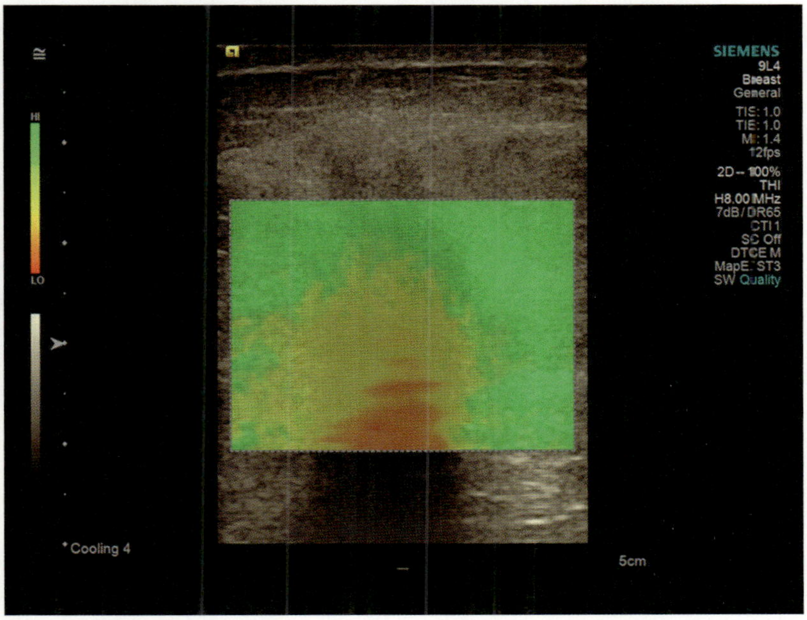

Fig. 5.28 Same lesion as Fig. 5.27. Using the VTIQ quality map, most of the breast lesion is coloured *yellow* and *red* which indicates that the shear wave velocity estimates in these areas may be unreliable or not possible. The surrounding breast tissue is coloured *green* indicating a high-quality generated shear waves and is the most reliable area to make the shear wave velocity measurements

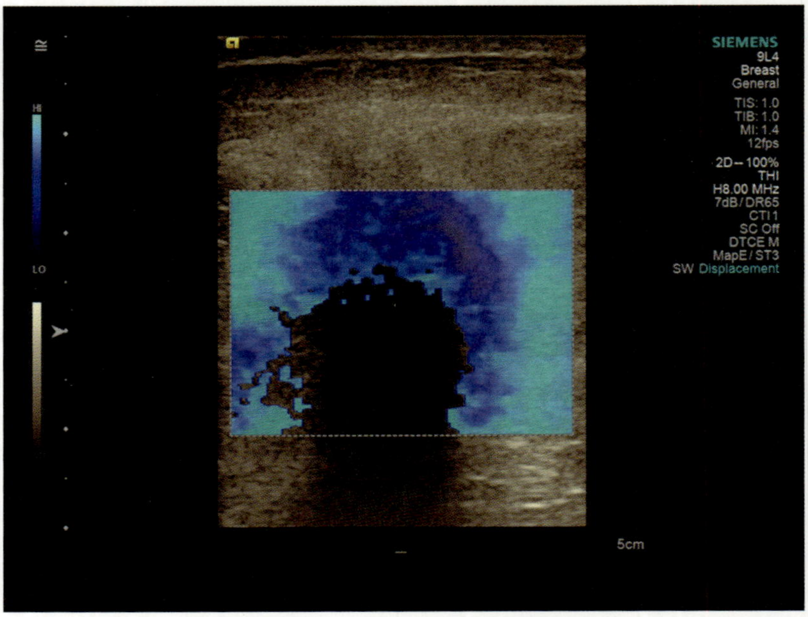

Fig. 5.29 Same lesion as Figs. 5.27 and 5.28. VTIQ displacement mode shows the central part of the lesion displayed as *black* which in this case indicates that the shear wave signal was not detected (as indicated in Figs. 5.27 and 5.28), whereas the tissue adjacent to the lesion is displayed as *dark blue* through to *light blue* as you get further from the lesion indicating moderate to good tissue displacement in the surrounding breast parenchyma

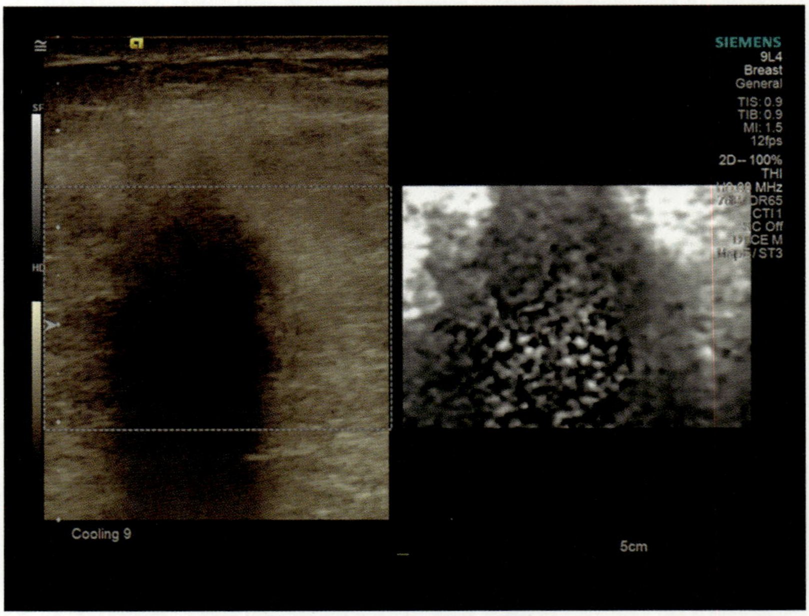

Fig. 5.30 In VTI elastography mode, the lesion has a *black* periphery with a mosaic appearance in the centre and is much larger in VTI-mode in comparison to the B-mode, indicative of a very stiff lesion

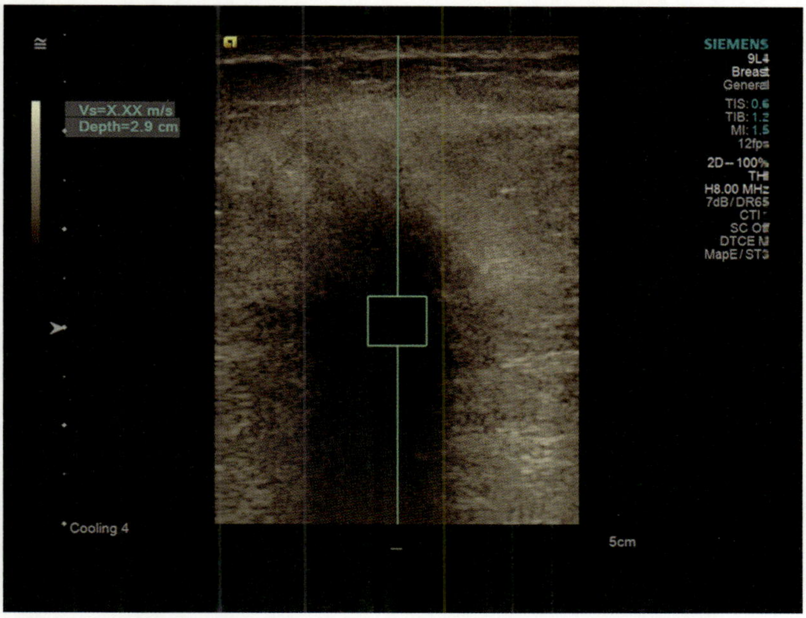

Fig. 5.31 In VTQ mode, the shear wave measurement in the centre of the lesion is displayed as X.XX m/s. This result is likely caused by the heterogeneity of the lesion making a large single point measurement unobtainable. VTIQ, particularly in the periphery of the lesion, is recommended in these cases where a measurement cannot reliably be made with VTQ

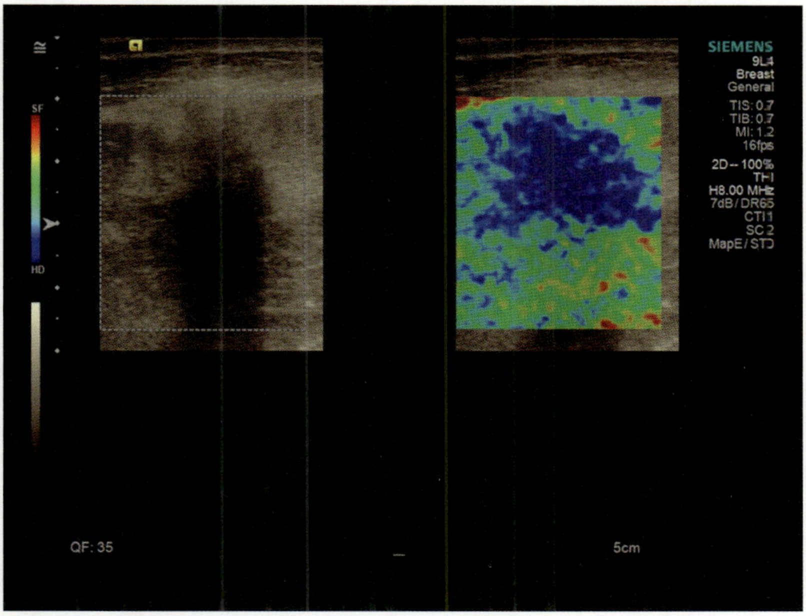

Fig. 5.32 In the strain elastogram, the lesion is shown as *blue* and is larger in comparison to the B-mode, indicative of a very stiff lesion

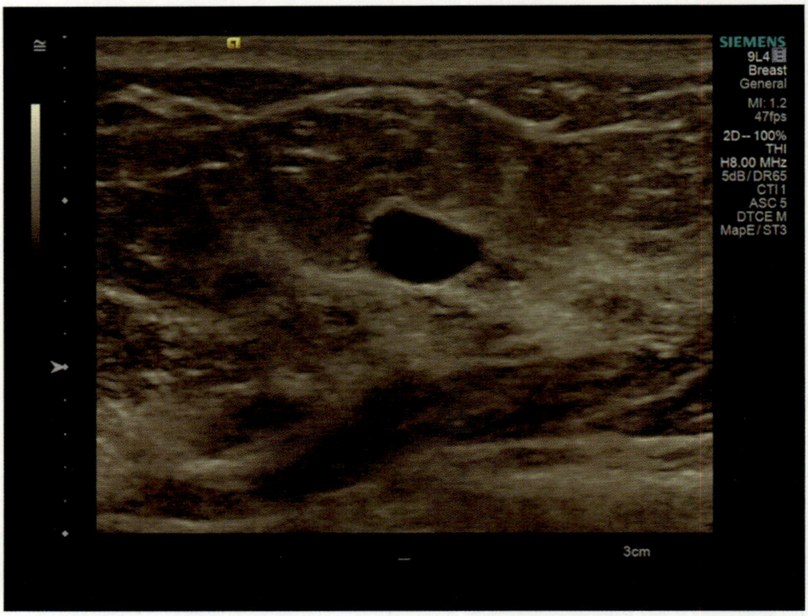

Fig. 5.33 Ultrasound images of a 43-year-old woman. B-mode sonography indicates an ovoid to round anechoic to hypoechoic lesion with a maximum diameter of 6 mm. The diagnosis was a haemorrhagic breast cyst

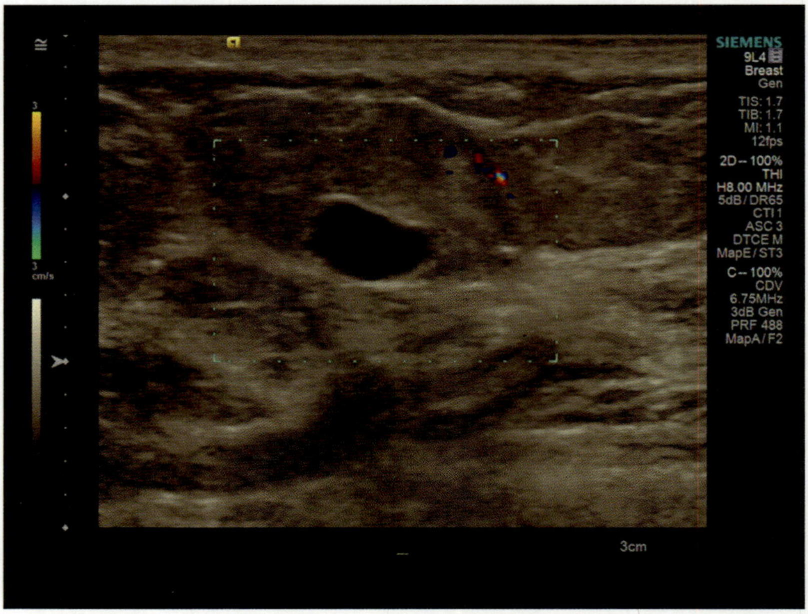

Fig. 5.34 Colour Doppler sonography indicates no vascularity in the lesion

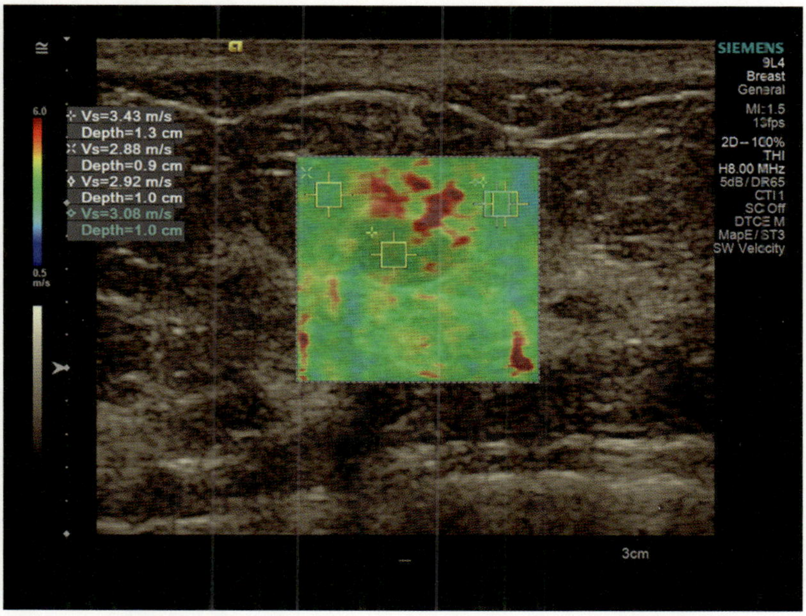

Fig. 5.35 VTIQ velocity colour overlay displayed relative shear wave velocities according to the adjacent colour spectrum, *red areas* corresponding to higher values and *green areas* corresponding to lower values. Shear wave velocity was measured in the lesion $v = 3.43$ m/s and in the surrounding tissue level between $v = 2.88–3.08$ m/s

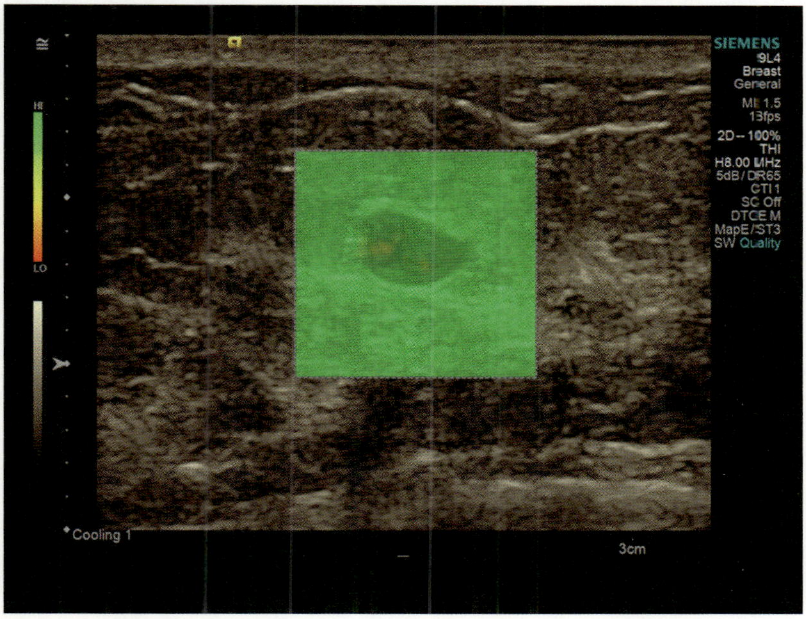

Fig. 5.36 Same lesion as Fig. 5.35. Using the VTIQ quality map, most of the breast lesion is coloured in *green* and *yellow* – an indicator of the reliable quality of the generated shear waves. The normal breast tissue is coloured *green* only indicating high reliability of the shear wave velocity estimations

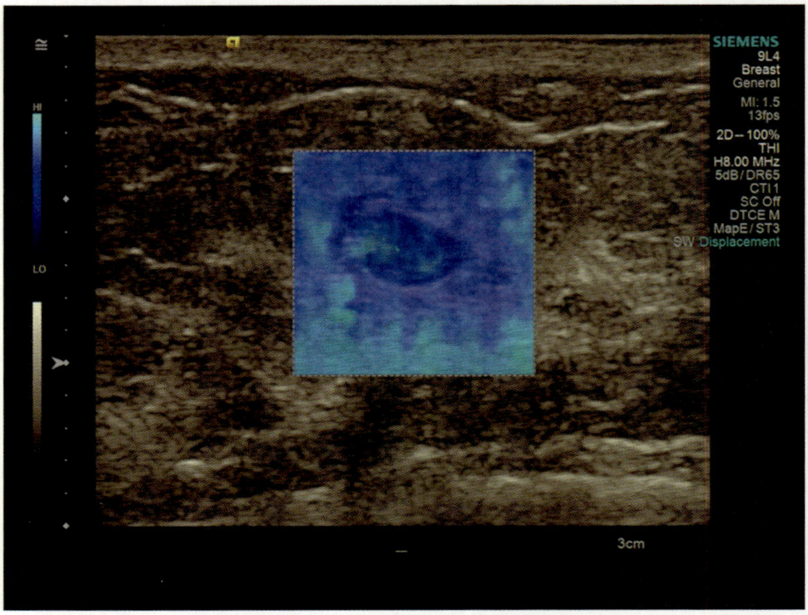

Fig. 5.37 Same lesion as Figs. 5.35 and 5.36. VTIQ displacement mode showed an intermediate deformation of the lesion displaying both *dark blue* and *bright blue* colours

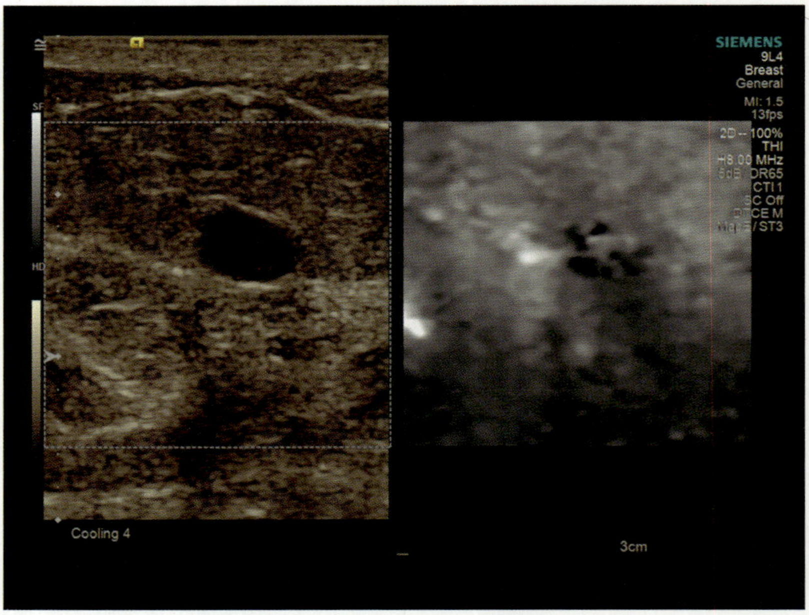

Fig. 5.38 In VTI elastography mode, the lesion appears as a ring of *small black dots*, with a *white centre*, indicative of a fluid-filled lesion

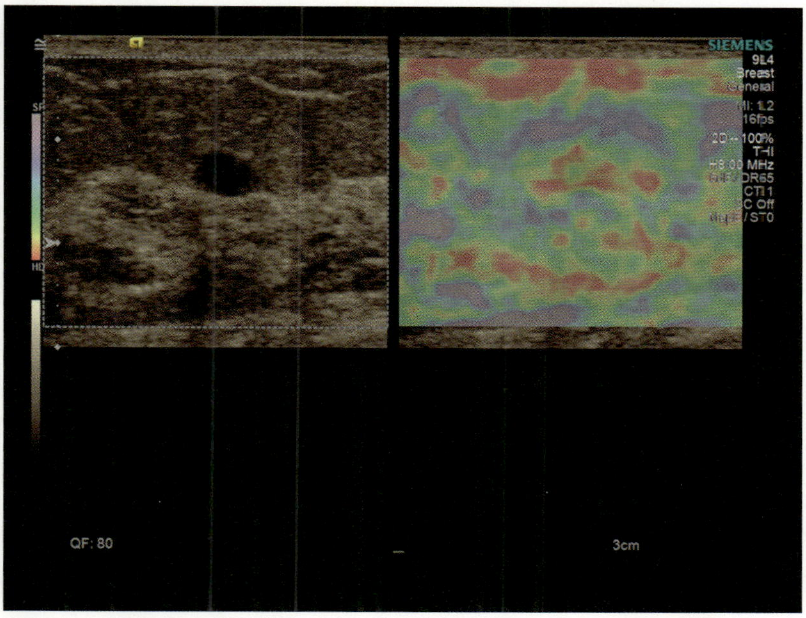

Fig. 5.39 In the strain elastogram, the lesion appears with bottom artefacts in *red* and *green*, indicating of a liquid lesion

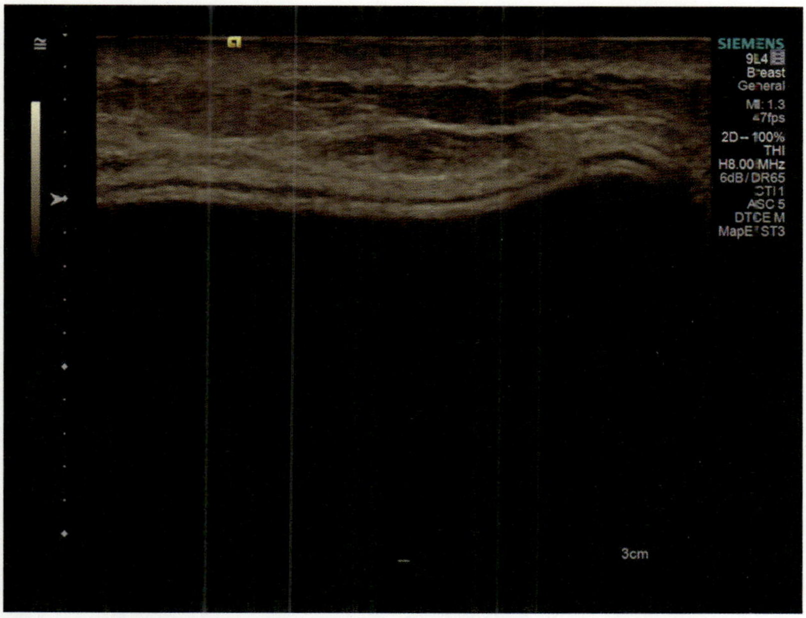

Fig. 5.40 Ultrasound images of a 42-year-old woman. B-mode sonography of a silicon breast implant

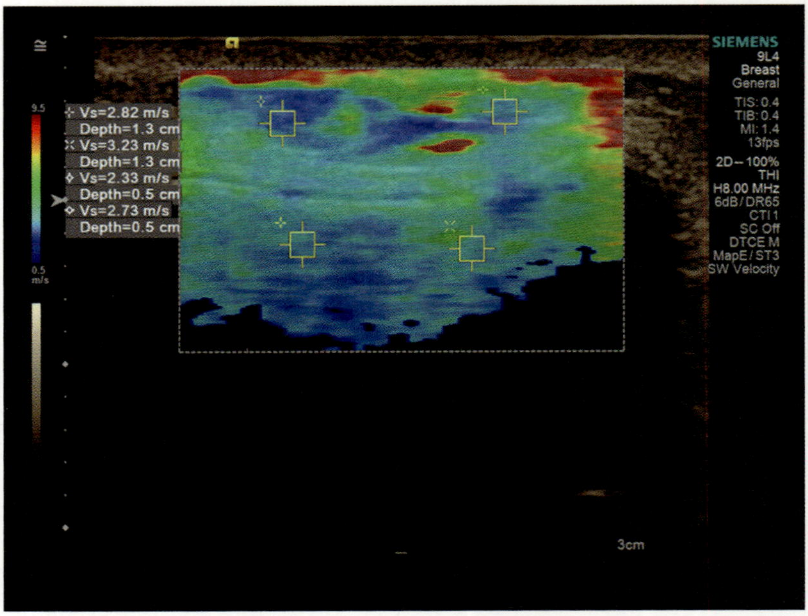

Fig. 5.41 VTIQ velocity colour overlay displayed relative shear wave velocities according to the adjacent colour spectrum. Shear wave velocity was measured in the silicon breast implant $v = 2.82$–3.23 m/s and in the surrounding normal breast tissue level between $v = 2.33$–2.73 m/s

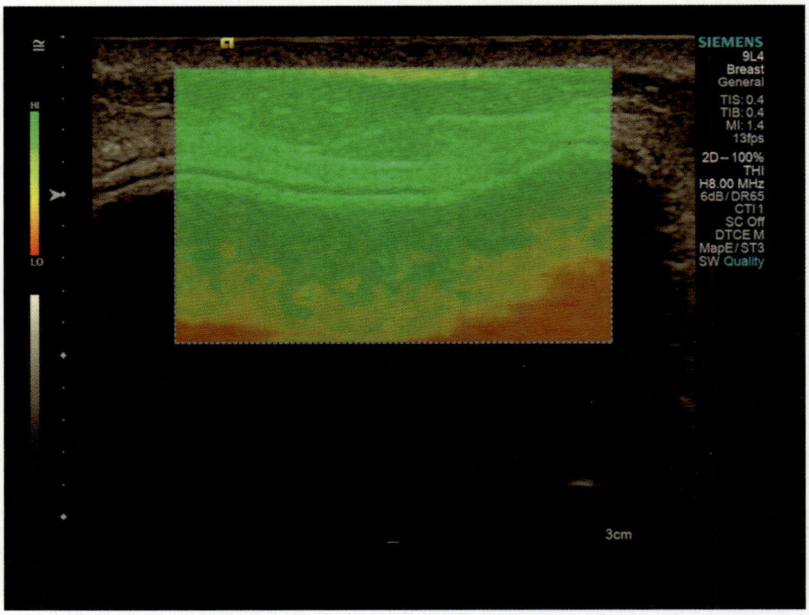

Fig. 5.42 Same lesion as Fig. 5.41. Using the VTIQ quality map, the normal breast tissue is coloured in *green* indicating a high reliability of shear wave measurements. The fluid-filled implant is displayed in *green*, *orange* and *red* colours indicating unreliable or no shear wave measurements possible

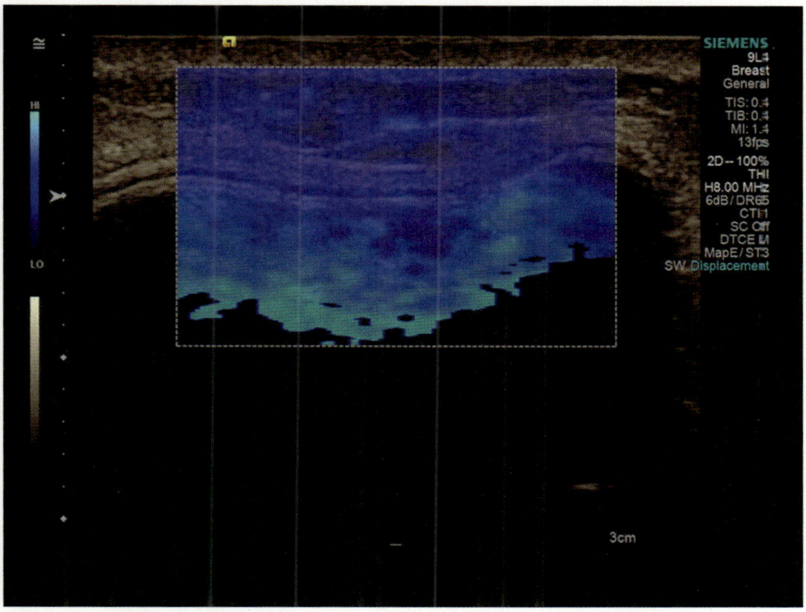

Fig. 5.43 Same lesion as Figs. 5.41 and 5.42. VTIQ displacement mode showed a *mid-blue colour* indicating intermediate deformation of the surface of the implant VTIQ displacement mode showed an intermediate deformation of the implant

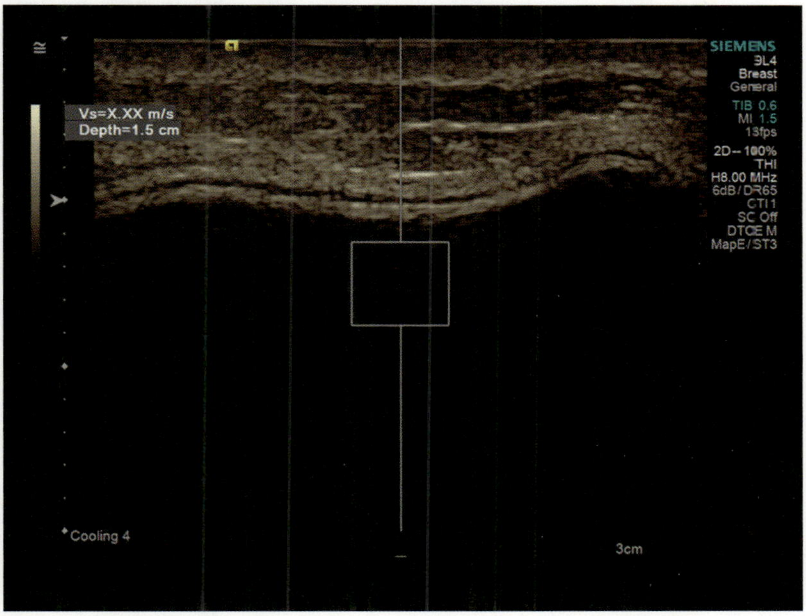

Fig. 5.44 In VTQ mode, the shear wave speed was measured in the implant, the system displaying v=XXX m/s. The result is X.XX because no shear waves are generated in the liquid (silicon)-filled implant. So a shear wave estimation is not possible in this area

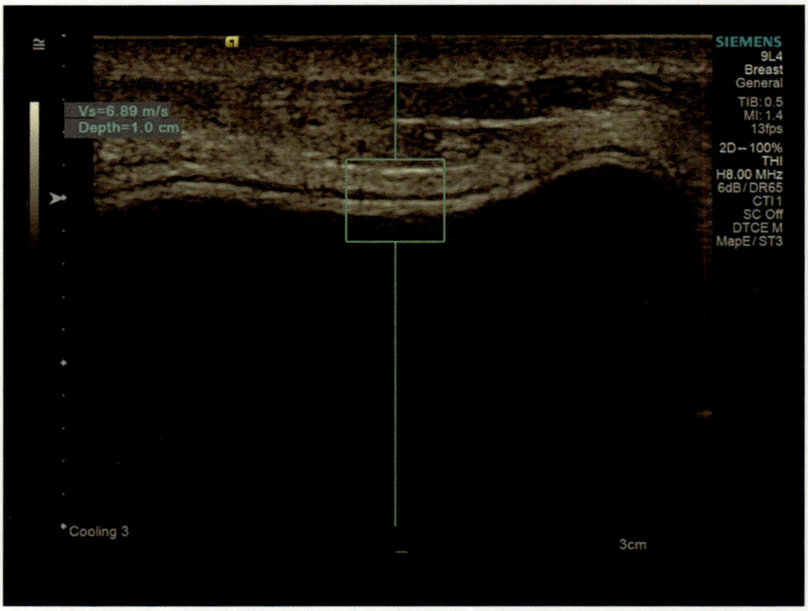

Fig. 5.45 In VTQ mode, the shear wave velocity was measured in the capsular of the implant as $v = 6.89$ m/s

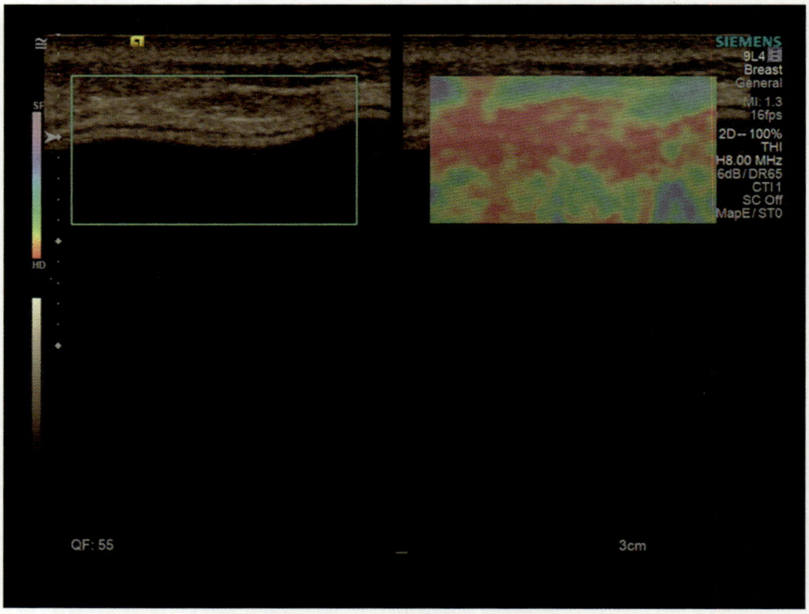

Fig. 5.46 In strain elastography mode, the capsule of the implant appears *red* and is much stiffer in comparison to the adjacent breast tissue

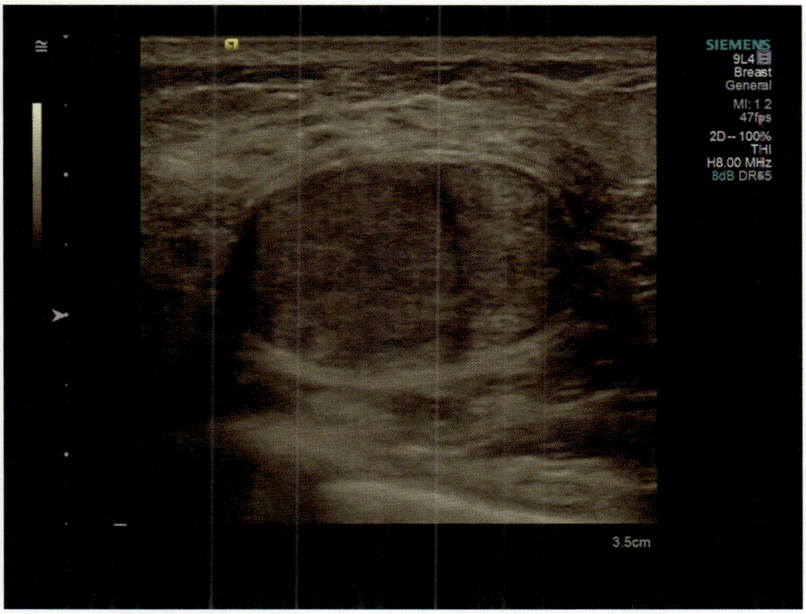

Fig. 5.47 Ultrasound images of a 37-year-old woman with a round fibroadenoma, histologically proven by core needle biopsy. B-mode sonography shows a round, well-circumscribed, hypoechoic mass with hyperechoic linear internal septa and absence of posterior shadowing, classified as BI-RADS 3

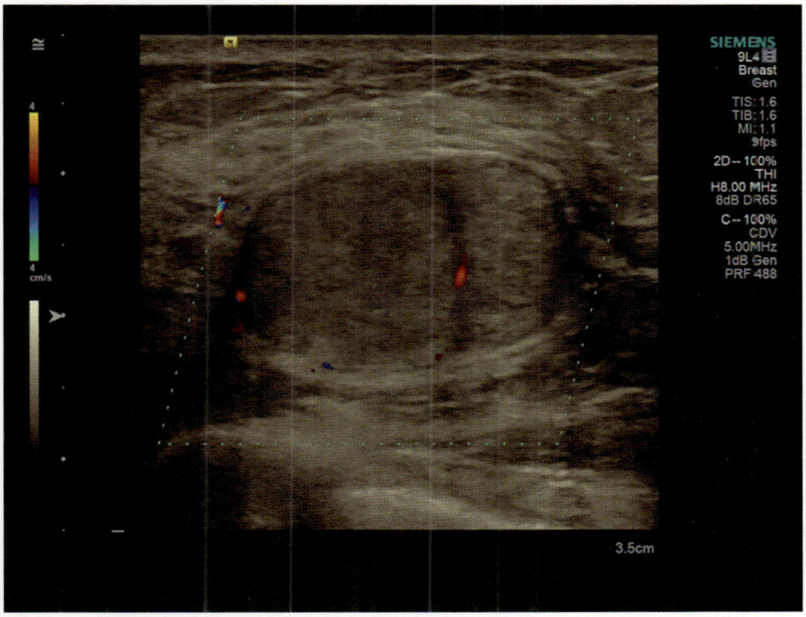

Fig. 5.48 Colour Doppler sonography indicates reduced vascularity

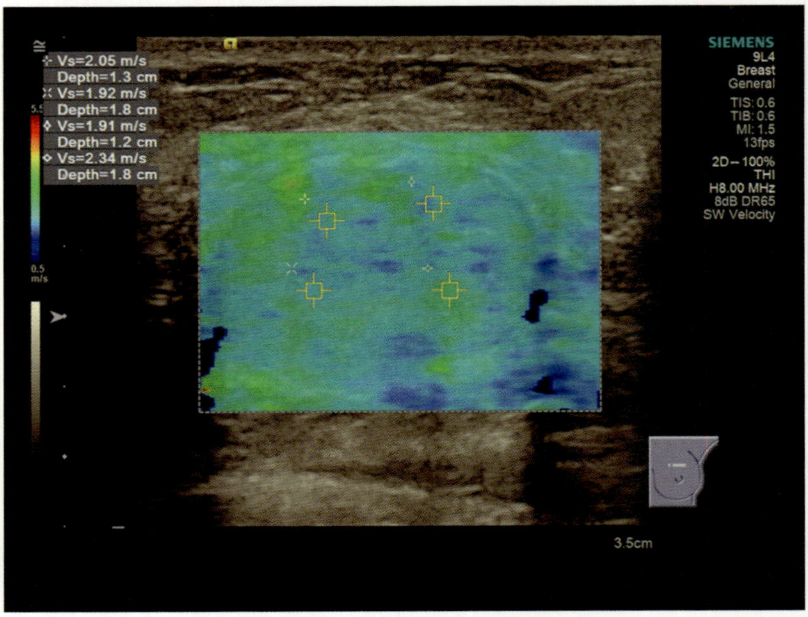

Fig. 5.49 VTIQ velocity colour overlay displayed relative shear wave velocities according to the adjacent colour spectrum, *red areas* corresponding to higher values and *blue areas* corresponding to lower values. Shear wave velocity was measured in the lesion $v = 1.92–2.34$ m/s

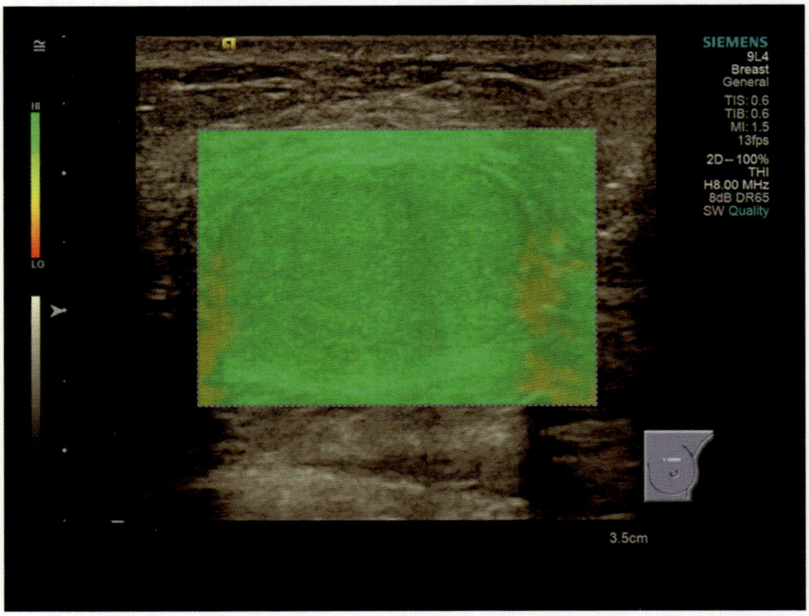

Fig. 5.50 Same lesion as Fig. 5.49. Using the VTIQ quality map, all of the breast tissue and lesion are coloured in *green*, an indicator of the high reliability of the generated shear wave measurements

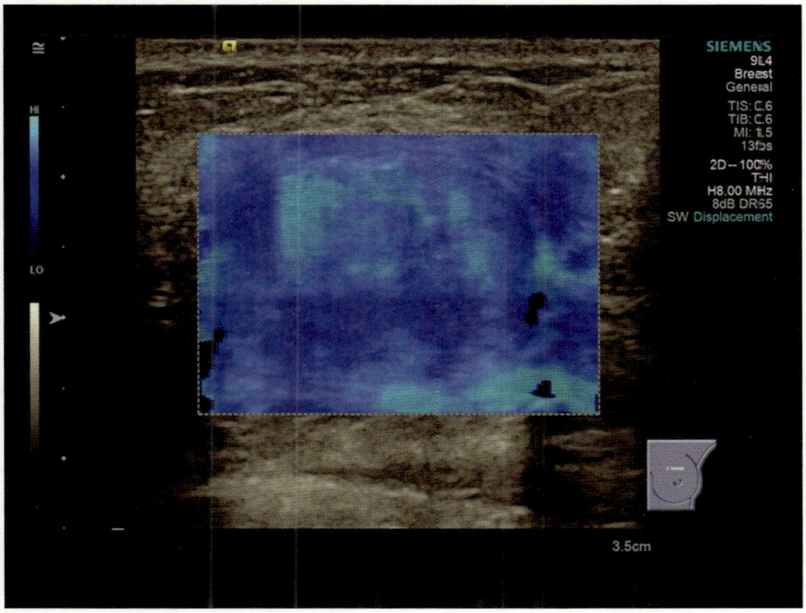

Fig. 5.51 Same lesion as Figs. 5.49 and 5.50. VTIQ displacement mode showed a moderate deformation of the lesion and the surrounding tissue displayed as *light blue*

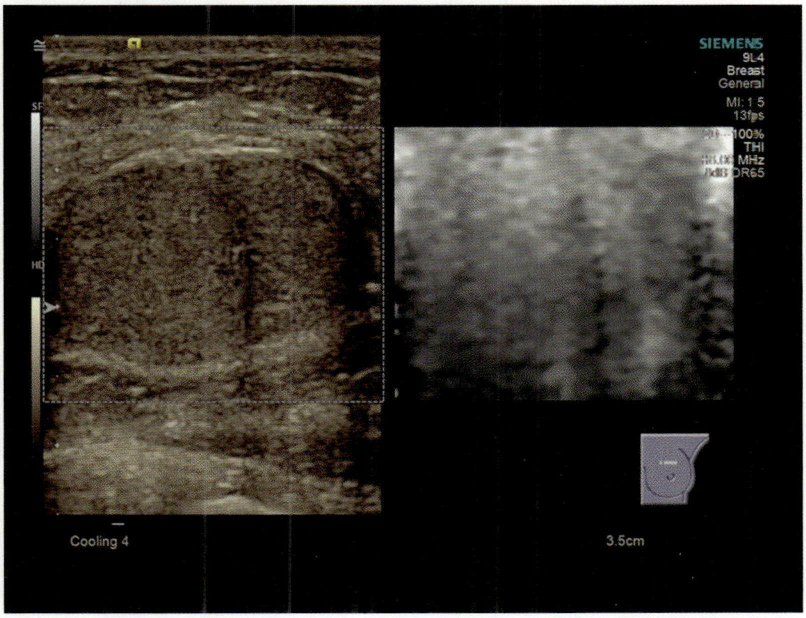

Fig. 5.52 In VTI elastography mode, the lesion appears *grey*, indicating an intermediate stiffness of the lesion. The lesion has the same size in the VTI-mode in comparison to the B-mode

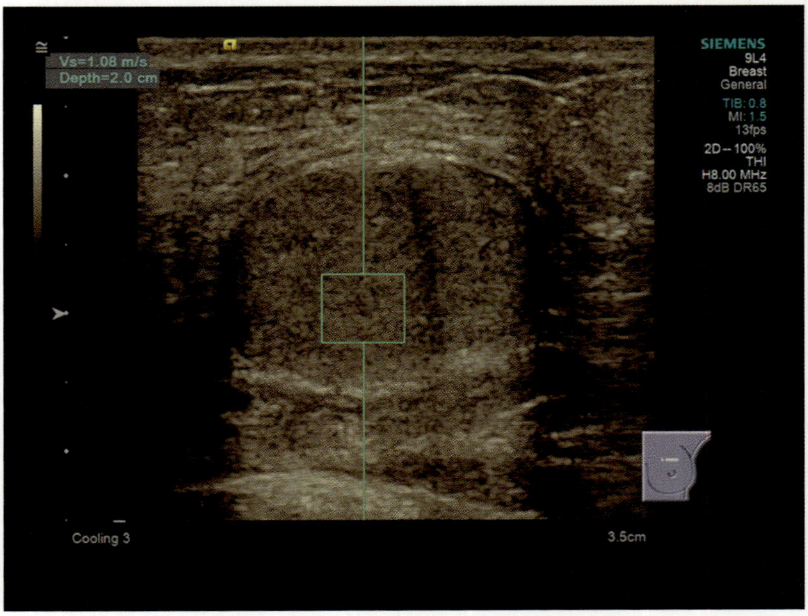

Fig. 5.53 In VTQ mode, the shear wave velocity was measured in the lesion, the system displaying $v = 1.08$ m/s

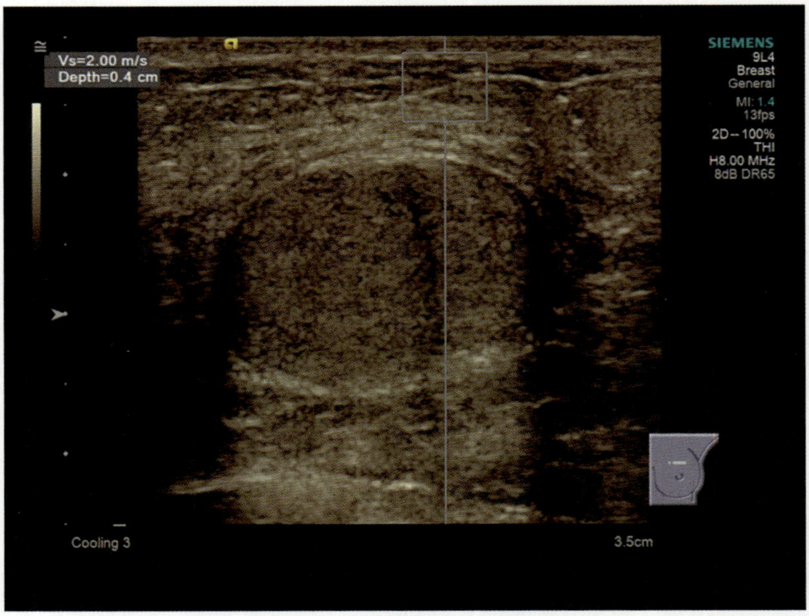

Fig. 5.54 In VTQ mode, the shear wave velocity was measured in the surrounding tissue, the system displaying $v = 2.00$ m/s

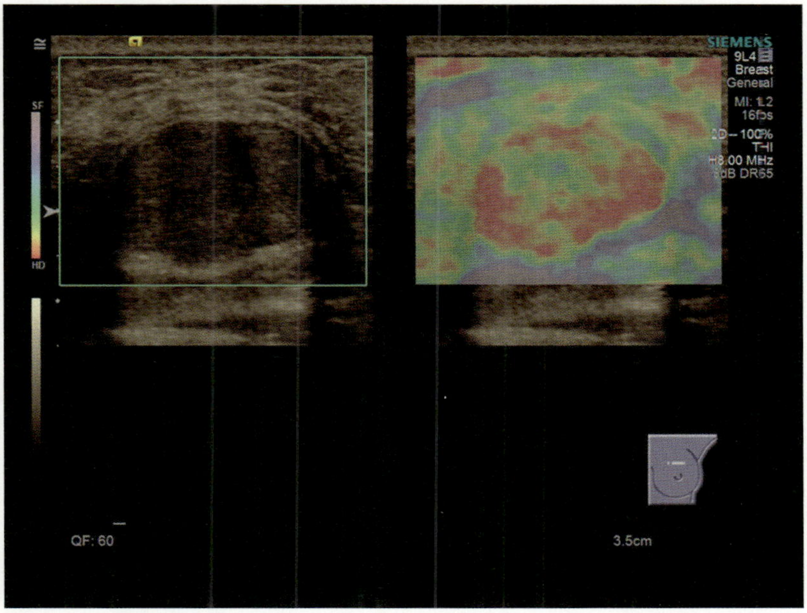

Fig. 5.55 The strain elastogram shows a mixture of *red* and *green colours*, indicating a moderately soft lesion. The lesion has the same size in the elastogram as in the B-mode image

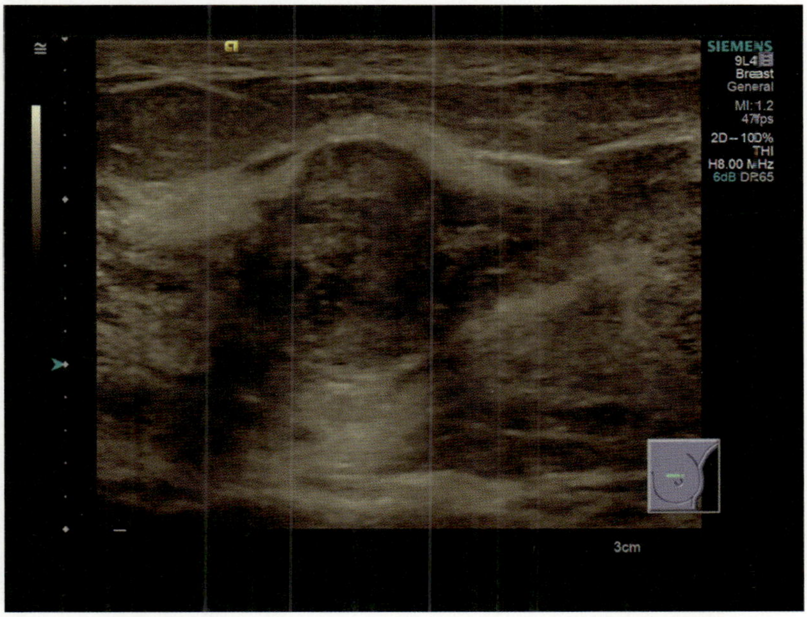

Fig. 5.56 Ultrasound images of a 41-year-old woman with fibroadenoma histologically proven by breast surgery, classified as BI-RADS 4a

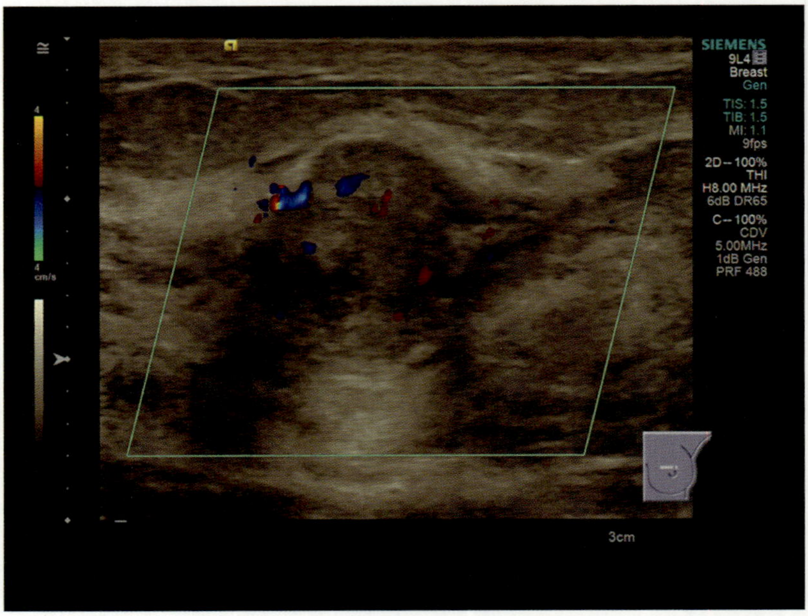

Fig. 5.57 Colour Doppler sonography indicates moderate vascularity of the lesion

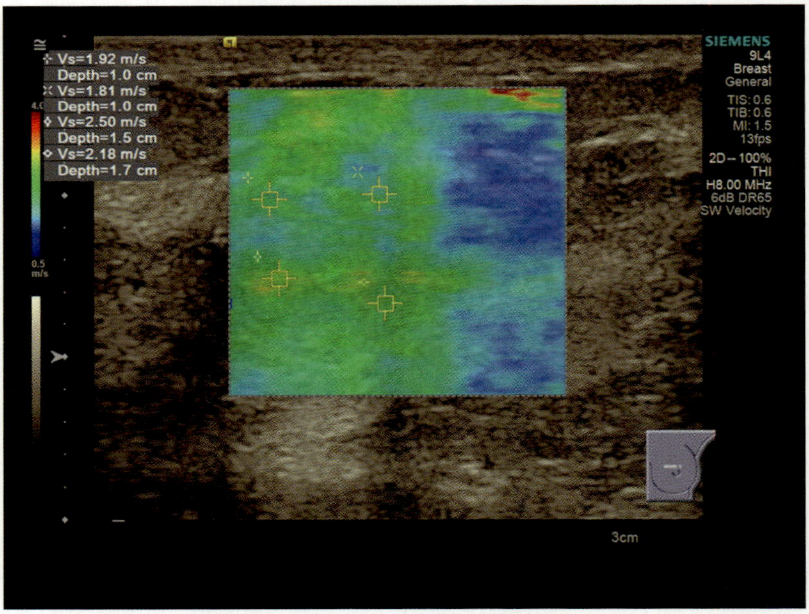

Fig. 5.58 VTIQ velocity colour overlay displayed relative shear wave velocities according to the adjacent colour spectrum, *red areas* corresponding to higher values and *blue areas* corresponding to lower values. Shear wave velocity was measured in the lesion $v = 1.81–2.50$ m/s

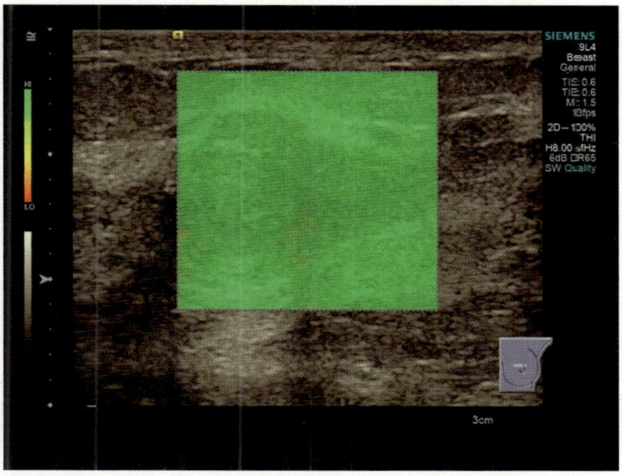

Fig. 5.59 Same lesion as Fig. 5.58. Using the VTIQ quality map, all of the breast tissue and the lesion are coloured in *green*, an indicator of the high reliability of generated shear wave measurements

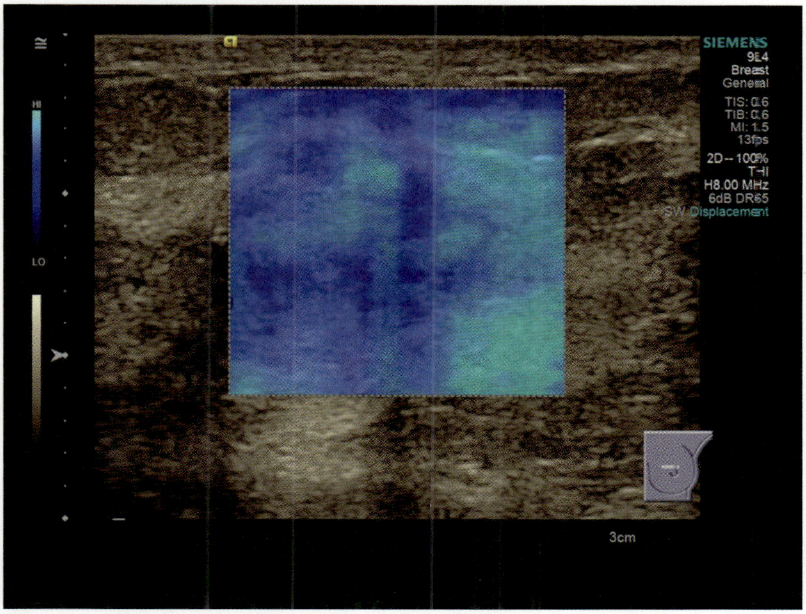

Fig. 5.60 Same lesion as Figs. 5.58 and 5.59. VTIQ displacement mode showed a moderate deformation of the lesion and the surrounding tissue displayed as *light blue*

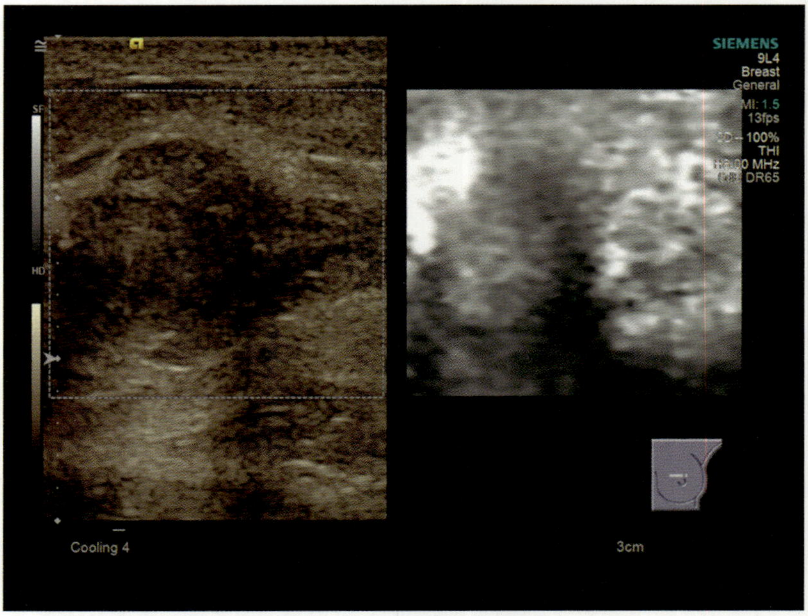

Fig. 5.61 In VTI elastography mode, the lesion appears *grey*, indicating an intermediate stiffness of the lesion. The lesion has the same size in the VTI-mode as in the corresponding B-mode

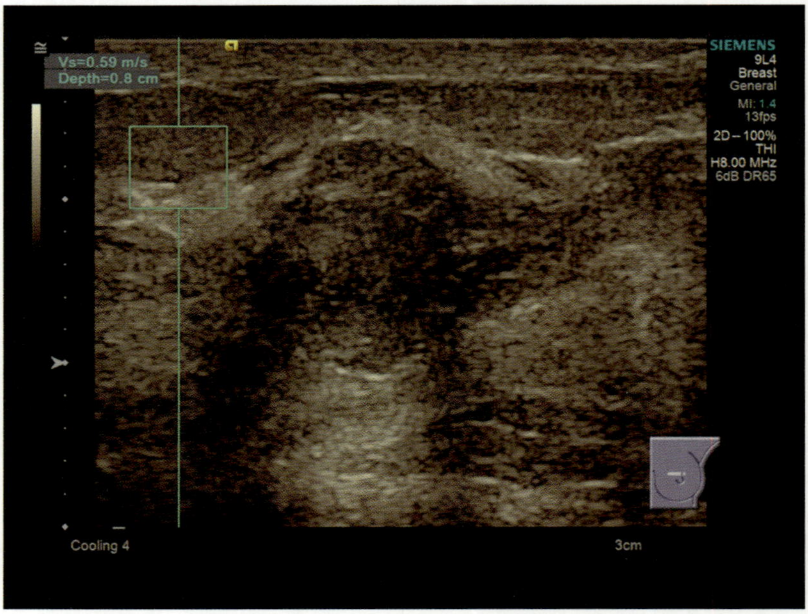

Fig. 5.62 In VTQ mode, the shear wave velocity was measured in the surrounding tissue, the system displaying $v = 0.59$ m/s

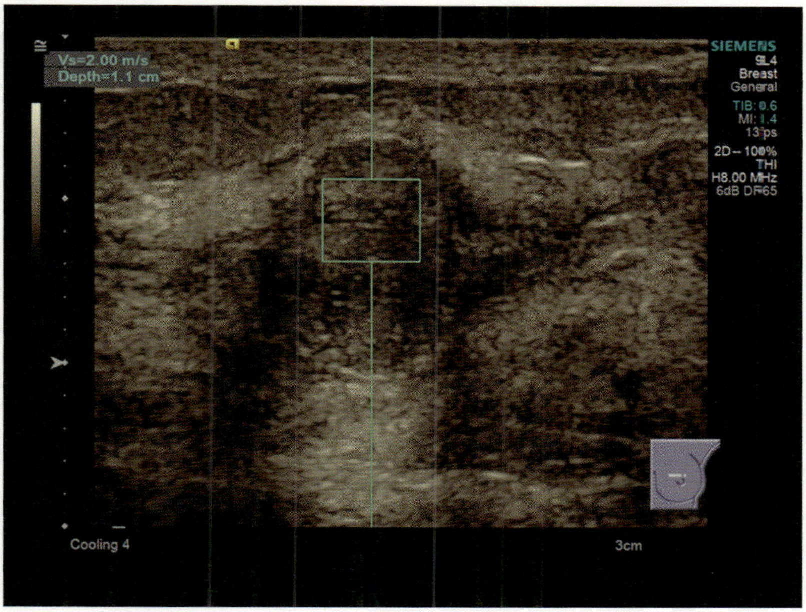

Fig. 5.63 In VTQ mode, the shear wave velocity was measured in the lesion, the system displaying $v = 2.00$ m/s

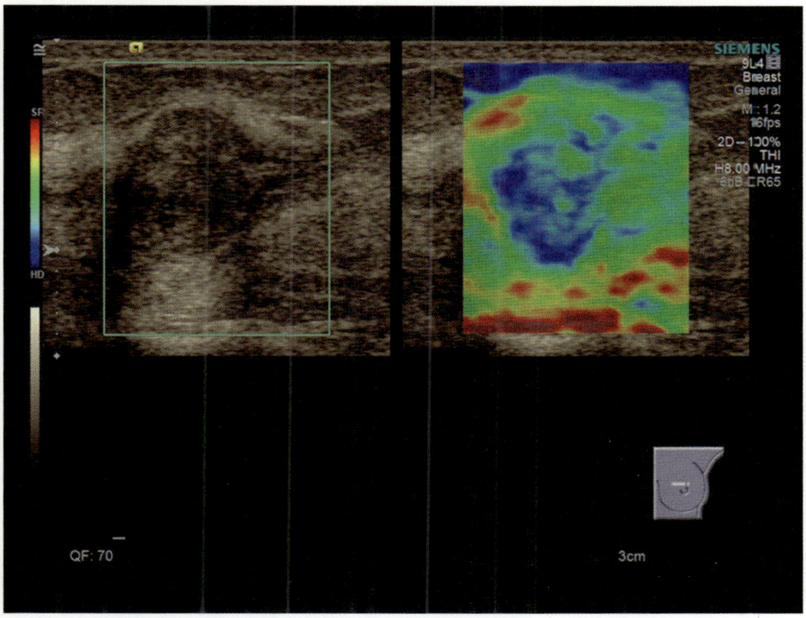

Fig. 5.64 The strain elastogram shows a mixture of *blue* and *green colours*, indicating a lesion that is stiffer than the surrounding tissue. The lesion has the same size in the strain elastogram as in the corresponding B-mode

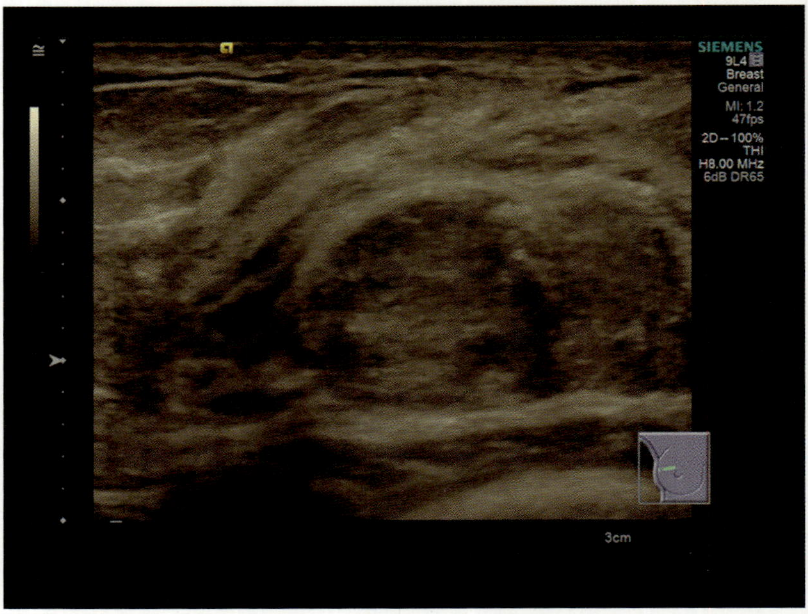

Fig. 5.65 Ultrasound images of a 43-year-old woman with smooth macrolobulated fibroadenoma histologically proven by breast surgery, classified as BI-RADS 4a

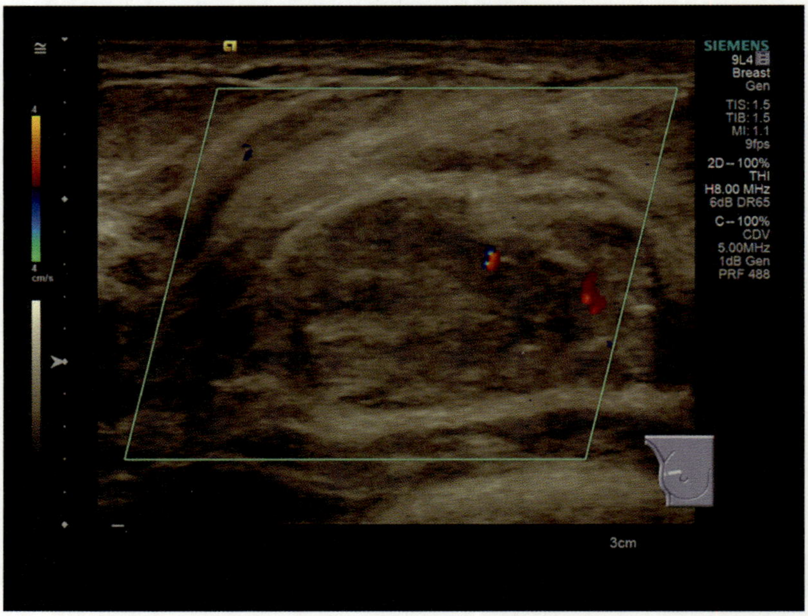

Fig. 5.66 Colour Doppler sonography indicates reduced vascularity

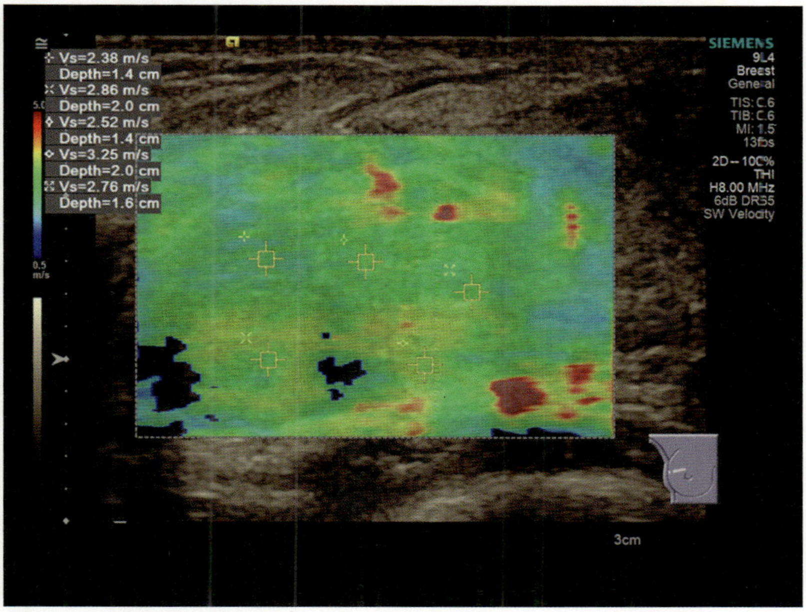

Fig. 5.67 VTIQ velocity colour overlay displayed relative shear wave velocities according to the adjacent colour spectrum, *red areas* corresponding to higher values and *blue areas* corresponding to lower values. Shear wave velocity was measured in the lesion $v = 2.38–3.25$ m/s

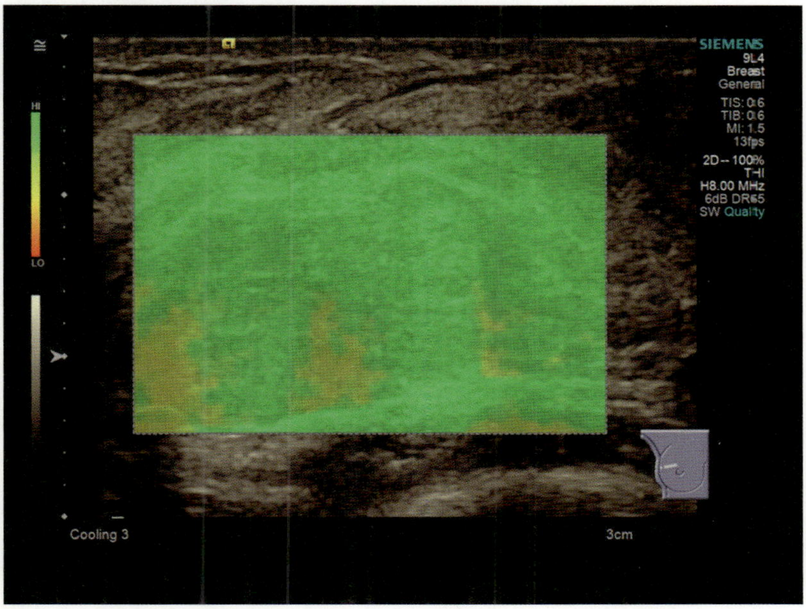

Fig. 5.68 Same lesion as Fig. 5.67. Using the VTIQ quality map, almost all of the breast tissue and the lesion are coloured in *green* as an indicator of the good reliability of the generated shear waves in those areas. The areas of *yellow* indicate that the shear wave estimates may be unreliable in this area (corresponding to the *black areas* of non-detectable shear waves in Figs. 5.67 and 5.69)

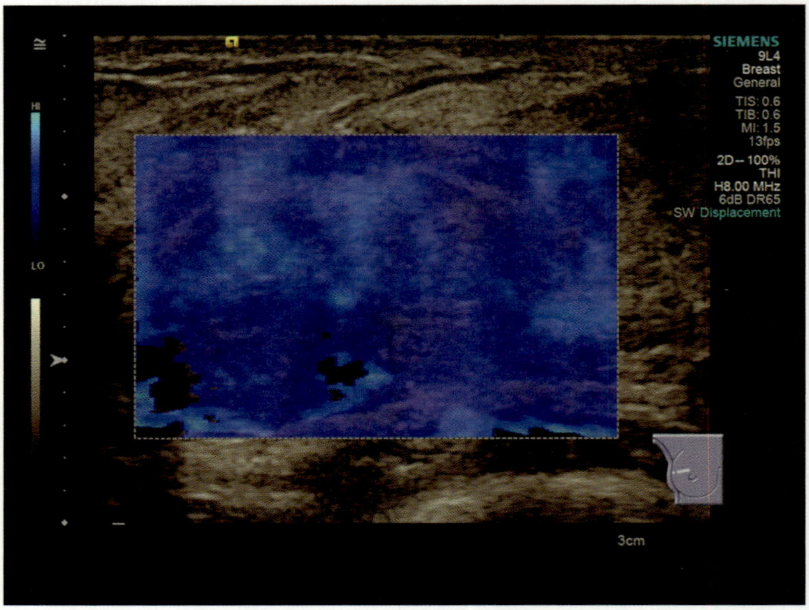

Fig. 5.69 Same lesion as Figs. 5.66 and 5.67. The *mid-blue colour* display of the VTIQ displacement mode indicates a moderate deformation of the lesion and the surrounding tissue

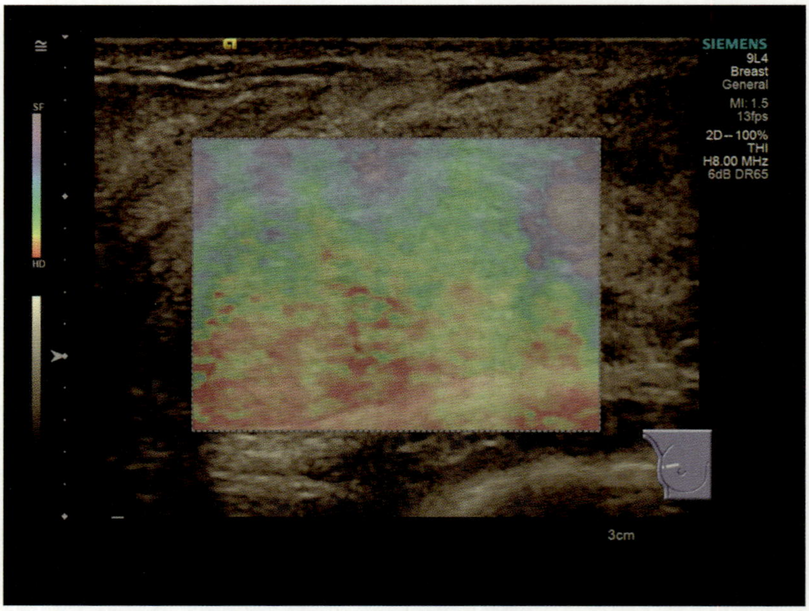

Fig. 5.70 In VTI elastography mode, the lesion is coloured both *green* and *red*, indicating an intermediate and increased stiffness in comparison to the superficial surrounding breast tissue. The lesion is the same size in the VTI-mode as in the comparison B-mode

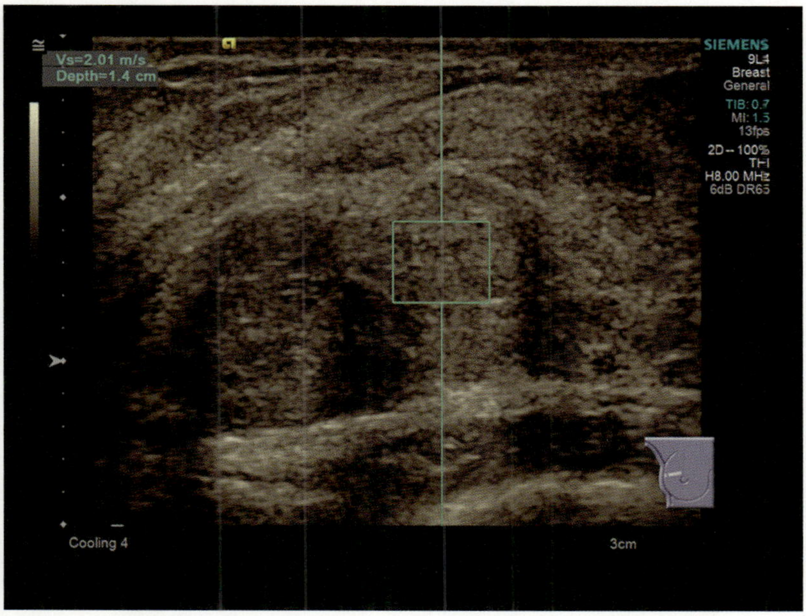

Fig. 5.71 In VTQ mode, the shear wave velocity was measured in the right side of the lesion, the system displaying $v = 2.01$ m/s

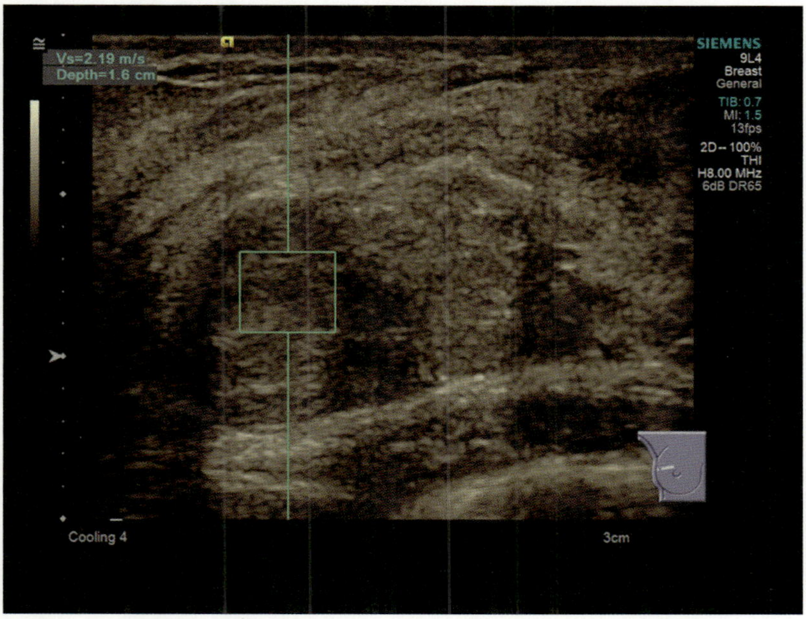

Fig. 5.72 In VTQ mode, the shear wave velocity was measured in the left side of the lesion, the system displaying $v = 2.19$ m/s

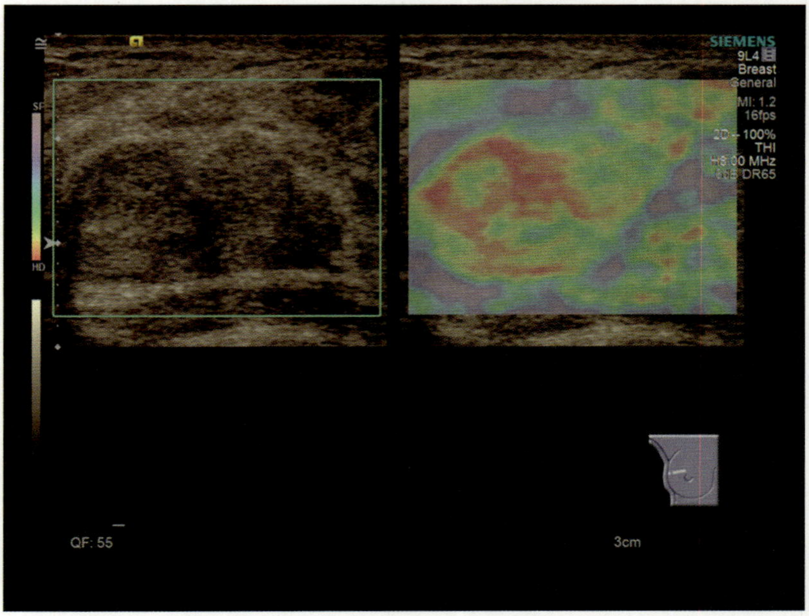

Fig. 5.73 The strain elastogram shows a mixture of *red* and *green colours*, indicating a lesion of intermediate stiffness. The lesion has the same size in the strain elastography mode as in the comparison B-mode

References

1. American College of Radiology. Breast imaging reporting and data system-ultrasound (BI-RADS). Reston: American College of Radiology; 2003.
2. Nothacker M, Duda V, Hahn M, et al. Early detection of breast cancer: benefits and risks of supplemental breast ultrasound in asymptomatic women with mammographically dense breast tissue – a systematic review. BMC Cancer. 2009;9:335.
3. Cho N, Jang M, Lyou CY, et al. Distinguishing benign from malignant masses at breast US: combined US elastography and color Doppler US – influence on radiologist accuracy. Radiology. 2012;262(1):80–90.
4. Lee SW, Choi HY, Baek SY, et al. Role of color and power Doppler imaging in differentiating between malignant and benign solid breast masses. J Clin Ultrasound. 2002;30(8):459–64.
5. Özdemir A, Özdemir H, Maral I, et al. Differential diagnosis of solid breast lesions: contribution of Doppler studies to mammography and gray scale imaging. J Ultrasound Med. 2001;20(10):1091–101.
6. Raza S, Baum JK. Solid breast lesions: evaluation with power Doppler US. Radiology. 1997;203(1):164–8.
7. Balleyguier C, Canale S, Ben Hassen W, et al. Breast elasticity: principles, technique, results: an update and overview of commercially available software. Eur J Radiol. 2013;82(3):427–34.
8. Itoh A, Ueno E, Tohno E, et al. Breast disease: clinical application of US elastography for diagnosis. Radiology. 2006;239(2):341–50.
9. Kim MY, Cho N, Yi A, et al. Sonoelastography in distinguishing benign from malignant complex breast mass and making the decision to biopsy. Korean J Radiol. 2013;14(4):559–67.
10. Rjosk-Dendorfer D, Gürtler VM, Sommer WH, Reiser M, Clevert DA. Value of high resolution compression elastography and color Doppler sonography in characterisation of breast lesions: comparison of different high-frequency transducers. Clin Hemorheol Microcirc. 2014;57(2):129–35.
11. Rjosk-Dendorfer D, Reichelt A, Clevert DA. Elastography as an additional tool in breast sonography. Technical principles and clinical applications. Radiology. 2014;54(3):211–6.
12. Rjosk-Dendorfer D, Reu S, Deak Z, Hetterich H, Kolben T, Reiser M, Clevert DA. High resolution compression elastography and color Doppler sonography in characterization of breast fibroadenoma. Clin Hemorheol Microcirc. 2014;58(1):115–25.
13. Thomas A, Fischer T, Frey H, et al. Real-time elastography – an advanced method of ultrasound: first results in 108 patients with breast lesions. Ultrasound Obstet Gynecol. 2006;28:335–40.
14. Yi A, Cho N, Chang JM, et al. Sonoelastography for 1,786 non-palpable breast masses: diagnostic value in the decision to biopsy. Eur Radiol. 2012;22:1033–40.

6 Musculoskeletal

Teresa Cammarota, Armanda De Marchi, and Simona Pozza

In recent years, elastosonography (ES) has become an important application in the study of the musculotendinous apparatus [1–4]; in fact, this method permits both a qualitative and quantitative evaluation of the elasticity properties of soft tissues and its alteration in traumatic lesions and degenerative pathology. In the field of rheumatology, in particular, it adds a complementary diagnostic element to the standard imaging studies represented by ultrasound (US) and magnetic resonance imaging (MRI). ES can therefore be considered a tool which provides additional and important information regarding certain functional characteristics of musculotendinous tissues.

When pressure is applied to a tissue surface, the force of compression is transmitted to the underlying tissue, producing a change in the mechanical stress of the tissue which will vary based on the tissue consistency: less change in rigid tissue and more in elastic tissue.

The elastosonographic methods, differentiated by modalities of force application to the tissue and modalities of measurement and visualization of the tissue response, are of two types: quantitative (shear wave imaging) and qualitative (strain imaging).

Shear wave ES evaluates the velocity of the transversal wave that is generated by the passage of the excitation wave, expressed as a number relative to the elasticity module.

Strain ES evaluates the deformation of the tissue along the propagation axis of the beam by means of analysis of the RF signal along each line of scanning, with a color-coded representation of the information where, by convention, red corresponds to elastic tissue, green to moderately elastic tissue, and blue to rigid tissue.

Both methods are used for the study of musculotendinous structures, though strain ES allows for a more immediate evaluation and better adapts itself to the structures in the region of interest.

In fact, it's a peculiarity that muscles and tendons have elastographic characteristics which differ not only from region to region but also based on the resting state or tension and/or contraction. Therefore, an elastographic study of musculotendinous structures is always a dynamic-type study.

Furthermore, it's important to be familiar with the elastographic aspect of normal muscular and tendon structures, both in the static and dynamic phases, in order to recognize the variations caused by different pathological conditions.

T. Cammarota (✉)
Department of Radiology, Azienda Ospedaliero-Universitaria Città della Salute e della Scienza di, Torino, Italy
e-mail: tcammarota48@hotmail.com

A. De Marchi • S. Pozza
Ospedaliero-Universitaria Città della Salute e della Scienza, CTO Hospital,
Via Zuretti 29, 10126 Torino, Italy

D.-A. Clevert et al. (eds.), *Atlas of Elastosonography*, DOI 10.1007/978-3-319-44201-3_6

Strain ES is performed with dedicated equipment using a linear transducer with which manual compressions and relaxations are applied in a vertical direction with a homogeneous and regular force which is quantified by an indicator on the screen.

Visualization of the tissue under examination occurs in real time using a double window on the monitor, which allows evaluation of the aspect both in basal condition and during elastosonography, with scans done parallel and perpendicular to the long axis of the tissue. The results are shown in a chromatic scale where blue represents maximum rigidity and red the maximum elasticity, passing through intermediate values going from light blue to green to yellow. This chromatic box, partially transparent, is superimposed on the basal ultrasound image, with the possibility to sample in regions of interest (ROI) the values of the ratio between pathological tissue and healthy tissue, adding therefore a quantitative evaluation to the exam.

Some authors use a "spacer" between the transducer and the skin to make the pressure exerted on the tissues more homogeneous and regular and also to reduce artifacts, especially in anatomical regions with irregular surfaces [3, 5].

Each tissue has, in normal conditions, mechanical properties and therefore a characteristic elasticity coefficient, which can undergo change in pathological conditions.

ES can be indicated when the ultrasound study is inconclusive, highlighting different elasticity between healthy and pathological tissue, especially when confronted with pain symptom when the ultrasound exam does not find any significant morphostructural tissue changes.

Healthy tissue and pathological tissue can, in fact, have the same echogenicity; it is this lack of tissue contrast that doesn't permit the recognition of alterations in certain pathological conditions [2, 6].

In the musculoskeletal field, the preliminary results in the study of tendinopathy and muscle disorders are encouraging [4].

Tendinopathies are frequent in athletes, but they are not easily treatable due to their multifactor etiology [7].

The alterations that tendons undergo, regarding both clinical findings, constituting thickening, and anatomopathological findings, are well known [8].

Continuous microtrauma, overload, and vascular alterations cause tissue damage which has repercussions on the elasticity of the fibrillary architecture [3].

ES has been used in some work groups to compare the behavior of healthy tendons with pathological ones in the rotator cuff, the elbow [9], and the Achilles tendon [8, 10, 11], with satisfying results in comparison to basal ultrasound.

Some authors have demonstrated that ES has detected alterations of the elastosonographic characteristics of tendons both in symptomatic and asymptomatic patients [10, 11]; this finding implies that this new method, combined with basal ultrasound, can increase the diagnostic accuracy given that it can detect alterations very early.

Healthy tendons and, in particular, the Achilles tendon, which is easy to study because of its size and location, have an elastosonographic pattern which is prevalently blue, expression of a certain rigidity and scarce deformability [10, 11].

In geriatric patients, however, the Achilles tendon has a prevalently green color with traces of blue, while when it's the site of tendinopathy, the color is predominately red due to the reduced consistency [4].

The supraspinatus tendon, according to the same author, has an analogous chromatic pattern in the same clinical conditions.

This finding has been confirmed by other authors who compared elastosonographic findings with those of magnetic resonance imaging which is the gold standard, highlighting a good sensitivity of ES [12].

ES has been used in the diagnosis of fatty degeneration of the rotator cuff with similar results also in this case with magnetic resonance imaging [12], demonstrating a reduced elasticity of the tendons in atrophy and providing useful information regarding prognosis and treatment.

Interesting applications have emerged in the study of *synovial pathology* where some authors were able to differentiate inflammatory synovial pathology from infectious synovial pathology, demonstrating a reduction in elasticity with predominant red color in areas with inflammatory disease in comparison to infectious complications, which present as areas of greater consistency with a green color [4].

An area of great interest is that of ES in the study of *muscle tissue* in different pathological conditions such as inflammation, trauma, and the rarer congenital dystrophies [13, 14].

Normal muscle tissue presents a chromatic pattern which is prevalently green. In this field, the exam of choice is magnetic resonance imaging, but the agreement that some authors have found between this method and ES could, in the future, lead to the substitution of MRI with ES due to MRI's limitations of claustrophobia, pacemakers, surgical clips, and higher cost [15].

In our study we used ES in muscle lesions following direct and indirect trauma, at a time interval of up to 6 months after the trauma, to allow for healing time in widespread lesions.

The criteria of inclusion are the traumatic event and pain.

We compared findings of basal ultrasound exam, ES, clinical examination, and MRI, which is considered the gold standard [16].

ES was able to demonstrate persistence of alterations even when basal ultrasound became normalized and allowed to correctly interpret the dynamics of tissue repair and eventual complications in the follow-up leading to the potential of the method to indicate the correct therapy or to modify the therapy enacted in order not to risk further damage.

The use of ES has also been extended to the study of space-occupying lesions of the skeletal muscle system in an attempt to characterize the tissue: confronted with the poor attendibility of the quantitative elastographic findings, the qualitative findings, expressed as a color-coded map, are useful in differentiating benign forms from malignant forms [17].

Preliminary studies of angiomatous lesions and of neurofibromatosis have shown an ES color pattern which is predominantly red for angiomas due to their soft consistency and predominantly green for neurofibromas due to their more rigid tissue structure [4].

ES has also been evaluated for *carpal tunnel syndrome*: the elasticity of the median nerve is decreased in pathological conditions with a blue chromatic pattern [18, 19].

ES has some limits; mainly it is operator dependent and therefore difficult to reproduce the findings; regarding this, it is indispensable to pay attention to the indicative scales on the screen during pressure application to the tissues during the examination.

At present, the imaging of the mechanical properties and of the elasticity of the tissues has arrived at a high technical level of development to make it clinically useful [20–22].

However, large-scale studies are necessary to define the indications and the role of the method in the diagnostic work-up of musculotendinous pathology, either as an exam associated with the basal ultrasound exam or as a substitute for less comfortable and more costly exams.

6.1 Image Gallery

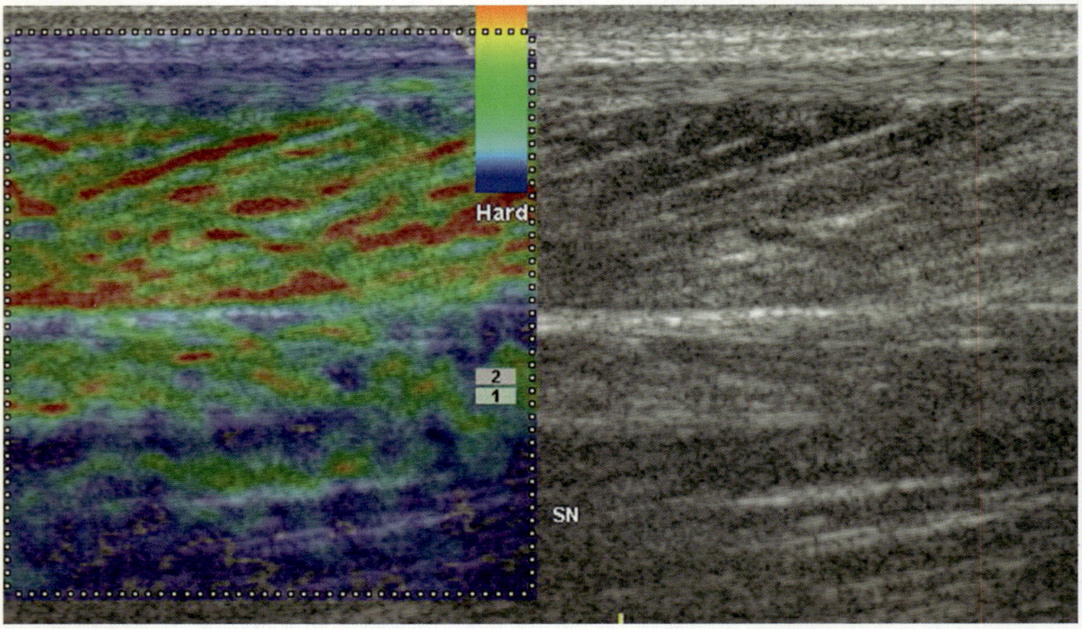

Fig. 6.1 Grayscale longitudinal image (*right*) of normal relaxed rectus femoris muscle. At sonoelastography (*left*), the muscle appears as a mosaic of intermediate stiffness *green color* with scattered softer (*red*) areas near muscle boundaries (ribbed elastic appearance)

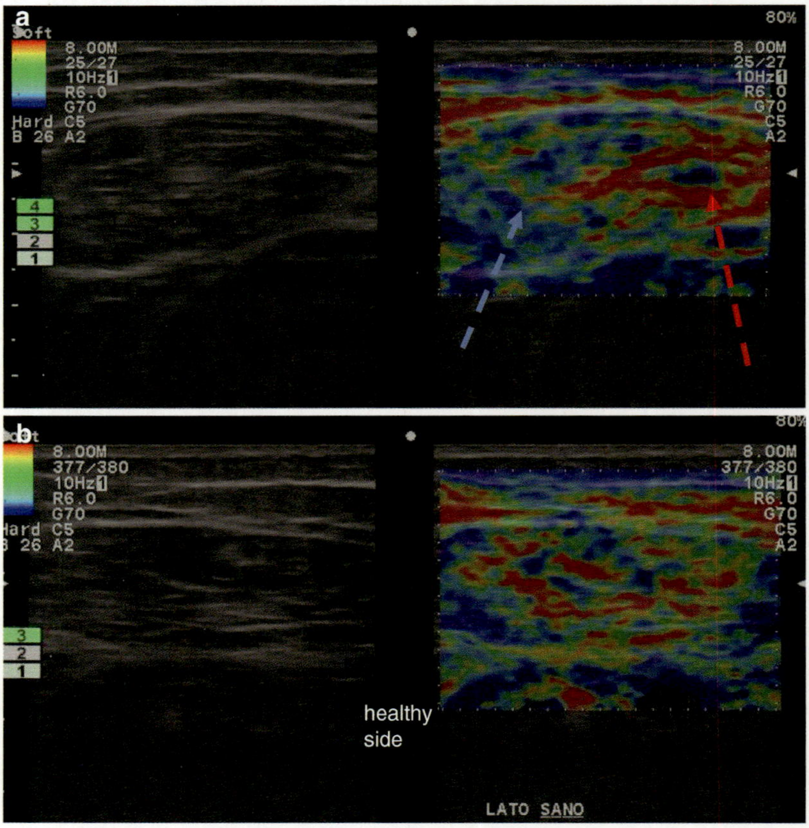

Fig. 6.2 (**a**) Grayscale axial scan (*left*) of the anterior rectus femoris shows a normal muscle aspect; at sonoelastography (*right*), an altered intrinsic elasticity with intramuscular stiffer areas (*blue dot arrow*) mixed with softer ones (*red dot arrow*) in patient with anterior thigh pain without trauma. (**b**) Contralateral healthy side. (**c**) MRI: SET2W and fat suppression images show a normal muscle aspect

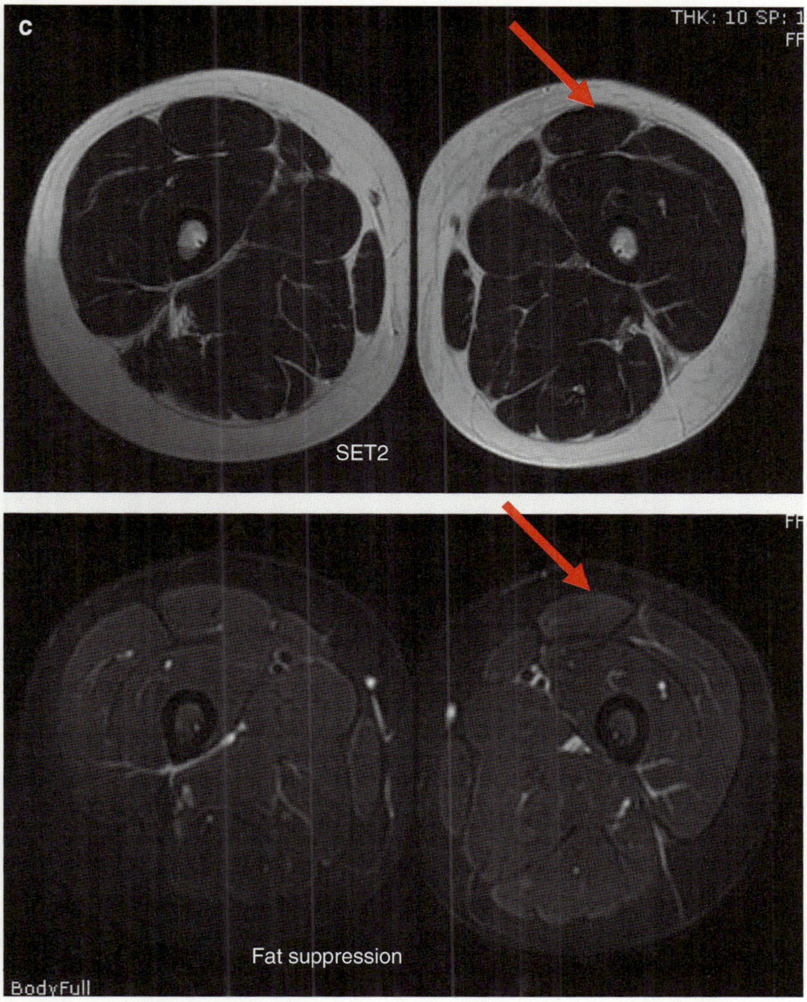

Fig. 6.2 (continued)

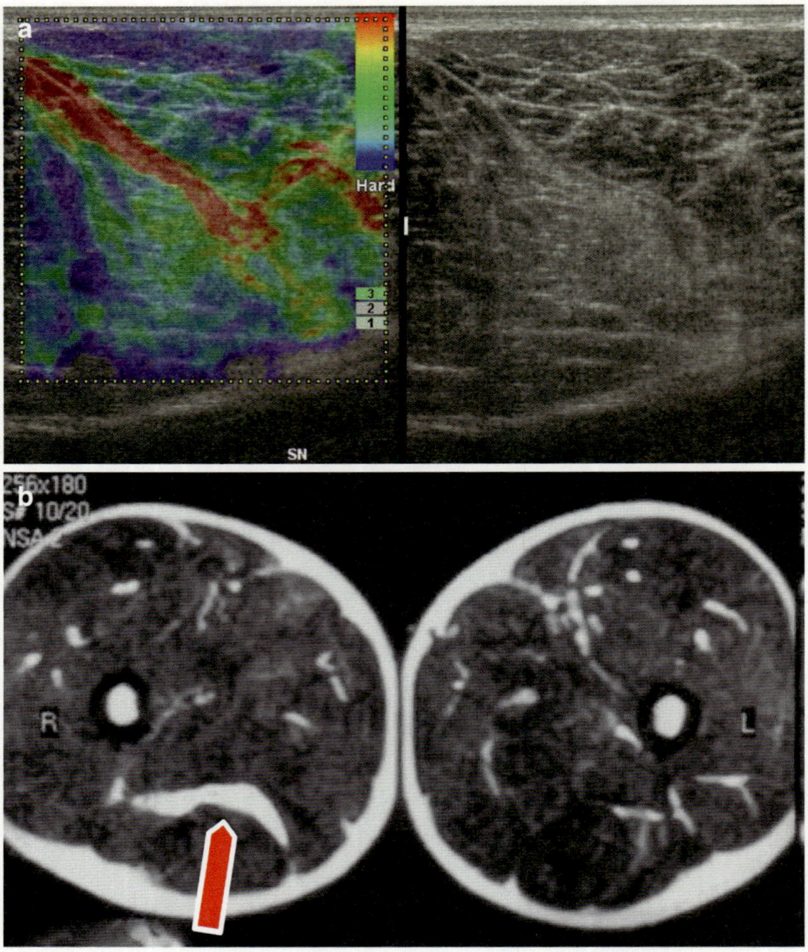

Fig. 6.3 (**a**) Grayscale axial images of the semimenbranosus and semitendinosus muscle (*right*): a post-traumatic intramuscular hyperechoic longitudinal area and corresponding elastogram (*left*) in neutral thigh position. The presence of a *red oblique area* between the muscles means a partial fluid collection. (**b**) Axial T2 W: fluid collection well defined with MRI

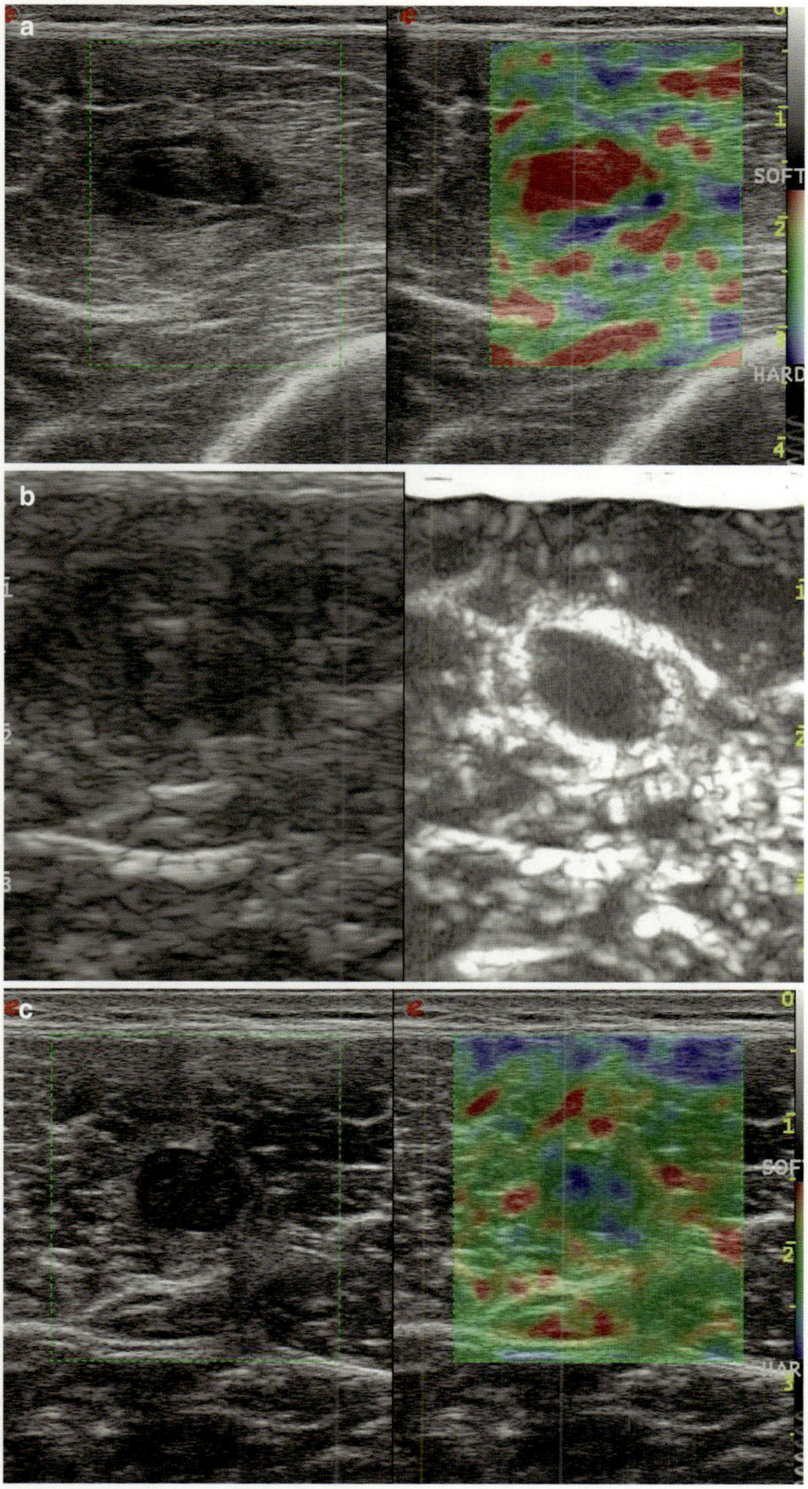

Fig. 6.4 (**a**) Grayscale axial image (*left*): partial quadriceps muscular rupture 10 days after trauma which appears like a hypo-anechoic round area; on the *right* a very soft aspect of the hemorrhage. (**b**) The contrast-enhanced US (CEUS) evidences the muscular lesion like a *black round area* without vascularization. (**c**) The lesion after 1 month appears stiff (*green/blue*) at sonoelastography due to the reparative process

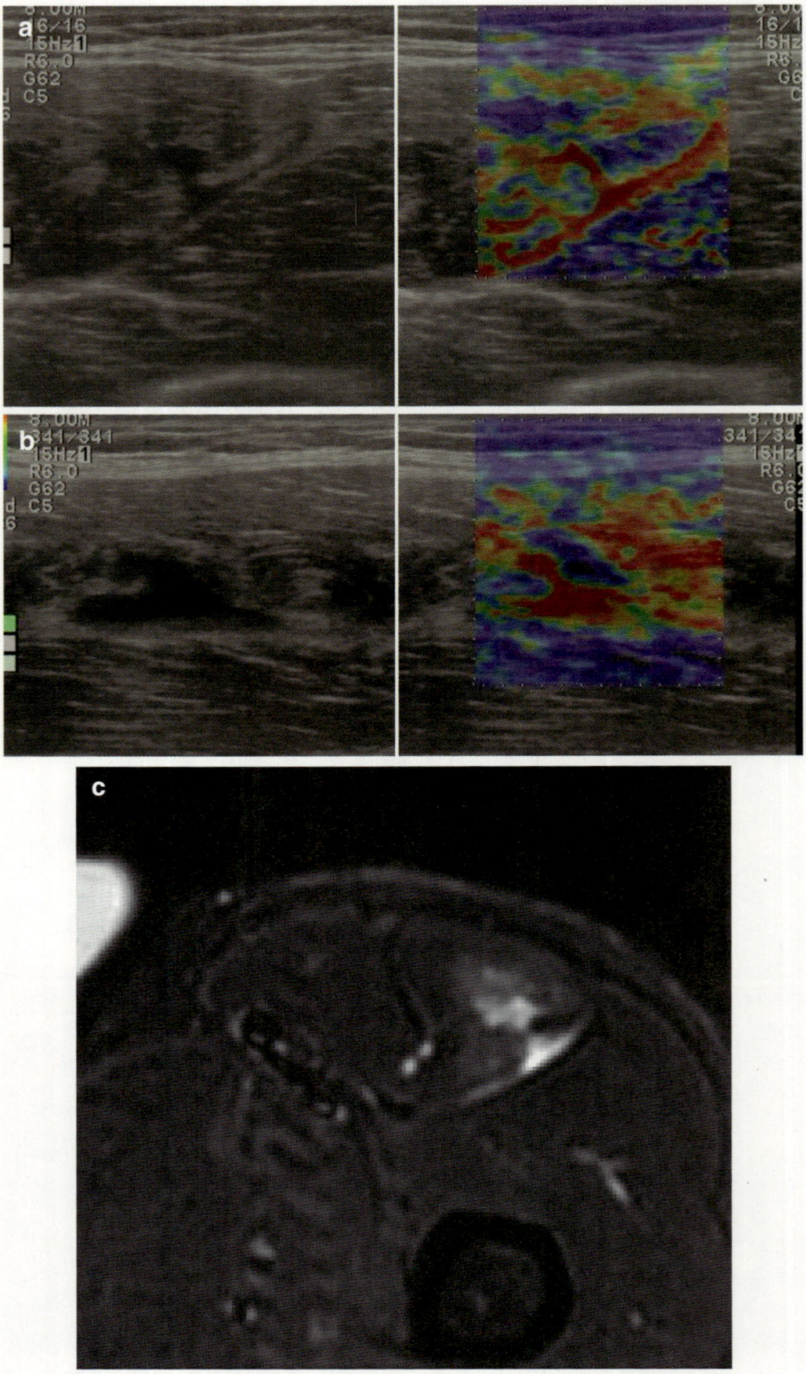

Fig. 6.5 (**a**, **b**) Grayscale axial (**a**) and longitudinal (**b**) images of the rectus femoris muscle (*left*): a post-traumatic intramuscular anechoic interfascial area. The corresponding elastogram (*right*) in neutral thigh position shows a *red soft area* that means a fluid interfascial collection and a soft aspect of the muscle because of the hemorrhage. (**c**) The MRI axial T2 fat suppression image confirms the interfascial liquid and the intramuscular hemorrhage

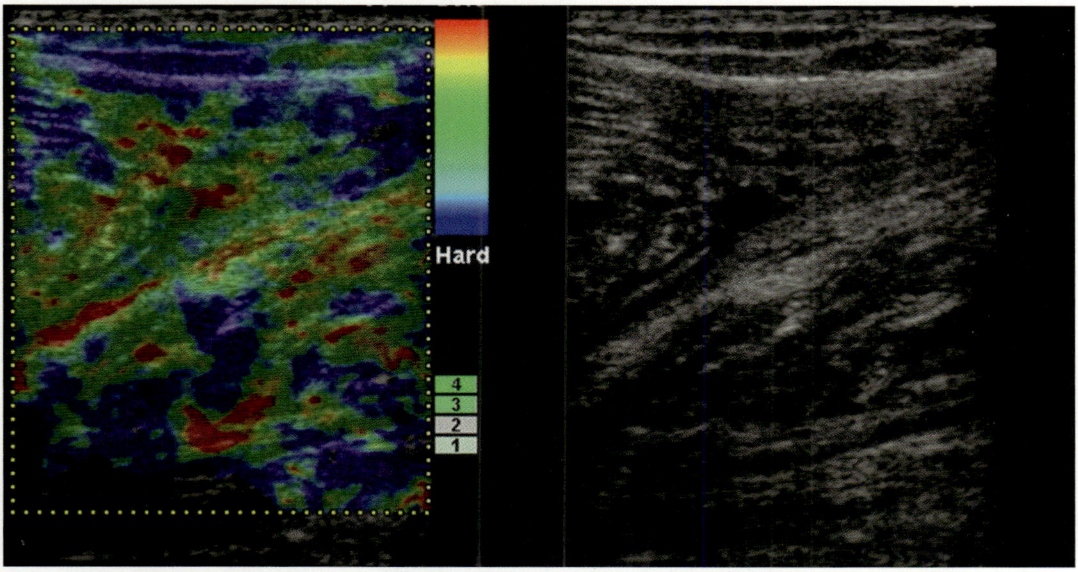

Fig. 6.6 Grayscale longitudinal images (*right*) of rectus femoris detachment; at elastosonography (*left*) very soft aspect of the hemorrhage in the distal portion of the muscle

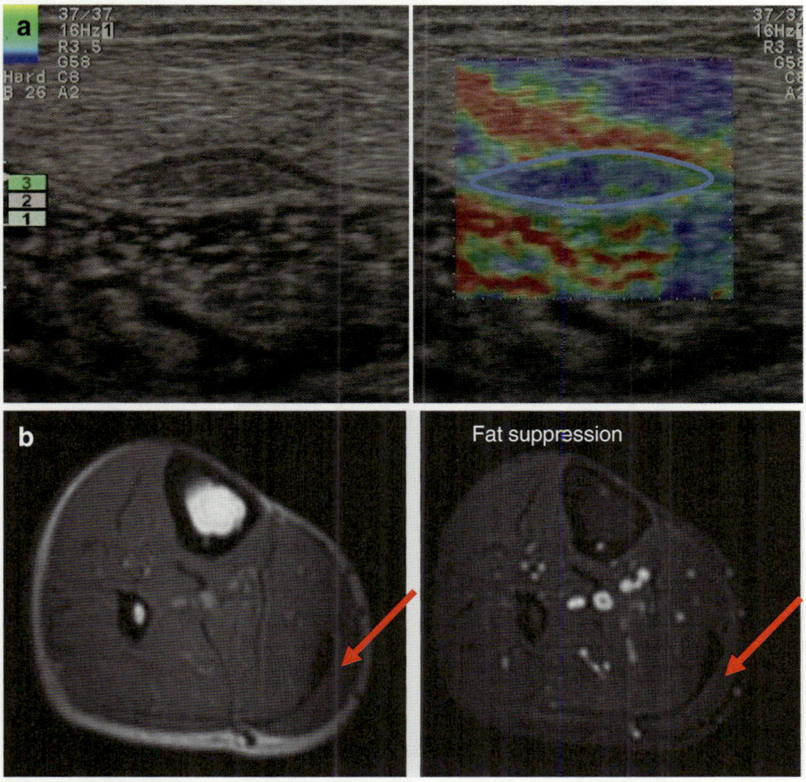

Fig. 6.7 (**a**) Axial grayscale (*left*) and sonoelastography (*right*) scan in patient with a fibrosis scar of the medial gastrocnemius muscle: the lesion appears hypoechoic at grayscale and *blue* like a stiff area at sonoelastography. (**b**) The MRI shows a fibrous tissue in SET2W and fat suppression images

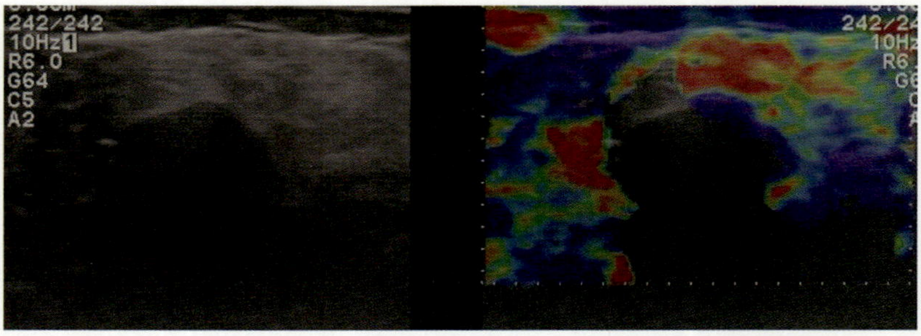

Fig. 6.8 Grayscale axial view (*left*) of the tibial anterior muscle which appears hyperechoic in patient with traumatic denervation; at elastosonography (*right*) shows a complex aspect characterized by an increase elasticity in the superficial region and low elasticity in the deep portion due to the fibrosis

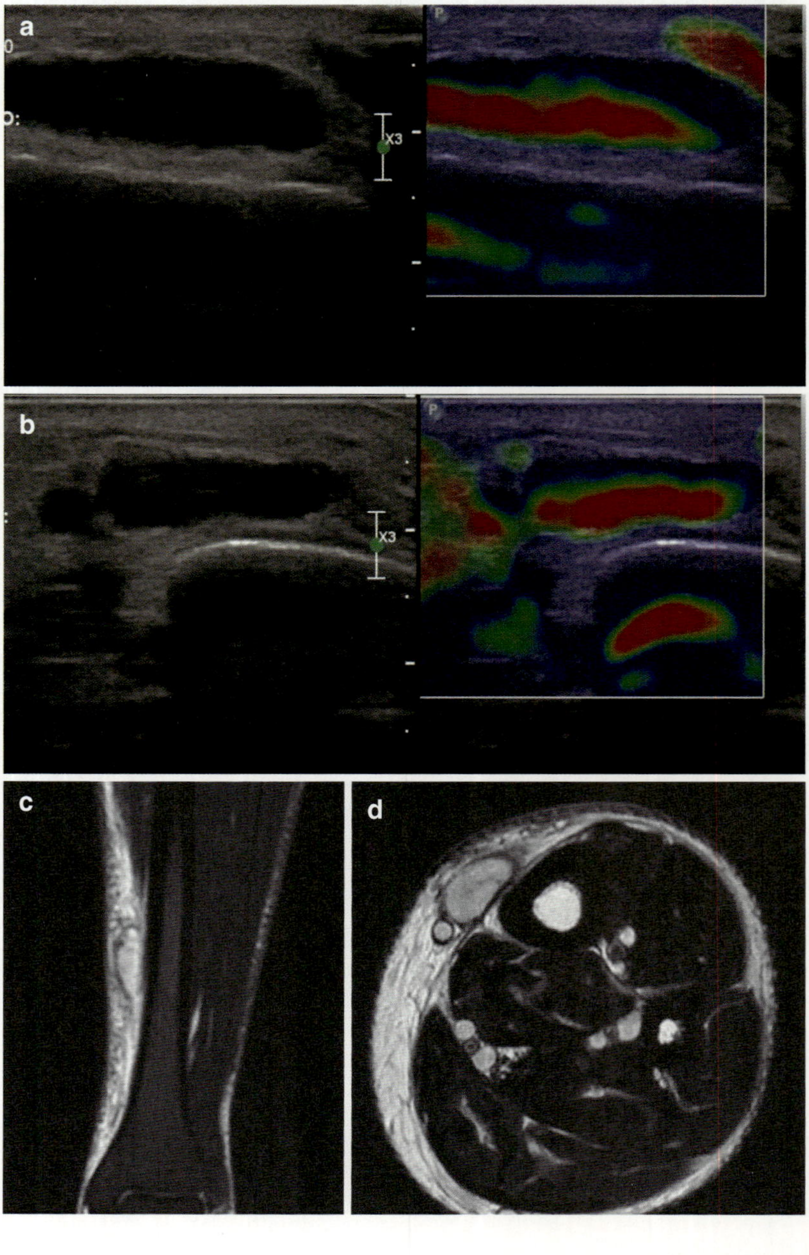

Fig. 6.9 (**a**, **b**) Grayscale longitudinal (**a**) and axial (**b**) scan of fluid homogeneous post-traumatic subcutaneous collection in the anterior tibial region on the *left*. At the sonoelastography (*right*), the collection appears as a typical *red-green-blue* aspect, like a cyst lesion. (**c**, **d**) Coronal T2FS (**c**) and axial T2 (**d**) view confirm the fluid collection

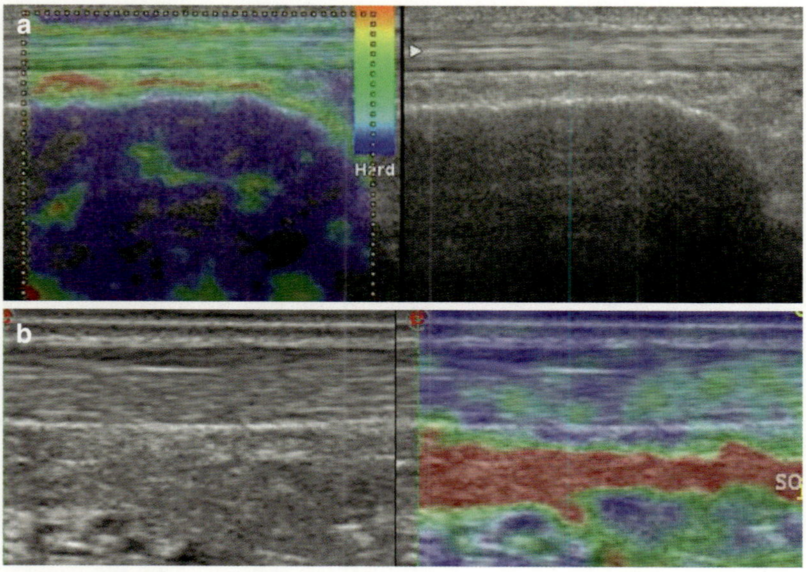

Fig. 6.10 (**a**) Grayscale longitudinal image of the normal anterior tibial tendon (*right*) and corresponding elastogram (*left*) in neutral ankle position. The tendons appear homogeneously stiff (*green-yellow*), with no distinct soft (*red*) areas. (**b**) Grayscale longitudinal image of the normal Achilles tendon (*left*) and corresponding elastogram (*right*) in extension position. The tendons appear homogeneously stiff (*green/blue*)

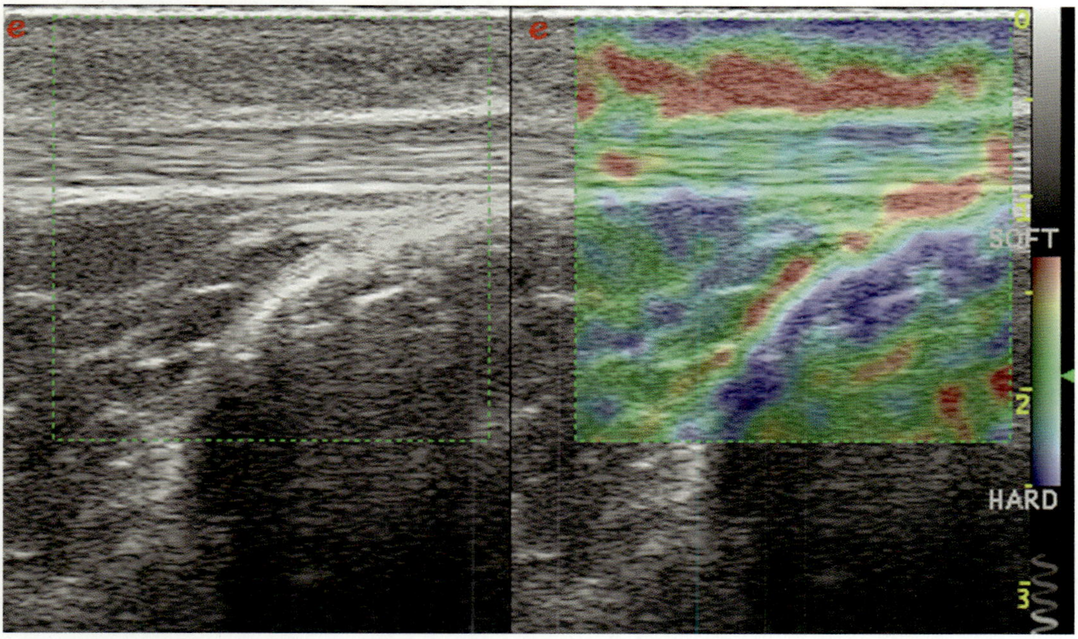

Fig. 6.11 Post-traumatic hypoechoic subcutaneous area in grayscale (*left*), at sonoelastography soft aspect of the hemorrhage near the Achilles tendon that is normal (*right*)

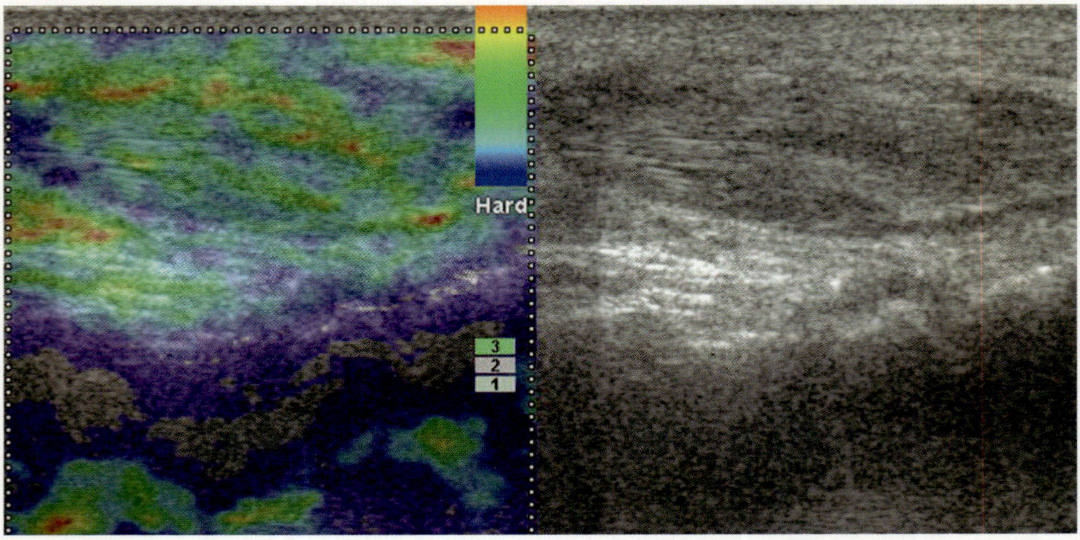

Fig. 6.12 Grayscale longitudinal image of the anterior tibial tendon (*right*) and corresponding elastogram (*left*) in neutral ankle position. Clinically the patient had difficulty to dorsiflexion. The tendon appears enlarged and inhomogeneous in grayscale with a prevalence of *blue* and *green area* with few *red spots* in superficial portion during the elastography: soft area alternating with areas of low elasticity which demonstrate small partial-thickness tear in tendinosis

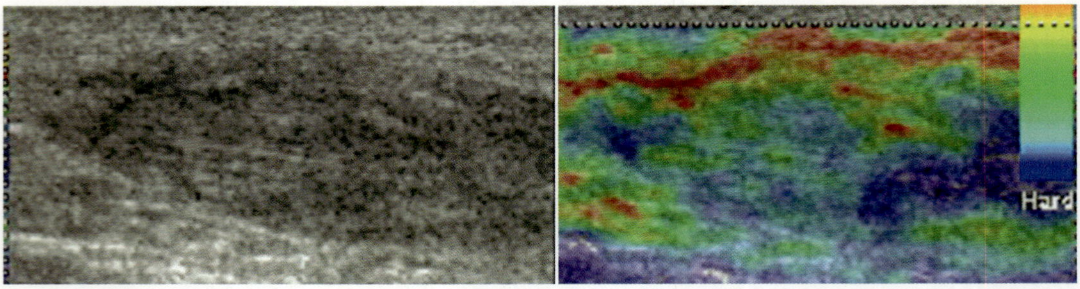

Fig. 6.13 Bis Longitudinal RTSE scan in patient with Achilles tendinopathy shows distinct superficial intratendinous softening and *blue areas* of reduced elasticity in the medial and deep portion (*right*)

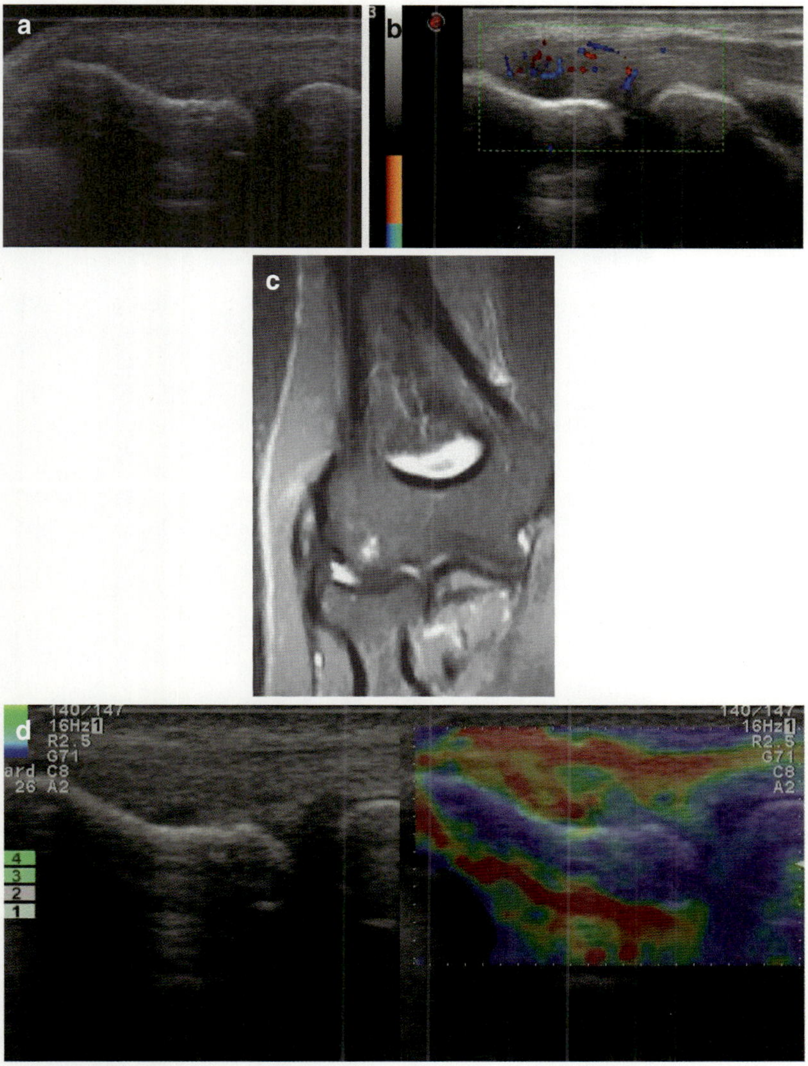

Fig. 6.14 (**a**) Grayscale sonographic image reveals swelling and intratendinous hypoechogenicity in common extensor tendon origin in patient with lateral elbow pain. (**b**) Color Doppler sonographic image shows increased vascularity epicondylitis. (**c**) MRI T2 FS coronal view shows a hyperintensity area in the proximal insertion of the common extensor tendon. (**d**) The elastosonography reveals a diffuse *red-coded area* in symptomatic common extensor tendon

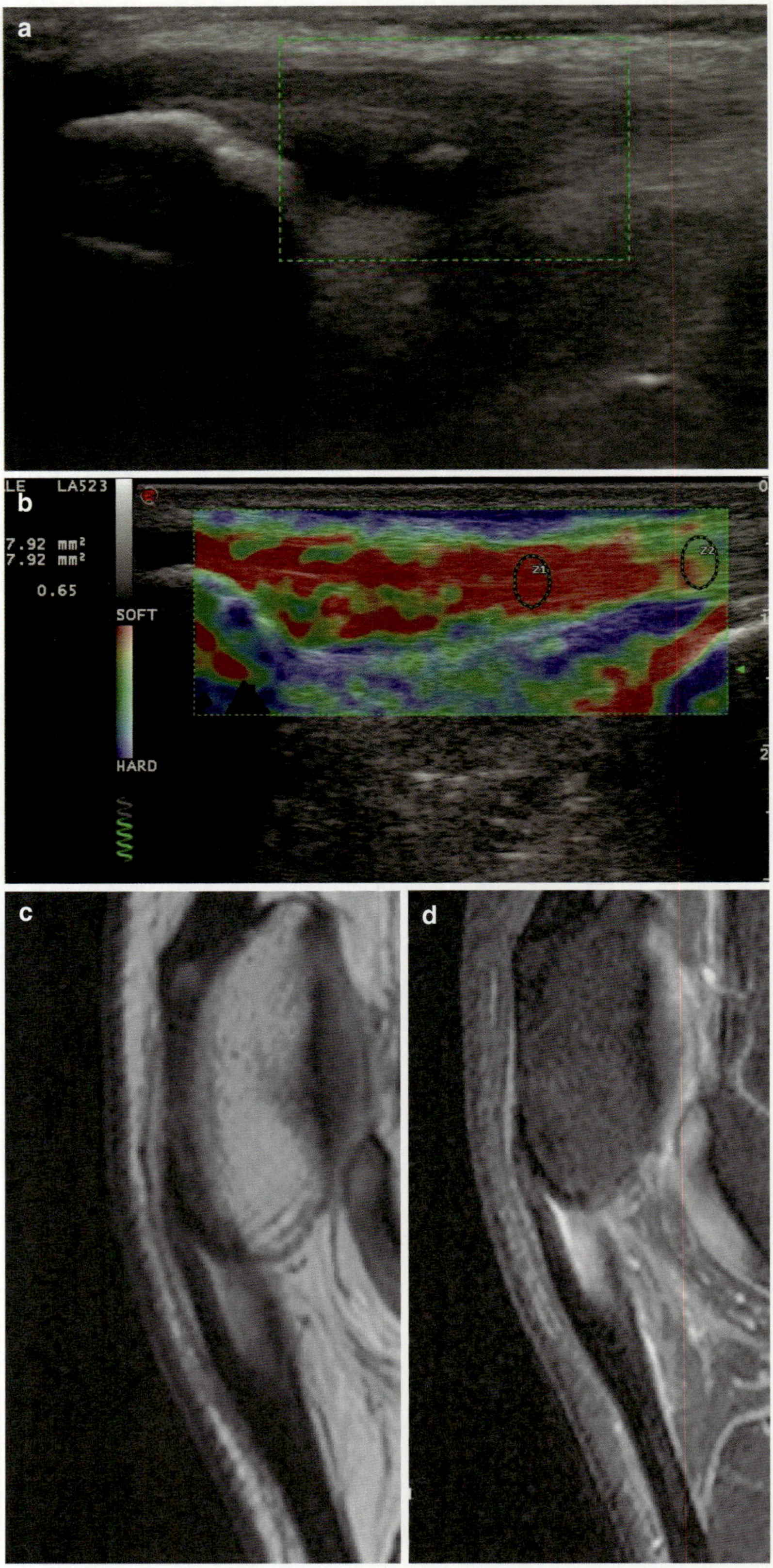

Fig. 6.15 (**a**) Longitudinal grayscale of the patellar tendon: the tendon appears thick and inhomogeneous with a small calcification in the proximal deep portion. (**b**) At the elastosonography the tendon reveals homogeneous increased elasticity in case of tendinopathy. (**c**) MRI sagittal view T2FSW (**d**) and T1SEW (**c**) images shows high signal intensity at the enthesis due to tendinosis

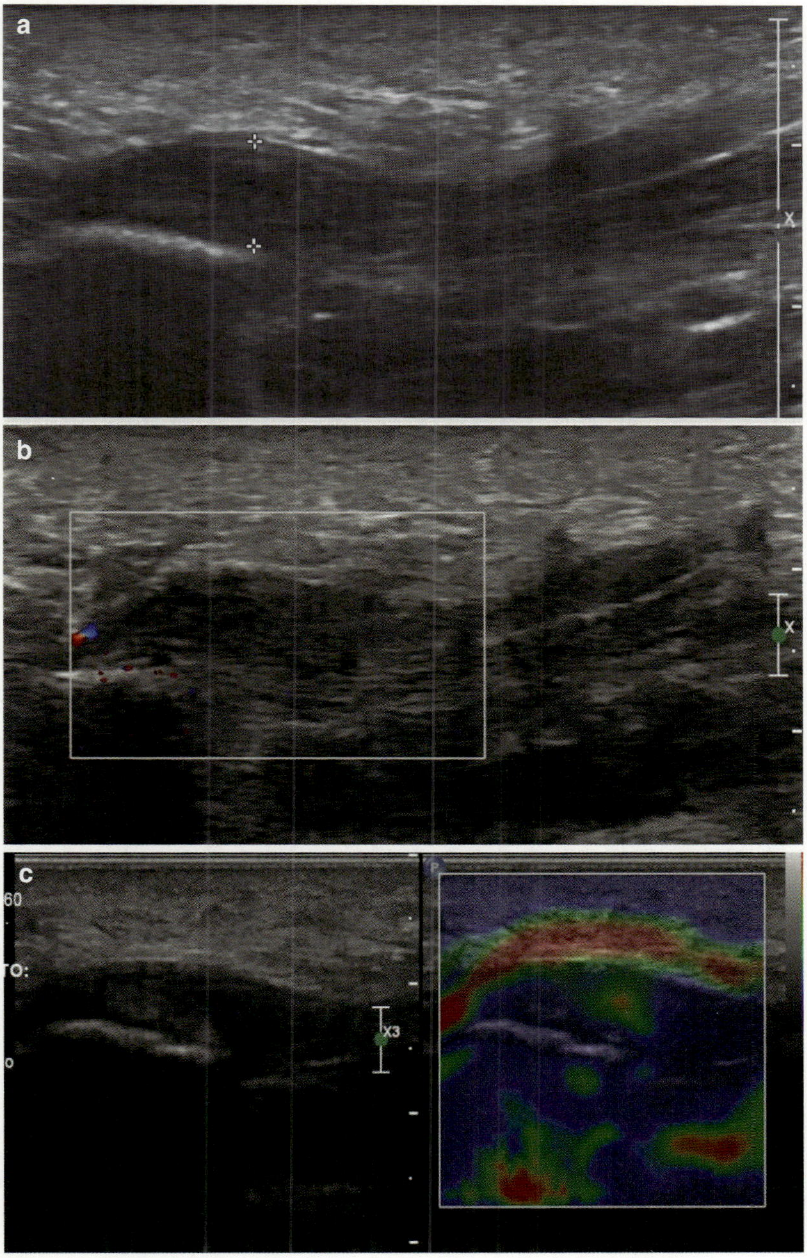

Fig. 6.16 (**a**, **b**) Grayscale longitudinal plane of the plantar fascial (**a**) and color (**b**). The plantar fascia appears ticked and hypoechoic in the insertion, in the intermediate and distal portion without spots of color. (**c**) Sonoelastography evidences focused softening of the plantar fascia in the intermediate region

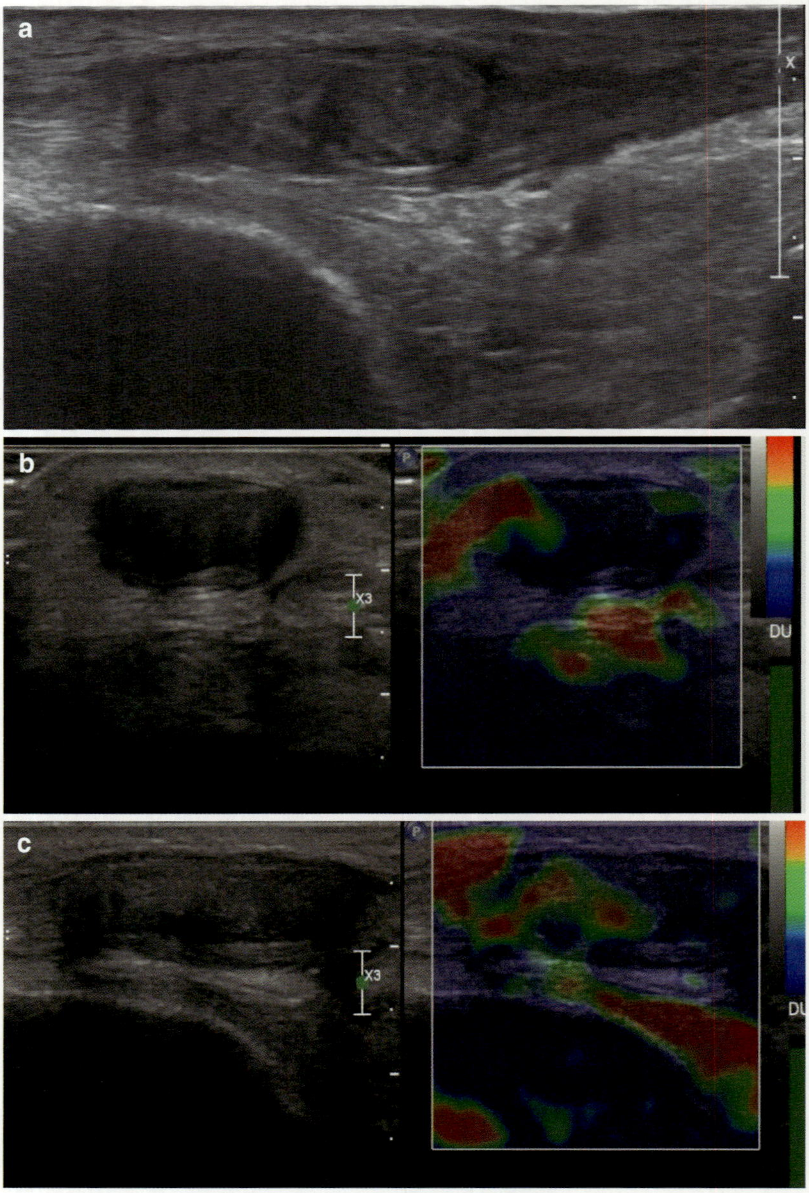

Fig. 6.17 (**a**) Grayscale longitudinal scan of anterior tibial tendon old rupture. (**b**, **c**) At elastosonography reduced elasticity of the tendon with area of fibrosis (*blue areas*) (**b** – transversal view, **c** – longitudinal view)

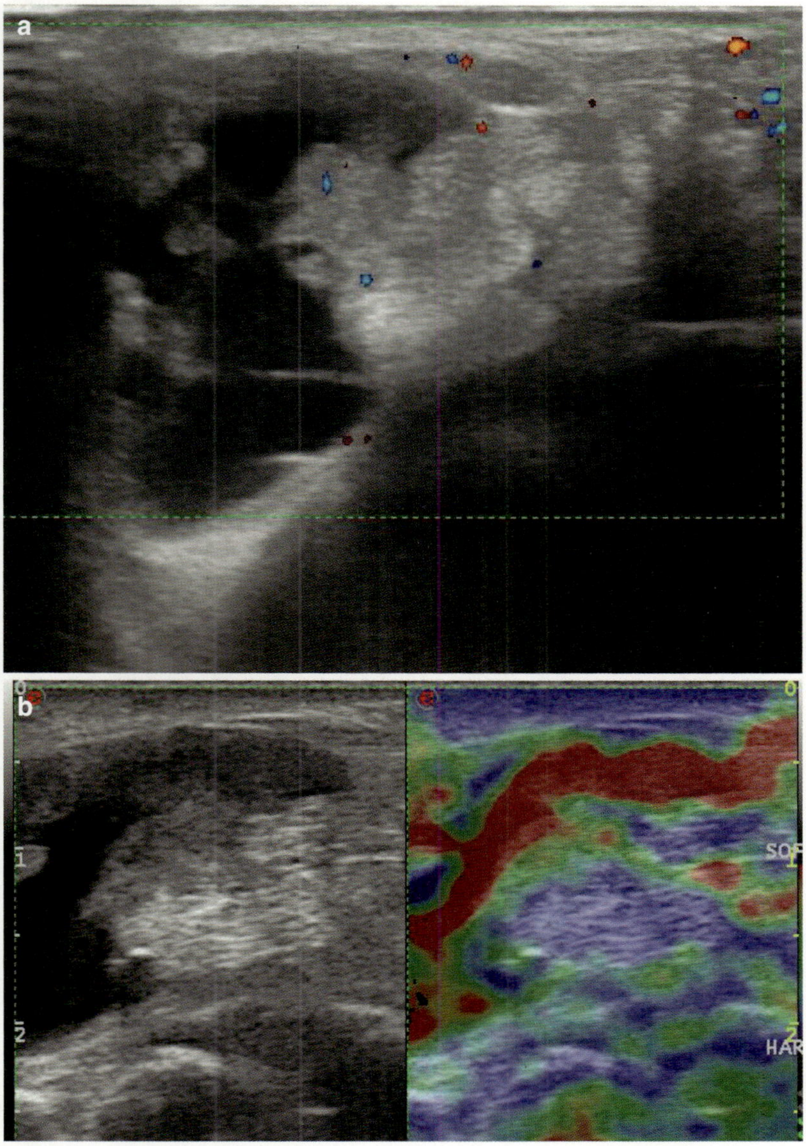

Fig. 6.18 Flexor tendons tenosynovitis in pregnant woman who had onset of pain. (**a**) US power axial scan of flexor tendons in the volar region of the hand: an evident anechoic area is visualized around the tendons which are increased in size as a result of edematous changes. (**b**) The anechoic area appears at elastosonography very soft and means an abundant effusion in the sheath

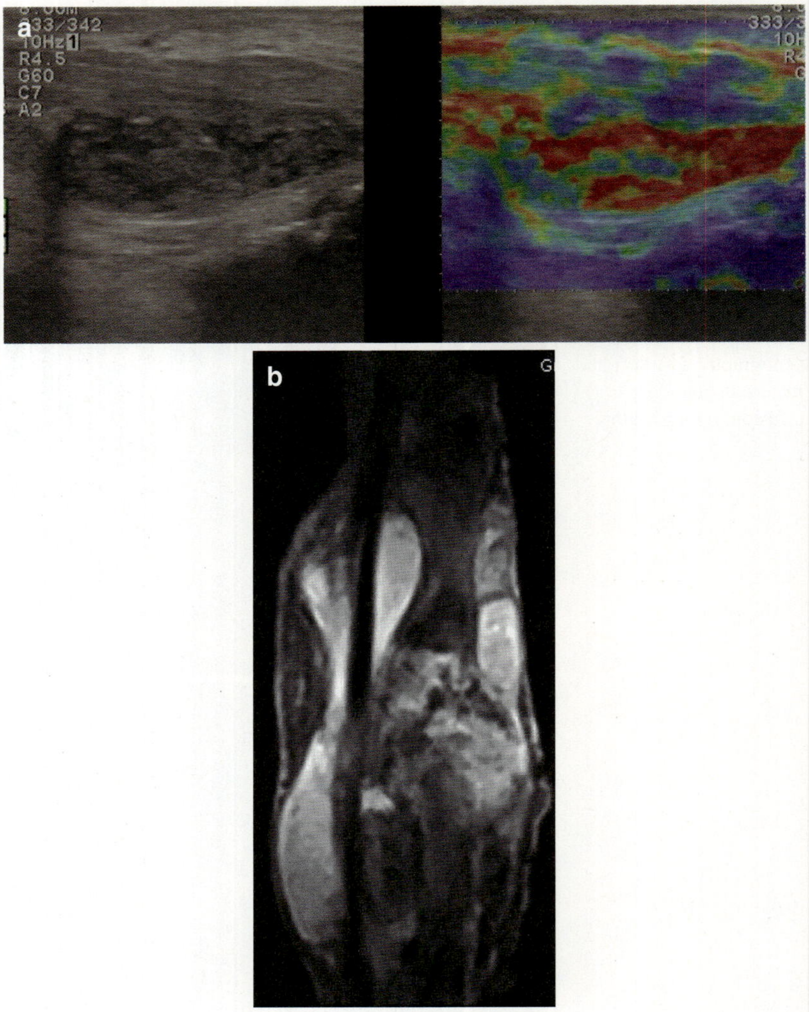

Fig. 6.19 Pigmented villonodular synovitis (PVNS). (**a**) Real-time sonoelastography view (*right*) and B mode image (*left*) in 74-year-old patient with pain and swelling of the wrist. Hypertrophied synovium shows predominant firm to soft nature, which is represented by predominant *red color* with patchy *blue areas*: (**b**) MRI gradient echo in sagittal plane confirms a heterogeneous synovial mass with decreased signal intensity caused by hemosiderin

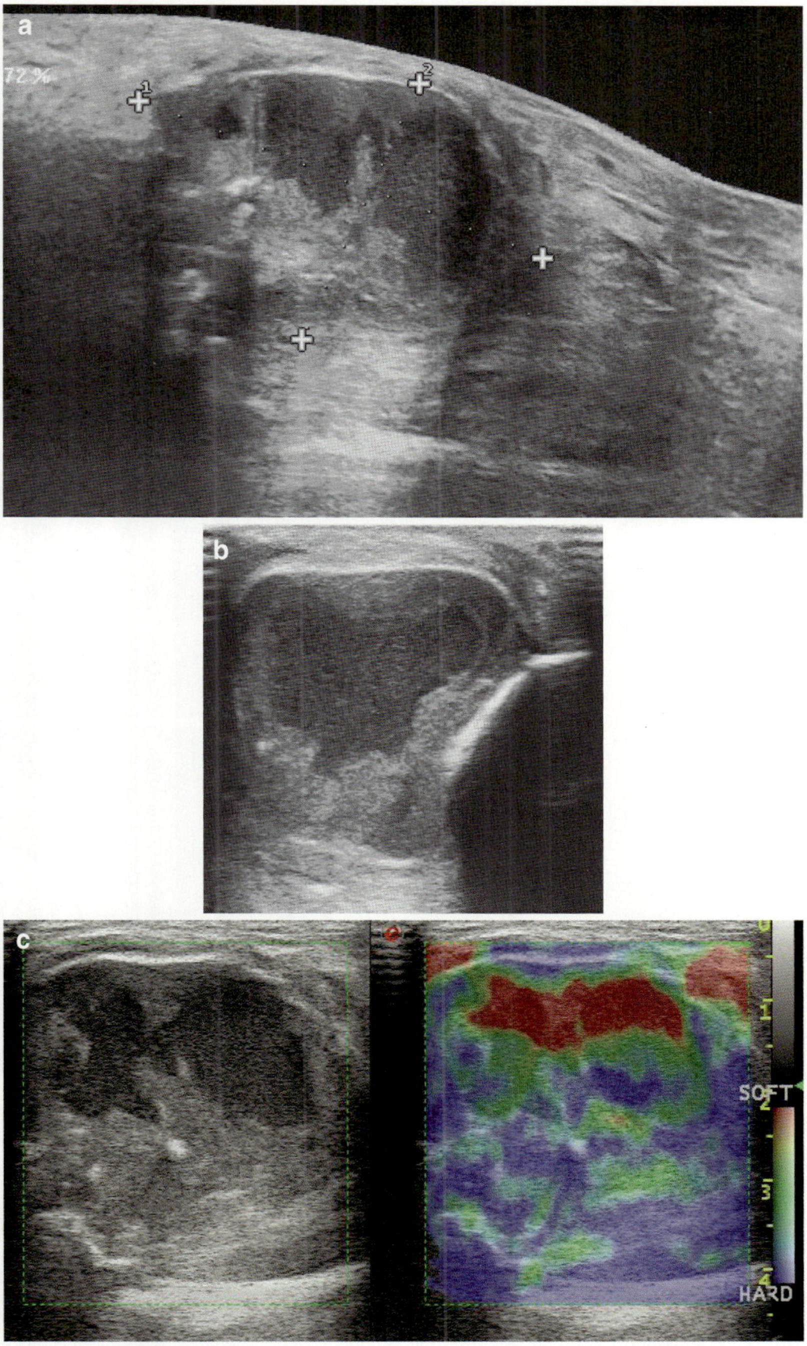

Fig. 6.20 (**a**, **b**) US grayscale longitudinal view (**a**) and axial view (**b**) show a heterogeneous mass next to the bone in tibial fracture in patient with pain and fever. (**c**) At elastosonography the lesion appears almost completely *blue* with a small superficial component of high elasticity: the lesion was a localized collection of pus and inflammation

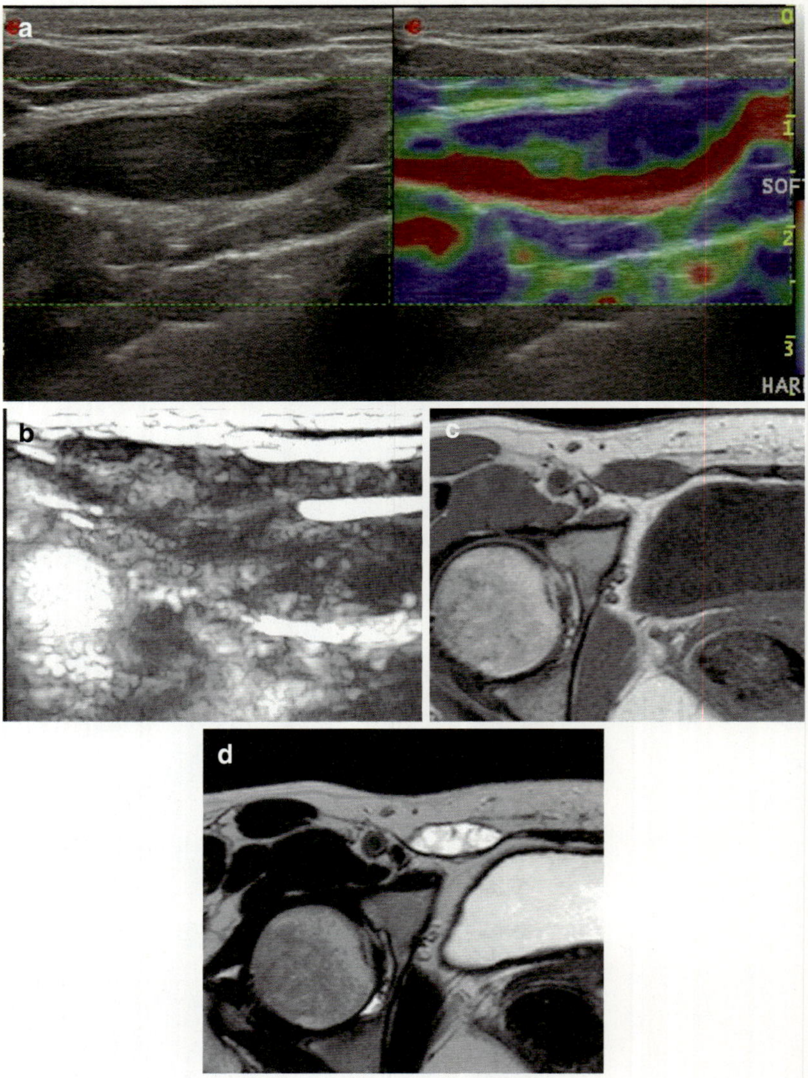

Fig. 6.21 Lymphangioma. (**a**) Grayscale (*left*) shows in the groin an oval-shaped mass anechoic between the fascia and subcutaneous tissue; at elastosonography (*right*), the lesion shows a cyst-like aspect (*red-green-blue*). (**b**) The mass evidences at CEUS a rich vascularization because of a lot of white spots inside. (**c**, **d**) MRI on axial SET1 and SET2W shows a liquid multiloculated mass with thin septa inside

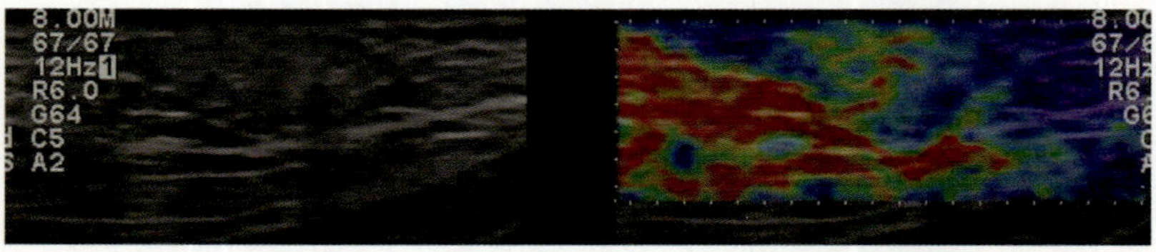

Fig. 6.22 Lipoma. Grayscale longitudinal images (*left*) of a little elliptical subcutaneous mass parallel to the skin surface hyperechoic relative to the adjacent muscle which contains linear echogenic lines; at elastography (*right*), the subcutaneous lipomas have a typical horizontally oriented striated pattern which is characterized as tricolor (*blue, green-yellow*, and *red*)

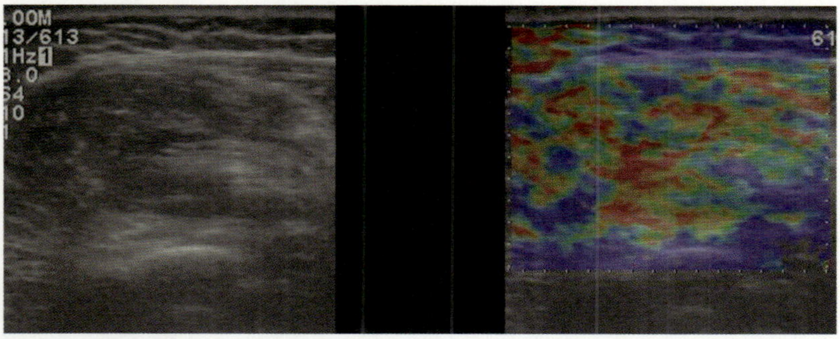

Fig. 6.23 Real-time sonoelastography view (*right*) and B mode image (*left*) of intramuscular lipoma; it has a mottled appearance without the horizontal striations. This probably is related to differences of elasticity in masses that are embedded in a muscle compartment surrounded by fascia

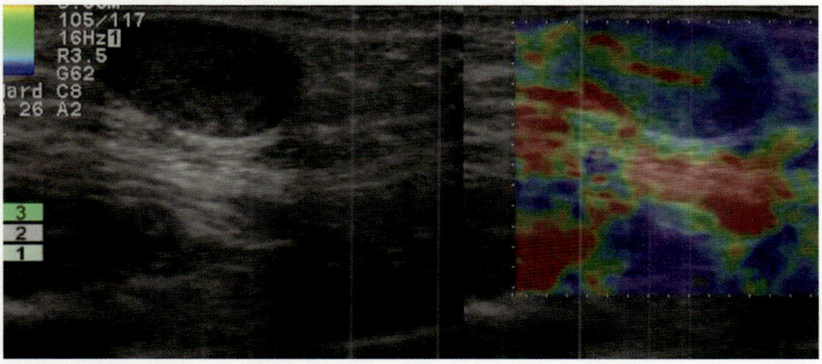

Fig. 6.24 Sebaceous cyst. B mode image (*left*) in longitudinal scan of subcutaneous mass, hypo-anechoic, inhomogeneous, with sharp margins and enhanced through-transmission deep to the lesion with refractive shadowing at the edges; real-time sonoelastography (*right*) shows a stiff and moderate elasticity in the mass due to different content of the cyst

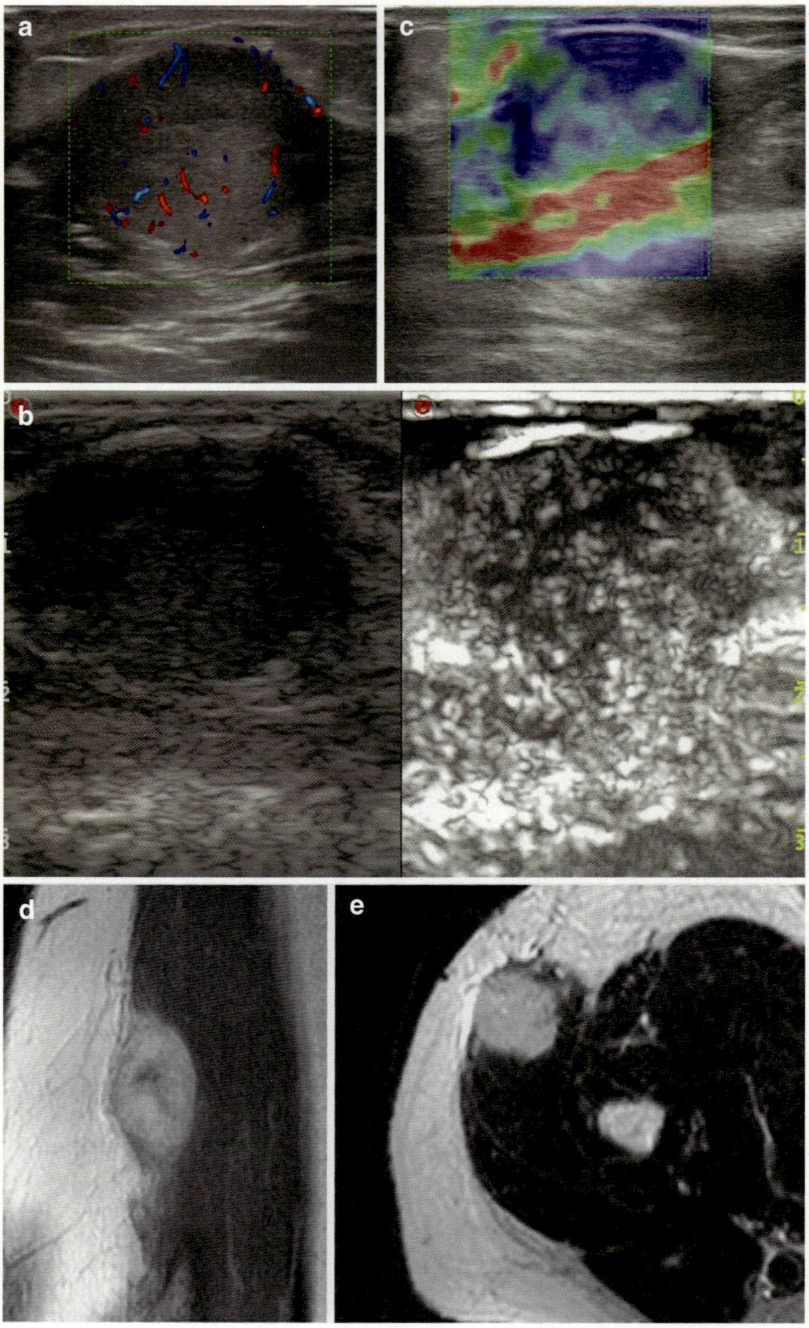

Fig. 6.25 Myxoid liposarcoma. (**a**) Longitudinal grayscale and *color* show an oval hypoechoic mass with regular edges and with some vessels inside. (**b**) The lesion studied with CEUS evidences a rich heterogeneous vascularization. (**c**) At sonoelastography in longitudinal view, the mass appears almost completely stiff. (**d**) MRI SET1 coronal plane image after intravenous gadolinium administration shows nonenhancing tissue central with peripheral enhancement. (**e**) MRI SET2 axial plane image shows a hyperintense lesion

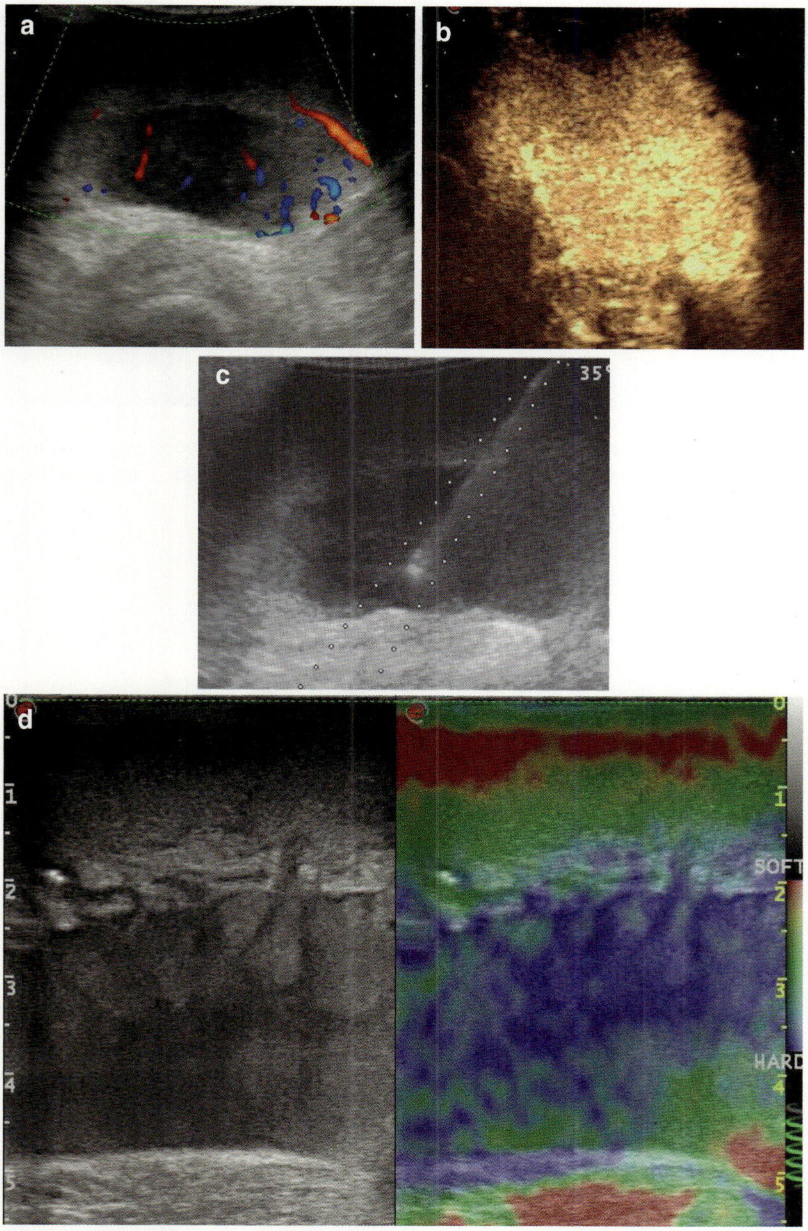

Fig. 6.26 Dermatofibrosarcoma protuberans (DFSP). (**a**) US color shows a huge hypoechoic hynomogeneous mass in the anterior region of the thigh with some vessels inside. (**b**) At CEUS the mass appears completely full of vessels. (**c**) The biopsy procedure. (**d**) At elastosoncgraphy the lesion appears very stiff in the half deep portion and with high elasticity in the other superficial part

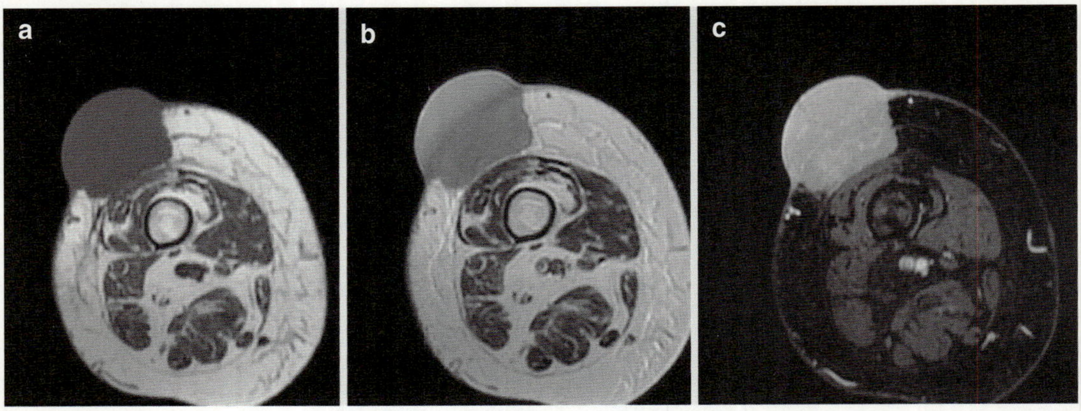

Fig. 6.27 MRI image evidences a large exophytic DFSP involving the skin, and subcutaneous fat of the medial anterior thigh shows in axial T1W image (**a**) low signal intensity, a homogeneous enhancement after gadolinium injection (**b**), and high signal intensity on the long TR images (**c**)

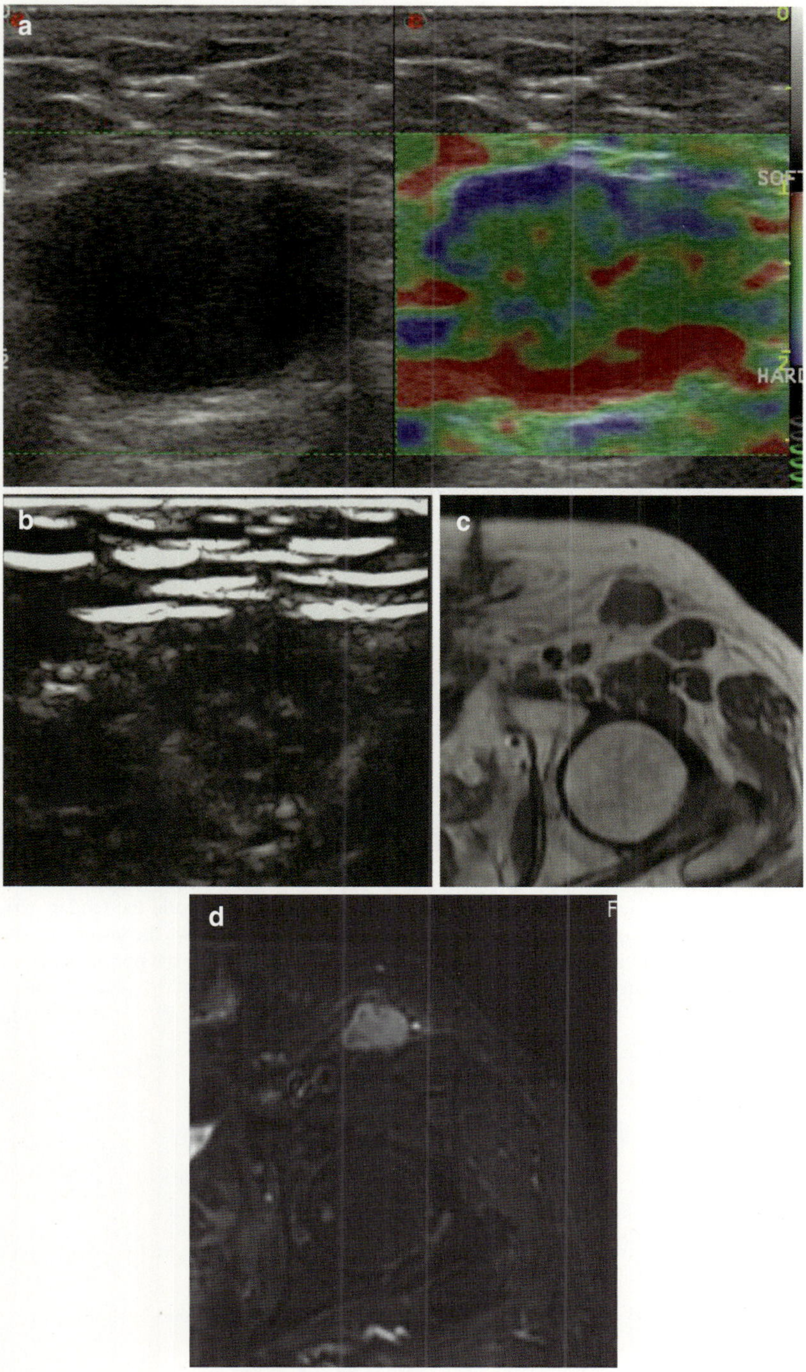

Fig. 6.28 Neuroendocrine carcinoma. (**a**) Grayscale axial view (*left*) shows a homogeneous hypoechoic mass in the groin which at elastosonography (*right*) evidences a moderate elasticity with a layer of low elasticity in superficial region. (**b**) At CEUS the lesion shows some vessel in the middle region. (**c**) MRI T1W axial image shows low enhancement of the lesion. (**d**) MRI T2 fat suppression shows inhomogeneous high signal

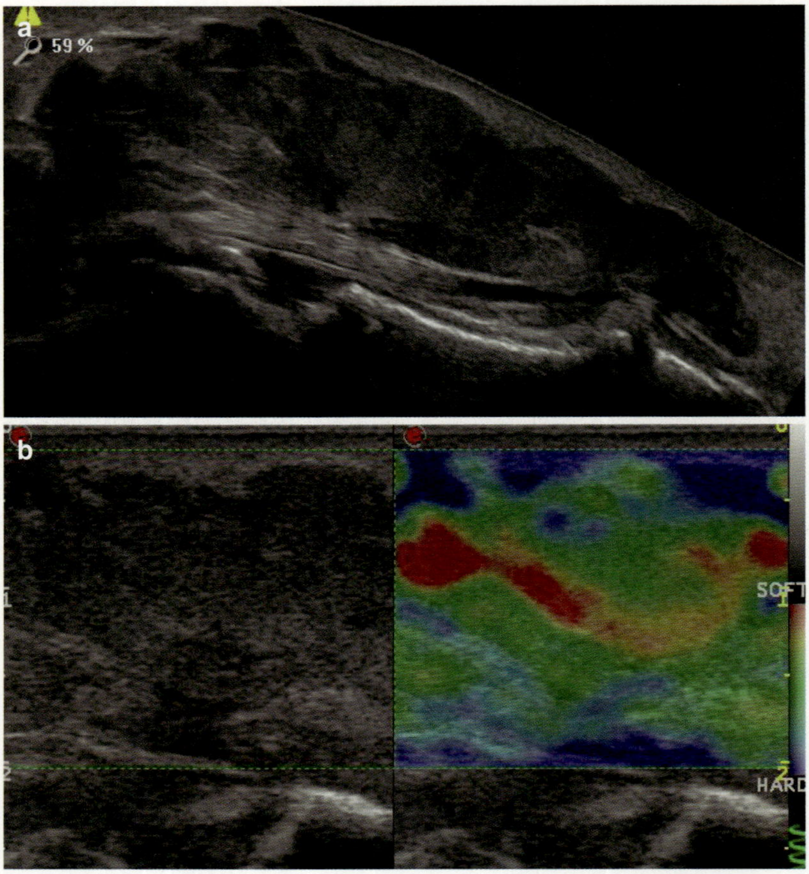

Fig. 6.29 Giant cell tumor of tendon sheath (nodular tenosynovitis) in woman with a slightly painful finger mass. (**a**) Grayscale longitudinal view of the volar region of the hand shows a lobulated and well-defined, hypoechoic lesion around the tendon. (**b**) Corresponding elastosonography shows the lesion as a mosaic of various levels of stiffness over the normal tendon which is *blue*

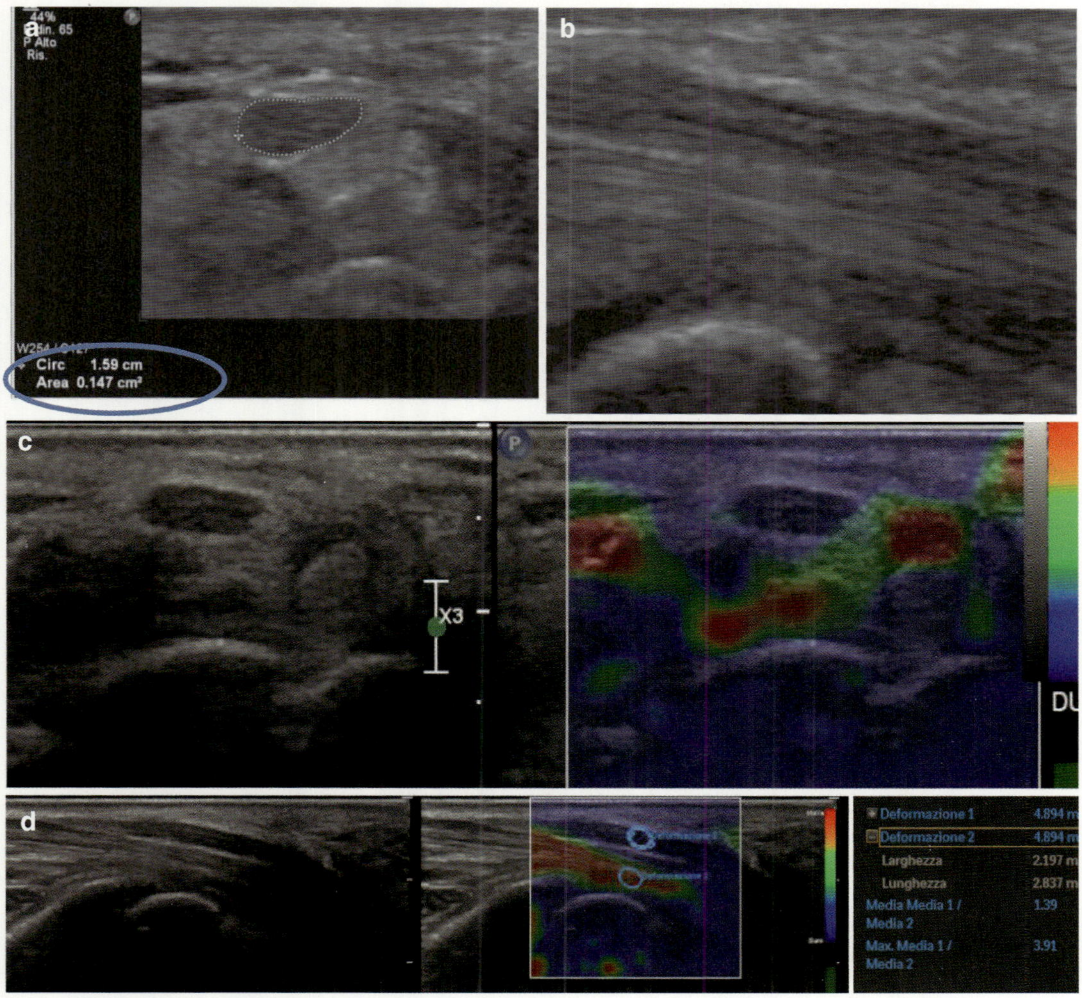

Fig. 6.30 (**a**, **b**) Grayscale axial (**a**) and longitudinal (**b**) view of the median nerve at the proximal carpal tunnel level evidences the enlargement of the median nerve cross-sectional area. The nerve is hypoechoic with a reduced fascicular pattern. (**c**, **d**) At sonoelastography in axial (**c**) and longitudinal view (**d**), the nerve appears significantly stiffer in patients with carpal tunnel syndrome

References

1. Varghese T, et al. Tradeoffs in elastographic imaging. Ultrason Imaging. 2001;23(4):216–48.
2. Frey H. Realtime elastography: a new ultrasound procedure for the reconstruction of tissue elasticity. Radiologe. 2003;43(10):850–5.
3. Klauser AS, et al. Sonoelastography: musculoskeletal applications. Radiology. 2014;272(3):622–33.
4. Lalitha P, et al. Musculoskeletal applications of elastography: a pictorial essay of our initial experience. Korean J Radiol. 2011;12(3):365–75.
5. Kjaer S, et al. EULAR 2011. London.
6. Niitsu M, et al. Muscle hardness measurement by using ultrasound elastography: a feasibility study. Acta Radiol. 2011;52:99–105.
7. Kannus P, Natri A. Etiology and pathophysiology of tendon ruptures in sports. Scand J Med Sci Sports. 1997;7(2):107–12.
8. Sconfienza LM, et al. Sonoelastography in the evaluation of painful Achilles tendon in amateur athletes. Clin Exp Rheumatol. 2010;28(3):373–8.
9. De Zordo T, et al. Real-time sonoelastography of lateral epicondylitis: comparison of findings between patients and healthy volunteers. AJR Am J Roentgenol. 2009;193(1):180–5.
10. De Zordo T, et al. Real-time sonoelastography: findings in patients with symptomatic achilles tendons and comparison to healthy volunteers. Ultraschall Med. 2010;31(4):394–400.
11. De Zordo T, et al. Real-time sonoelastography findings in healthy Achilles tendons. AJR Am J Roentgenol. 2009;193(2):W134–8.
12. Schreiber V, et al. Real-time sonoelastography in rotator cuff imaging and comparison to magnetic resonance imaging as gold standard. RSNA. 2009.
13. Drakonaki EE, Allen GM. Magnetic resonance imaging, ultrasound and real-time ultrasound elastography of the thigh muscles in congenital muscle dystrophy. Skeletal Radiol. 2010;39(4):391–6.
14. Monetti G, Minafra P. Elastosonography in the evaluation of the post-traumatic muscular pathology Musculoskeletal Ultrasound Society Meeting, Paris. 2007.
15. Adler RS, Garofalo G. Ultrasound in the evaluation of the inflammatory myopathies. Curr Rheumatol Rep. 2009;11(4):302–8.
16. De Marchi A, et al. EUROSON 2012. Madrid. 2012.
17. Park SK, et al. Diagnostic performance of ultrasound elastography in the evaluation of benign and malignant soft tissue tumors. RSNA. 2013.
18. Miyamoto H, et al. Carpal tunnel syndrome: diagnosis by means of median nerve elasticity- improved diagnostic accuracy of US with sonoelastography. Radiology. 2014;270:481–6.
19. Orman G, et al. Ultrasound elastographic evaluation in the diagnosis of tunnel carpal syndrome: initial findings ultrasound. Med Biol. 2013;39:1184–9.
20. Wells PN, Liang HD. Medical ultrasound: imaging of soft tissue strain and elasticity. J R Soc Interface. 2011;8(64):1521–49.
21. Brandenburg JE, et al. Ultrasound elastography: the new frontier in direct measurement of muscle stiffness. Arch Phys Med Rehabil. 2014;95(11):2207–19.
22. Eby SF, et al. Validation of shear wave elastography in skeletal muscle. J Biomech. 2013;46(14):2381–7.

Thyroid Gland

7

Vito Cantisani, Hektor Grazhdani, Emanuele David, Christoph Frank Dietrich, Maija Radzina, Antonio Pio Masciotra, Chandra Bortolotto, Fabrizio Calliada, and Ferdinando D'Ambrosio

Abbreviations

ARFI	Acoustic radiation force impulse technology
ECI	Elasticity contrast index
FNAB	Fine-needle aspiration biopsy
MNSR	Muscle-to-nodule strain ratio
PNSR	Parenchyma-to-nodule strain ratio
p-SWE	Point shear wave elastography
ROI	Region of interest
SE	Freehand strain elastography
SR	Strain ratio
SSI	Supersonic shear imaging
SWE	Shear wave elastography
SWS	Shear wave speed
TI-RADS	Thyroid Imaging Reporting and Data System
TSI	Thyroid stiffness index
US	Ultrasound
USE	Ultrasound elastography

V. Cantisani (✉) • F. D'Ambrosio
Department of Radiological Sciences, Policlinico Umberto I, Sapienza University of Rome, Rome, Italy
e-mail: vito.cantisani@uniroma1.it

H. Grazhdani
Associazione dei Cavalieri Italiani, Sovrano Militare Ordine di Malta, Poliambulatorio Roma Eur, Rome, Italy

E. David
Department of Biomedical Sciences and Morphological and Functional Imaging, University of Messina, Messina, Italy

C.F. Dietrich
Department of Internal Medicine 2, Caritas Krankenhaus, Bad Mergentheim, Germany

M. Radzina
Diagnostic Radiology Institute, Paula Stradins Clinical University Hospital, Riga, Latvia

A. Masciotra
Casa di Cura Villa Maria, Campobasso, Italy

C. Bortolotto
Radiology Institute, IRCCS Policlinico San Matteo Foundation, University of Pavia, Pavia, Italy

F. Calliada
Department of Radiology, University Hospital S.Matteo, Pavia, Italy

7.1 Introduction

Ultrasound elastography (USE) is used mainly to improve ultrasound efficacy for the characterization of thyroid nodules, e.g., detection of malignancy, and less commonly for evaluation of diffuse diseases, e.g., chronic thyroiditis. The stiffness of the gland depends on the structural properties of the matrix of tissues (cells, membranes, extravascular matrix, microvessels), whereas in conventional ultrasound (US), it is the microscopic structure that determines reflectivity. Thus, elastography provides correlation with

D.-A. Clevert et al. (eds.), *Atlas of Elastosonography*, DOI 10.1007/978-3-319-44201-3_7

histologic tissue structure, enabling differentiation of the normal gland from nodules and parenchymal diseases. Tissue stiffness is a feature that reflects the nature of the thyroid nodule; neoplasia and inflammation alter the tissue composition and structure and increase the stiffness [1, 2].

Thyroid nodules are ubiquitous in the general population, encountered with a prevalence of 20–67 % and of about 50 % in the individuals older than 40 years of age. People affected by the disease are mostly living in iodine-sufficient parts of the world [3–6]. The incidence increase is partly due to the widespread use of ultrasound (US), and as most of these nodules are clinically irrelevant during the lifespan of the individuals, they are termed "incidentalomas" as incidentally found during the US examination. Most of them are hyperplastic nodules and not clinically relevant neoplasms [7]. However, part of them are malignant and/or become clinically significant and even fatal for the individual [8–11] with a 2.4 times of increase in thyroid malignancy in the last 30 years [11]. Multinodular thyroids have the same likelihood of malignancy for each nodule as the thyroid with a solitary nodule [12].

US examination, although accurate in the detection of the nodules, presents a discrete diagnostic performance for the differentiation of benign from malignant nodules [13] with sensitivity and specificity reported to range in the various studies between 52 and 97 % and 27 and 83 %, respectively [14, 15]. US features that would prompt the need for fine-needle aspiration biopsy (FNAB) are microcalcification, marked hypoechogenicity, taller-than-wide shape, and thick irregular or lobulated margins [16, 17]. The American Thyroid Association guidelines state that, in the cases with normal thyroid-stimulating hormone level, FNAB may be performed in nodules greater than 10 mm [8, 15]. The currently evolving Thyroid Imaging Reporting and Data System (TI-RADS) is attempting to standardize the description of signs and eventual malignancy probability [8, 18, 19].

However, FNAB is mostly carried out in benign nodules, due to the great prevalence of the thyroid nodules in the population, with economic costs and emotional implications for the patient. The performance of this tool is not as high as necessary, reported in various studies with a specificity of 60–98 % and sensitivity of 54–90 % [20–22]. Indeed repetition of FNAB procedure is often requested.

As a consequence of limited diagnostic accuracy of US and FNAB, a significant number of patients receive unnecessary thyroid surgery. Considering that thyroid surgery implies inherent risks, with costs, and complications, improvement in the diagnosis of thyroid cancer is needed.

7.2 Thyroid Elastography

Ultrasound elastography (USE), which offers elasticity assessment, can detect a firm or high stiffness nodule which is a sign of thyroid malignancy, mostly of the papillary cancer. More than 170 articles have been published on this topic, and USE has recently been used as an additional tool for thyroid nodule differentiation, in the context of US and FNAB diagnostic algorithm.

USE in the thyroid is applied with the two different techniques, according to the type of compression force utilized: the freehand strain elastography (SE) and the quantitative method of transducer-induced excitation with an acoustic wave the pulse shear wave elastography (SWE). SE is utilized with its qualitative variant and semiquantitative variant called the strain radio (SR) elastography, whereas SWE measures the speed of the shear wave generated; therefore, it can be performed using the acoustic radiation force impulse (ARFI) technology either in a small region of interest (ROI) (point shear wave elastography, p-SWE) or over a larger field of view using color coding to visually display the stiffness values, also named two-dimensional shear wave elastography (2D-SWE). A small ROI can be placed at the site of interest during 2D-SWE and the stiffness value is determined. In addition, some 2D-SWE can be performed in a real time such as Aixplorer of SuperSonic Imagine or the Aplio 500 of Toshiba. There is also a thyroid-specific variant of SE with no external pressure required, called in vivo quasi-static elastography which takes advantage of the pulsations of the carotid artery and which induces the displacement necessary to assess thyroid elasticity. This technique is applied with a semiquantitative evaluation.

7.2.1 International Guidelines

The guidelines of the European Federation of Societies for Ultrasound in Medicine and Biology (EFSUMB) [1] and the World Federation of Societies for Ultrasound in Medicine and Biology (WFUMB) [2], based on a systematic and updated review of current literature, have provided clinical recommendations and limitations of the USE in thyroid nodule evaluation. Elastography is recommended as an additional tool to conventional ultrasound for a better characterization of thyroid nodules, especially to guide follow-up of lesions previously diagnosed as benign at fine-needle aspiration biopsy.

Regarding the techniques of USE applied in the thyroid and their physical principles, the reader can refer to these valuable resources for detailed description, especially when facing the variety of denominations of the manufacturers. However, we would like to focus in this chapter on the thyroid applications of the various USE techniques, referring to the description of signs, the current role of elastography in thyroid nodule characterization, the results of literature reports, practical advice with tips and tricks, and limitations and pitfalls for each technique and variant.

7.2.2 Examination Technique

SE and SWE are performed with no patient preparation; a state-of-the-art ultrasound equipment that supports elastography is required [1, 2], equipped with a 12–15 MHz linear probe. During B-mode US, thyroid nodules are identified and a region of interest for elastography is selected [23]. For shear wave elastography (SWE), some systems require the use of a lower-frequency transducer (9 MHz). In these cases, the high-frequency transducer should be used to evaluate the B-mode findings, and the lower-frequency probe is used to perform SWE [2].

The thyroid gland is superficially located and the local anatomy is relevant for the USE examination. It is surrounded by a sheath derived from the pretracheal layer of the deep fascia, which attaches the gland to the trachea and the larynx. Anterior and lateral to the lobes lie the strap muscles (sternohyoid, sternothyroid, sternomastoid, and omohyoid). Posterior and lateral are the common carotid arteries, internal jugular veins, and vagus nerves. More medial and posterior to the lobes are the larynx, trachea, esophagus, and long muscles of the neck [24].

SE is somehow problematic in the case of a superficial protuberant mass combined with sparse overlying subcutaneous and deep cervical connective tissue, which produce difficulties in applying a uniform freehand pressure over the entire region of interest. On the other hand, lesions adjacent to the carotid arteries have lateral displacements from its pulsations, which can result in mistracking artifacts [1, 2]. For the latter, placement of the transducer in the longitudinal plane parallel to the long axis of the adjacent artery appeared to improve the consistency, hence the quality of elastograms [25]. The longitudinal scanning also offers more thyroid gland as reference tissue.

7.2.3 Strain Elastography

Strain elastography defines the stiffness in the tissues by calculating the change in length dimension during compression and dividing it by the pre-compression length. As it is not possible to measure the external applied stress, quantification is not possible [26] and strain elastograms only show relative stiffness. The external stress in SE is the freehand compression with the transducer. A few manufactures have devised the use of the carotid artery pulsations as compression force (quasi-static elastography).

Stress with the transducer is applied by uniform light compressions and decompressions on the skin of the patient by oscillatory movements of only a few millimeters [1, 2]. The elastogram depicting the strain change in the ROI is displayed in a split screen with a side-by-side image of the conventional B-mode and the respective elastogram. An alternative display shows the elastogram as a color overlay on the B-mode image which is also denominated as real-time SE.

The tissue stiffness is depicted in the elastogram box in a continuum of colors from red through green to blue, in order to depict soft (high strain), intermediate (equal strain), and hard (no strain) pattern respectively. A manufacturer uses, in his system, a gray-scale display of strain in the ROI box. The lack of color standardization between brands of devices is still an issue with no established color standard for stiff and soft, with some manufacturers using an inverse color scale. Furthermore, the user can customize the color in the display preferences. The operator should refer to the color coding that their US system uses.

However, lately, most manufacturers (>80%) display stiff tissues in blue, soft tissues in red, and the intermediate tissues in green and the array of hues in between. This is also the color coding we will refer to in this chapter.

To monitor the quality of the compression, SE systems provide a color bar or scale to allow the user to optimize the amount of external force applied. An invalid compression as shown by the indicator is discarded and repeated, and only the optimal compressions are utilized as valid.

SE allows for a qualitative and a semiquantitative assessment of elasticity.

7.2.3.1 Qualitative Strain Elastography of Thyroid Nodules

On SE, classic benign nodules present as soft, represented in the elastogram box as red or green, and nodules suspicious for malignancy present as hard (high stiffness), depicted in the elastogram as a pattern of blues or mostly blues (stiff) [27–31]. Scoring systems are devised in an attempt to standardize the visual evaluation of strain and its significance. Subjective scoring of the predominant color in a nodule, which originated from breast nodule research, has been adopted for the thyroid nodules [32, 33].

The method first reported by Itoh [32] uses a 5-point scale:

- Score 1: indicates deformity of the entire lesion.
- Score 2: deformity of most of the lesion with some small stiff areas.
- Score 3: deformity of the peripheral portion of the lesion with stiff tissue in the center.
- Score 4: the entire lesion is stiff.
- Score 5: the entire lesion and surrounding tissue are stiff.

When the nodule is scored between 1 and 3, it is assigned benignity, whereas scoring 4 or 5 are suspicious for malignancy. A large number of studies have used this scoring system, finding the score above 4 highly predictive for malignancy [34, 35].

A similar scoring scale was developed by Rubaltelli et al. [30] as follows:

- Score 1: homogenously soft
- Score 2: heterogenously soft
- Score 3A: mixed with peripheral stiff areas
- Score 3B: mixed with central stiff areas
- Score 4: homogenously stiff

For the Rubaltelli scale, scores of 1 and 2 are indicative of benign nodules, and scores of 3 and 4, of malignant nodules, with higher scores having a higher probability of malignancy [30]. Other authors have found that assigning benignity to score 3 further increases the specificity of the method for cancer detection [36].

Neither of the scoring systems appears to be superior. The subjectively determined score combined with the operator-dependent freehand compression may contribute to interobserver variability [27, 37, 38].

Some researchers have tested the utility of a simplified two-pattern scoring system in which combining the Itoh patterns as follows: score 1 defined less than 50% blue meaning mainly soft nodules and score 2 as more than 50% blue related to mainly stiff nodules [39]. With the use of this score, researchers found excellent sensitivity and specificity [28].

7.2.3.2 Semiquantitative Strain Elastography-Strain Ratio (SR) Elastography

Semiquantitative measurements in SE are feasible by comparing the strain of the nodule to the normal thyroid parenchyma or muscle. It is an automated generation in real time by the device of a strain ratio (SR) when the operator places a region of interest (ROI) in the normal thyroid and a ROI inside the nodule; thus, a ratio is acquired by dividing the strain of the normal thyroid parenchyma by that of the nodule [27, 40, 41]. As strain decays proportionally with the depth investigated, it is necessary that the two ROIs are positioned at the same or similar depths, with a maximum difference in depth of 10 mm [42]. It is understood that the SR assessment does not directly represent the elasticity (i.e., Young's modulus), but it does show how much stiffer the nodule is in comparison to the normal thyroid parenchyma with low SR referring to benign nodule as having little difference in strain in comparison with the normal parenchyma and higher values above a cutoff are related to malignancy [42].

The literature reports show with this technique very good results, however, with a range of different cutoff values for SR, from 2 to 4 [27, 43–45], with no agreement being reached so far on the critical cutoff point to differentiate between benign and malignant nodules [45–49]. In a study, the best cutoff point was found at 4.22, which resulted in a sensitivity of 81.8 %, specificity of 82.9 %, and accuracy of 88 % [36], whereas another report, with a cutoff SR 3.79, found sensitivity of 97.8 % and specificity of 85.7 % [45], respectively. In the literature, cutoff SR as low as 1.5 and as high as 5 were reported as useful.

Some researchers have studied the distinction between two types of SR: parenchyma-to-nodule strain ratio (PNSR), which is the strain in the normal thyroid parenchyma divided by the strain in the thyroid nodule, and the muscle-to-nodule strain ratio (MNSR) defined as the strain in an adjacent strap muscle divided by the nodule strain [44]. No significant difference were found between the PNSR and MNSR in the distinction between benign and malignant thyroid nodules which suggests that MNSR could be used in situations where PNSR could not be assessed, e.g., when a large nodule occupies the whole thyroid gland or in the presence of abnormal thyroid parenchyma (e.g., thyroiditis) [50].

7.2.3.3 Strain Elastography Using Carotid Artery Pulsation

Few US systems are set up with software that detects the strain in the thyroid induced by the carotid artery pulsation SE. Similar to the SR, an automated calculation of a semiquantitative measure, called elasticity index, is calculated [51]. The examination technique entails holding the transducer motionless with slight contact to the skin over the thyroid in the transverse scan plane, and the carotid artery pulsations are the sole strain inductors. The patient is asked to perform a breath hold and strain data are obtained in about 3–4 s. The systolic push of the carotid artery compresses the thyroid against the trachea, and an anteroposterior deformation that results is detected and used for strain measurements. US signals in pre- and postcarotid expansion-compression are tracked and measured [27, 52, 53]; at the same time, the ratio of the strain near the carotid artery (a high strain area) is divided by the thyroid nodule strain, called the thyroid stiffness index (TSI) or a different calculation used by another manufacturer, the elasticity contrast index (ECI) [27, 54–56]. The manufacturer states that to maximize the efficacy, the system considers the highest strain near the carotid artery in comparison with the lowest strain in the nodule for TSI calculation. In this type of system, the operator draws two ROIs, one close to the area of the highest strain adjacent to the carotid artery in the surrounding muscle and another in the nodule at the region of the lowest strain (highest stiffness as shown by the elastogram), and the device calculates the TSI [52]. Differently, in the other system, only one ROI is drawn inside the borders of the nodule, and ECI is measured by the device with co-concurrence matrix comparison of benign and malignant features in a nodule, using complex calculations [51].

7.2.3.4 Limitations and Artifacts in SE

Macrocalcifications in the nodule alter stiffness assessment as they are hard and can produce a stiff image of the nodule. Fibrosis inside longstanding benign nodules or associated with subacute or Hashimoto thyroiditis may also induce stiff areas within nodules [57, 58].

Furthermore, colloid and cystic fluids impair stiffness assessment, as liquid is a limit in strain measurement [Bibliog21, 29, 44, 45]. In the elastogram, the color inside a cyst is random as it is noise due to fluid movement during compression; the result is low-quality strain estimates [1, 27]. RGB (red/green/blue), or the three-color layer artifact, may appear in the elastograms of cystic lesions in some US systems, while the bull's-eye artifact can be seen in others [59]. Thus, if the ROI is placed in a mixed solid and cystic area, the strain measurement is altered.

Nodules larger than 3 cm or large enough to replace an entire lobe of the thyroid cannot be assessed with SE because of the lack of reference tissue and the depth of their deeper portions [60]. Also coalescent nodules are unsuitable for SE [61].

It has been shown that experienced sonographers in elastography have greater specificity in their measurements than those without experience [62]. The pressure of the freehand of different operators cannot be standardized. Nonuniformity is the rule, and strain variations due to changes in the amplitude and velocity of compression are unavoidable [27]. This seems to be the main reason for the intraobserver and interobserver variability [37].

For all elastographic methods, the fact that tissue becomes stiffer as it is stressed by focused compression is an important factor: precompression can result in misleadingly high stiffness readings, especially in superficial tissues [27, 62, 63].

The color-coded scoring systems involve at least some inevitable subjectivity in evaluation, as seen by the wide variability of performance of SE in different literature reports [64].

Nodules in the isthmus, as those close to the carotid artery or deeply located, may be more difficult for SE [63]. Isthmic nodule evaluation with SE is markedly limited as these nodules are compressed between the transducer and the trachea, both hard structures, and with very little normal thyroid or strap muscle, which is necessary to be regarded as the reference tissue of comparison. Carotid artery pulsations adjacent to the thyroid induce periodic deformations in the thyroid that interfere with the freehand compression-decompression cycle and degrade the strain measurements. This effect is more pronounced with nodules that are adjacent to the carotid artery, especially those that are positioned anterior to the carotid artery. Thyroid nodules deep in the posterior thyroid are subject to impaired transmission of compression and provide less strain, which may make them appear artificially stiff [65]. Trying to optimize the displacement of deep tissues of interest with more stress applied with the transducer may result in poor quality elastograms in the near field.

A certain amount of mottled noise is often present in the elastogram due to some inevitable errors in the estimation of tissue displacement by the US system [62]. The areas, where accurate strain values cannot be computed, are not color coded on the elastogram. Noise on elastograms can be a cause for further increase of the interpretation subjectivity [27].

The limitations of qualitative SE also apply to strain ratio SE. Furthermore in SR, in situations where the thyroid nodule or multiple nodules are so large that they occupy the whole thyroid lobe, there may not be enough normal thyroid left in the scan for placement of the second ROI to calculate the strain ratio. Also thyroid tissue outside a nodule may not be normal but may present with multinodular goiter or lymphocytic thyroiditis, both conditions with a hard tissue consistency that would alter the strain ratio [27]. These limitations also apply to thyroid stiffness index (TSI) SE with carotid artery pulsations. The use of the strap muscles as the reference tissue can obviate this limitation.

When a group of waves of different color surrounds a lesion in the elastogram, this means that it was moving in and out of the imaging plane during freehand compression. This can be corrected by repeating a correct compression in the right plane [66].

The additional time needed to complete the elastography evaluation after the conventional US examination is variable with the different techniques and in certain situations can become a limitation [27].

7.2.3.5 How to Improve the Examination

1. As SE displays relative elasticity within a ROI, in order to have a reference for comparison of strain, it is advisable to set an ample ROI, preferably covering the whole nodule together with a good portion of adjacent normal thyroid tissue. Some authors advise at least 5 mm of parenchyma around the borders of the nodule [67]. The box for elasticity assessment in SE should be placed ideally as close as possible to the transducer, as strain diminishes with distance from the transducer.
2. Exclude from the elastogram box the carotid artery and hard tissues, such as the trachea and bones, and, if possible, also non-thyroid tissue, as they notably alter the contrast and the displayed color scale of the SE image [42].
3. The US devices provide a real-time quality control indicator during the freehand compression that can be a numeric scale or an elasticity color bar or a cycle compression bar. The operator must observe in real time whether the compressions are within a range, considered reliable, or there is a need to repeat it.
4. A number of publications advocate the need for three different compressions and SR measurements, and an average result should be considered for elasticity assessment [36, 61]. The WFUMB guidelines require at least two compressions [2].
5. An extended neck position and good breath hold with no swallowing during the examination are the prerequisites for performing a valid compression.
6. As always during the US exam, also for SE, the B-mode focus needs to be positioned at the level of the nodule or slightly below it.
7. Select a strain elasticity scale preset for the thyroid, or modify the elasticity scale if a preset for the thyroid is not available.
8. Operator experience is required for a good compression technique. Correct measurements depend on the quality of the compression, i.e., slight and uniform compressions produce adequate elastograms. One study found that stronger pressure with the freehand altered results; thus, light and uniform compression for all measurements is important [44].
9. Large nodules and multiple ones as multinodular goiter are difficult for SE assessment as there may be no surrounding reference thyroid tissue. Enlarge the elastogram box and include the strap muscles in an attempt to obviate the lack of the thyroid parenchyma in the scan.
10. Sometimes the displayed elasticity scale should be adjusted according to the stiffness of the tissue. Similar to the manipulation of the Doppler scale when assessing high- or low-velocity flow, for a very stiff nodule, the scale can be changed to increase the upper limit of display to allow differentiation between relatively very stiff and soft areas; similarly in a very soft nodule, the scale should be lowered to enable the display of the relatively hard regions in a nodule.
11. Finally, one should remember that what is displayed in SE color is merely a representation of the relative stiffness, a mere comparison between strains of the tissues in the elastogram box. SE is by no means capable of measuring absolute values of strain or elasticity. The deformation of tissues is dependent on the amount of compression; hence, the measured strain is always variable with freehand SE, but the color contrast is similar between compressions, because it shows the comparisons in strain values inside the elastogram box.

7.2.4 Shear Wave Elastography (SWE) Imaging of Thyroid Nodules

7.2.4.1 Examination Technique

In SWE external acoustic (ultrasound) push pulses generated by the probe are sent into the tissue which induce transverse shear waves inside the tissue. This minute transverse motion travels away from the push pulse lines and its speed can be measured. The induced shear wave speed is directly proportional to the stiffness of the tissue, stiffer tissue conducting shear waves faster. Using pulse echo US, the ultrasound machine is able to measure the shear wave speed in meters per second (m/s), and high stiffness values correspond to high velocities. Moreover, making some assumptions regarding the tissue properties, the machine calculates the stiffness as Young's modulus in kilopascals (kPa). Most systems allow the user to choose whether the stiffness value is displayed as shear wave speed or Young's modulus.

Most of the US systems measure the shear wave speed within a preselected fixed-size small ROI that the operator positions at the desired site. This technique is denominated point shear wave elastography (p-SWE), and it provides a numerical result of the SWS of the tissue in the ROI box either in m/s or kPa and in some systems together with the depth of the ROI (which is a relevant parameter considering the decay of the push pulse in the depths of the tissues). High stiffness values correspond to high velocities. Acoustic radiation force impulse (ARFI) technology is the brand name of the software that used p-SWE technology for the first time.

On the other hand, some systems are capable of displaying a color-coded representation of shear wave measurements in a large ROI box, practically a velocity map, also called elasticity image or elastogram. The size of the elastogram box can be controlled manually by the operator, and it is displayed as superimposed on the reference B-mode image. This is called 2D shear wave elastography (2D-SWE). One or more measurement ROIs can then be placed in the color-coded elastogram box. 2D-SWE can be performed as a "one-shot" technique or as a "real-time" technique. US systems that are capable of real-time 2D-SWE assessment are those of SuperSonic Imagine (SSI). Opposite to SE elastograms, in SSI soft tissue is shown as blue and stiff (hard) tissue is shown as red.

With both p-SWE and 2D-SWE techniques, it is important that there is no motion during the acquisition to obtain a stable elastogram. Breath hold is necessary. Moreover, with real-time 2D-SWE, several seconds of stationary positioning of the probe on the area of concern are important in order to obtain an accurate evaluation.

The transducer should only lightly contact the skin of the neck. With increasing pressure of the transducer, the stiffness increases rapidly, due to nonlinear elastic effects [42], especially relevant in the isthmic nodules as they are easily compressed against the tracheal cartilages. Similar to SE, a strain ratio can be calculated using either normal thyroid tissue or muscle as the reference.

Malignant nodules appear stiff, and also as observed with velocity map elastograms, they tend to be more heterogeneous than benign lesions. Furthermore, often the stiffness seems to be most marked at and around the periphery of the malignant nodules.

The quantitative nature of SWE (unlike SE evaluation) and the fact that a consistent acoustic pulse moves the tissue (not the freehand compression with its variability) may improve inter- and intraobserver agreement and accuracy.

7.2.4.2 Diagnostic Value of SWE for Thyroid Nodules

Literature publications report, for p-SWE, shear wave velocity of the normal gland at 1.60 ± 0.18 m/s [68, 69]. At 2D-SWE using SSI, reports of normal thyroid values are at 2.6 ± 1.8 m/s and 20.8 ± 10.4 kPa [70–72].

For nodule benignity-malignancy differentiation, studies using SWE reported cutoff values ranging from 3.65 m/s to 4.70 m/s (34.5–66 kPa). Different studies report various cutoff values associated with different diagnostic performance, ranging from best cutoff at 34.5 kPa [73] to 65 kPa [74] and 66 kPa [70, 75]. The sensitivities for SWE range from 0.80 to 0.86 (95 % CI 0.73, 0.92), while the specificities range from 0.84 to 0.90 (95 % CI 0.80–0.94). The AUROC values range from 0.91 to 0.94. Shear wave speed (SWS) was found to be significantly higher in the malignant than benign lesions, with a value higher than 2.87 m/s strongly suggestive of malignancy [27, 76].

A group of researchers found that by increasing the cutoff value from 10.3 to 132 kPa, the specificity changed from 8.9 to 100 % [73]. Noteworthy is that two studies report that SSI can differentiate thyroid nodules, even in the presence of autoimmune thyroiditis [77, 78]. A recent research found that SWE (with both forms: p-SWE and 2D-SWE) may be useful in selecting patients with thyroid nodules for surgery [79].

A meta-analysis noted significant heterogeneity in reported sensitivity and specificity ($p<0.001$) [80]. However, overall, both p-SWE and 2D-SWE, in all reports, show good sensitivity and specificity for the differential diagnosis of thyroid nodules. Furthermore, as shown in a number of researches, the interobserver and intraobserver repeatability of both p-SWE and 2D-SWE are high, with reported interclass correlation of 0.90–0.97 [70, 71, 76, 81, 82]. All studies and meta-analyses suggest that SWE (p-SWE and 2D-SWE) may be a useful complementary tool to conventional US in differentiating between benign and malignant nodules.

7.2.4.3 How to Improve the Examination

1. In all SWE techniques, for accurate measurements, a slight contact of the probe to the skin is essential, as pressure applied by the probe alters the measurements and causes artifacts of increased stiffness [76]. For this reason experience is required to perform reliable examinations and SWE quantification [27, 73, 76]. Liberal use of ultrasound coupling gel can help maintain only slight contact with the skin. The patient should perform adequate breath hold.
2. If you encounter a pattern of red in the near field, also called a vertical artifact, you may reduce it by minimizing probe compression [27, 73]
3. The isthmic nodules, compressed against the trachea, are the most at risk to effect of probe pressure. To avoid the artifactually increased measured stiffness, some authors advise the use of paracoronal scanning in order to avoid compressing the nodules against the trachea [77].
4. The ROI should include as much as possible of the area of the nodule. Normal thyroid parenchyma should not be included in the ROI.
5. ROI must be placed in the nodule avoiding cystic or calcified areas as these alter the measurements. However, the use of the standard size ROI in p-SWE sometimes makes it impossible to exclude fluid and calcified areas of a nodule.
6. Choosing a correct preset is important to acquire accurate measurements, and the preset should be 0–180 kPa for the thyroid application [42]. Increase the elasticity color gain to its maximum till the noise starts to appear in the elasticity image, because this will aid in acquiring good color sensitivity elastograms.
7. With 2D-SWE in order to obtain the most significant quantitative readouts, ROIs should be placed on the stiffest part of a lesion as shown in the velocity map (2D-SWE elastogram). Malignancy is often very heterogeneous in stiffness; it is useful to choose the stiffest site for the measurement.
8. In the elasticity image, there can be areas with no color that may be due to fluid content, calcification, or impossible velocities' measurements due to technical problems [42]. In some systems the displayed measurements show "X.XX" or "0.00" because these nodules contain cysts and calcifications [76, 83]. Cysts, when containing nonviscous fluids, do not support shear waves, and so they appear as color voids, usually seen as black regions where the anechoic B-mode layer shows through. On the other hand, when the cyst fluid is viscous, shear wave signals may be seen and would display a soft region [1].
9. With p-SWE, sometimes the system cannot calculate an accurate measurement due to a variety of factors such as motion or noise or probably a too low amplitude of the generated shear wave or even too high stiffness in the nodule with a too high shear wave speed that cannot be sampled [42, 84]. ARFI for example, when it cannot yield a measurement, displays "X.XX m/s" instead of the expected numeric value. In such an occurrence, slightly change the position of the probe and repeat the evaluation.

10. With ARFI, in the experience of some researchers, ten measurements were needed to obtain an average which yielded a reliable accuracy [42, 84]. Another research group had good results with five measurements [68].
11. Always bear in mind that, as with strain elastography, malignancy may appear genuinely soft, albeit rarely. Follicular carcinomas, in particular, can be soft and difficult to distinguish from benign nodules.
12. For good documentation, some authors recommend, for every nodule, the acquisition of three cine loops, each of at least 10 s of duration [81].

7.3 Discussion

With 3–5 min of added time to the US exam time, strain elastography can easily be performed as an extension to the routine thyroid scanning. SE should always be interpreted in conjunction with the B-mode imaging since US signs have been shown to have a fair sensitivity in detecting suspicious nodules [33]. However, the use of SE in the routine clinical practice has still to be defined. Suspicious US findings in patients should override the SE information, i.e., if the nodule is suspicious on US, FNAB should be recommended. In case of the opposite findings, current literature does not sufficiently support active intervention. On the other hand, in the cases of benign findings with SE, more prospective studies are needed to understand if SE findings can avoid unnecessary FNAB. SE results have shown to be helpful in patients with non-diagnostic or indeterminate cytology to direct to a repetition of FNAB or follow-up. Operator experience is essential for SE since significant false-positive results can occur with lack of experience. Training that involves at least five SE examinations with expert guidance is a minimum requirement [85]. The quality indicator of the US device should guide the compression-relaxation cycle of the manual compression. Furthermore, the color-coded display scale should be optimized when needed. Documentation with static images and cine loops must be provided for eventual further review.

Nowadays, there are many and variable technological solutions, with nonuniformity and with different scoring systems and cutoff values, that make the comprehensive assessment of the SE in the thyroid still a matter of debate [86]. The technique is in a need for overall standardization.

Shear wave elastography appears to have the advantage of being less operator dependent: in addition, the learning curve for strain elastography seems to be short [85] and has improved significantly by the availability of real-time operator feedback. Some authors claim that SWS is an operator-independent and reproducible technique [74, 86]. However, only a small number of studies have been published; future multicenter studies are needed.

Conclusions

According to present literature and our personal experience, ultrasound elastography is a useful additional tool for thyroid nodule evaluation. Both strain and shear wave elastography may be used, but adequate training and observance of technical parameters are mandatory to obtain valid results.

7.4 Image Gallery

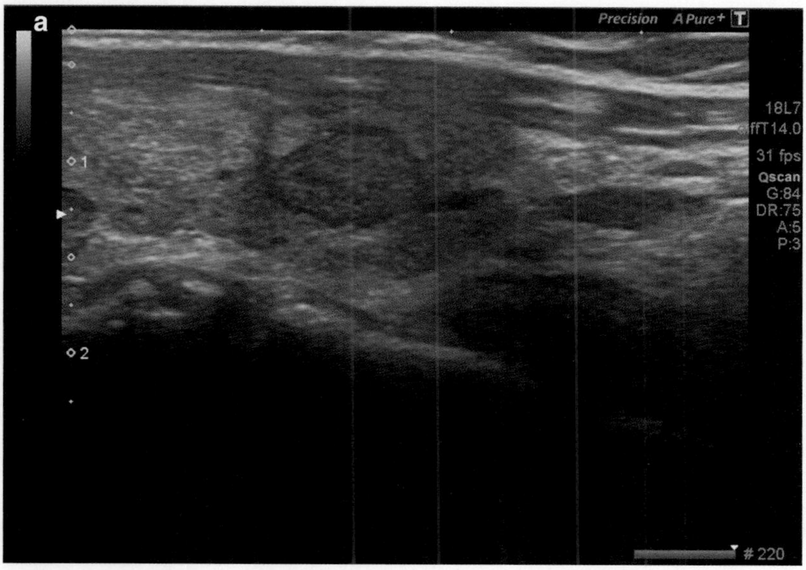

Fig. 7.1 Hyperplastic follicular lesion histologically proven. (**a**) At baseline ultrasound the lesion appears iso-hypoechoic with peripheral halo sign. (**b1**, **b2**) At power Doppler and at Advanced Dynamic Flow™ (*ADF*), the nodule shows pattern III. (**c**) Qualitative evaluation with SE shows score 1 by Itoh et al. and Rubaltelli et al. (**d**) At semiquantitative evaluation, nodule appears benign with a strain ratio of 1.05 under the cutoff value of 2.0

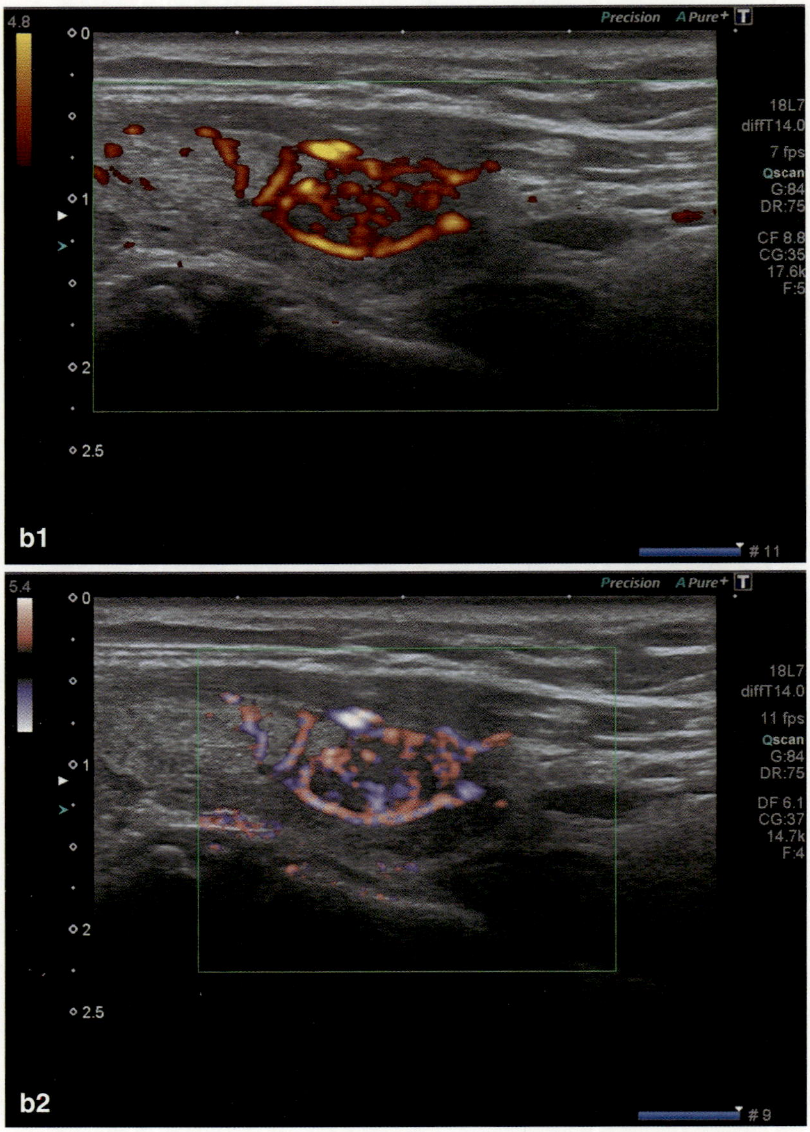

Fig. 7.1 (continued)

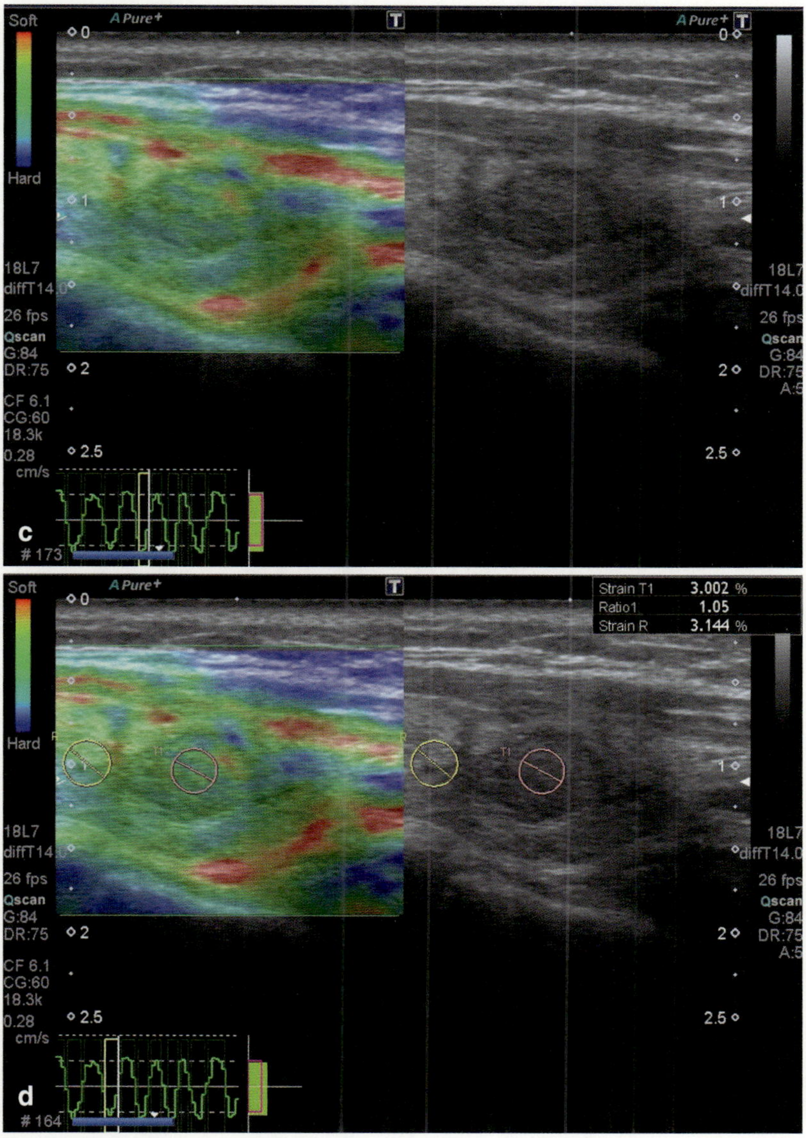

Fig. 7.1 (continued)

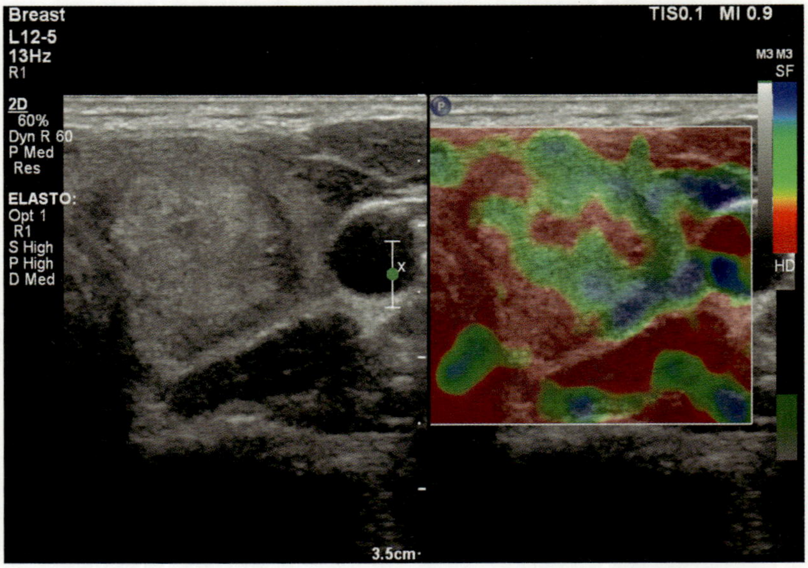

Fig. 7.2 Benign nodule at FNAC. Isoechoic nodule with halo sign which shows score 2 at qualitative evaluation

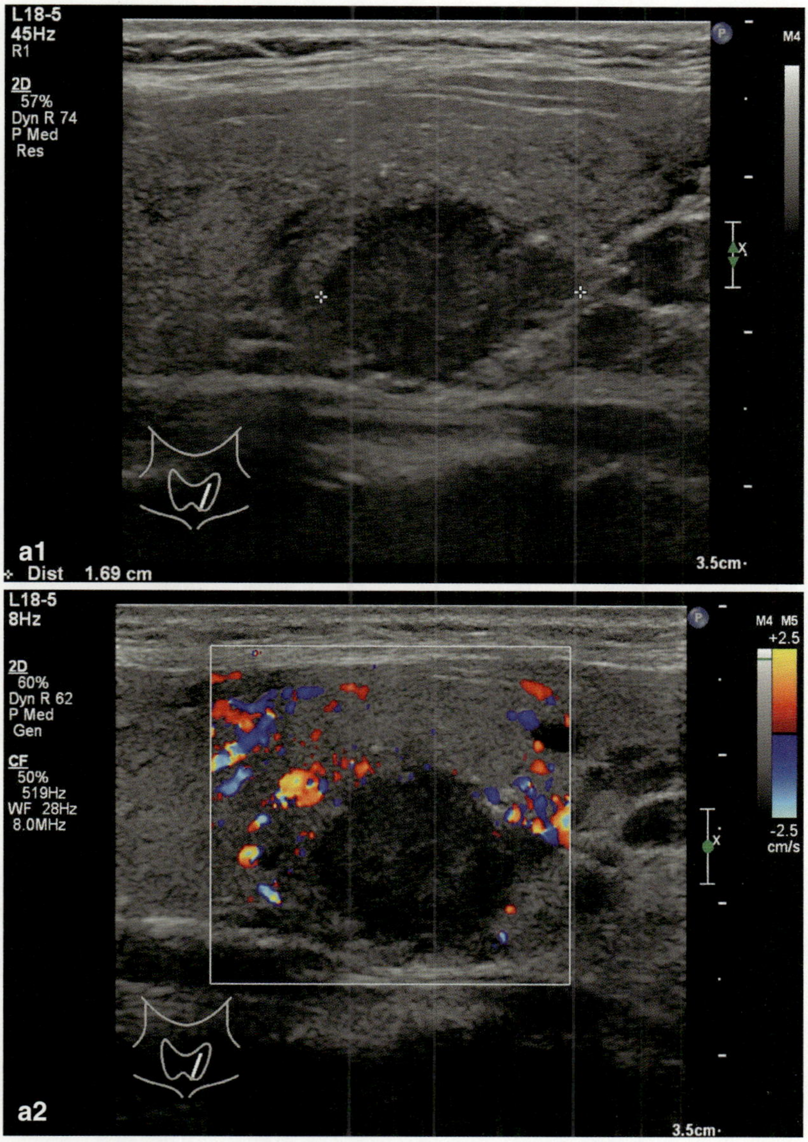

Fig. 7.3 Papillary carcinoma histologically proven. (**a1**, **a2**) Hypoechoic nodule with irregular margins and pattern I at color Doppler evaluation. (**b**) At qualitative evaluation the nodule appears hard

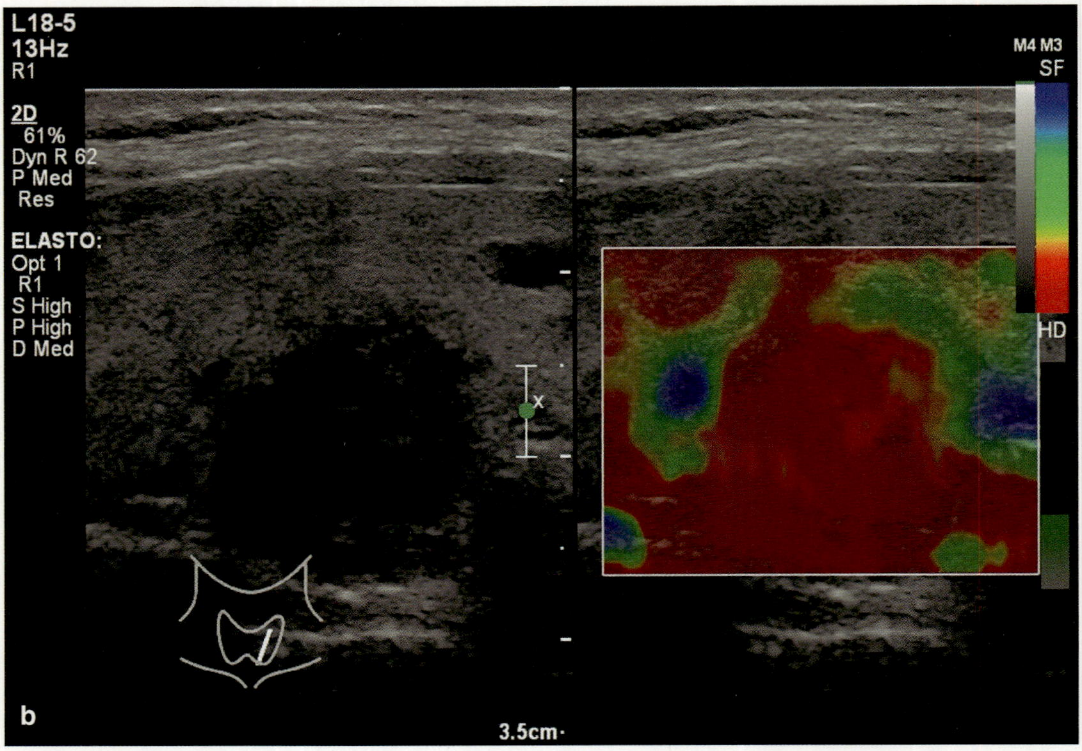

Fig. 7.3 (continued)

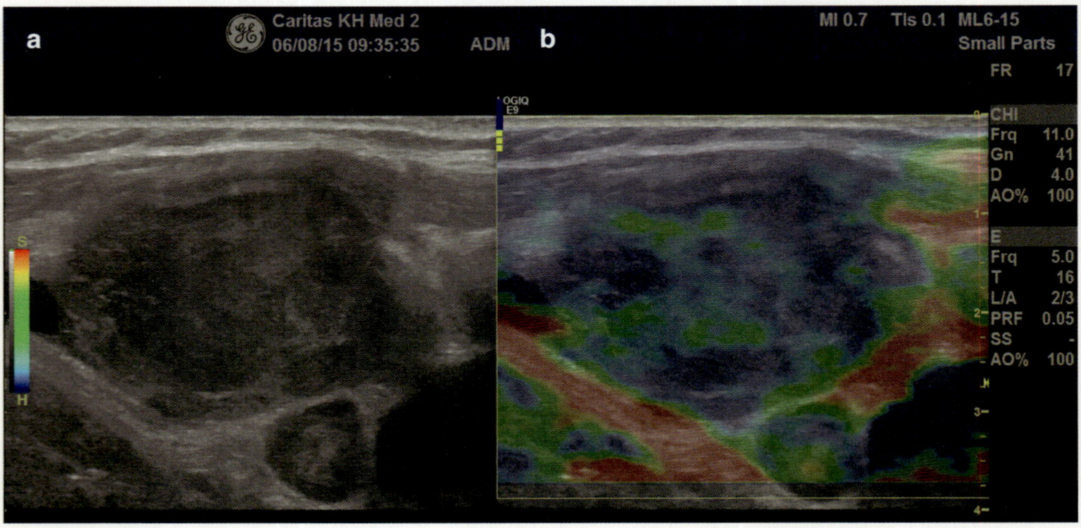

Fig. 7.4 Anaplastic carcinoma (histologically proven). (**a**) B-mode of the tumor revealed diffuse infiltration with cervical lymphadenopathy. (**b**) Elastography revealed stiff tissue

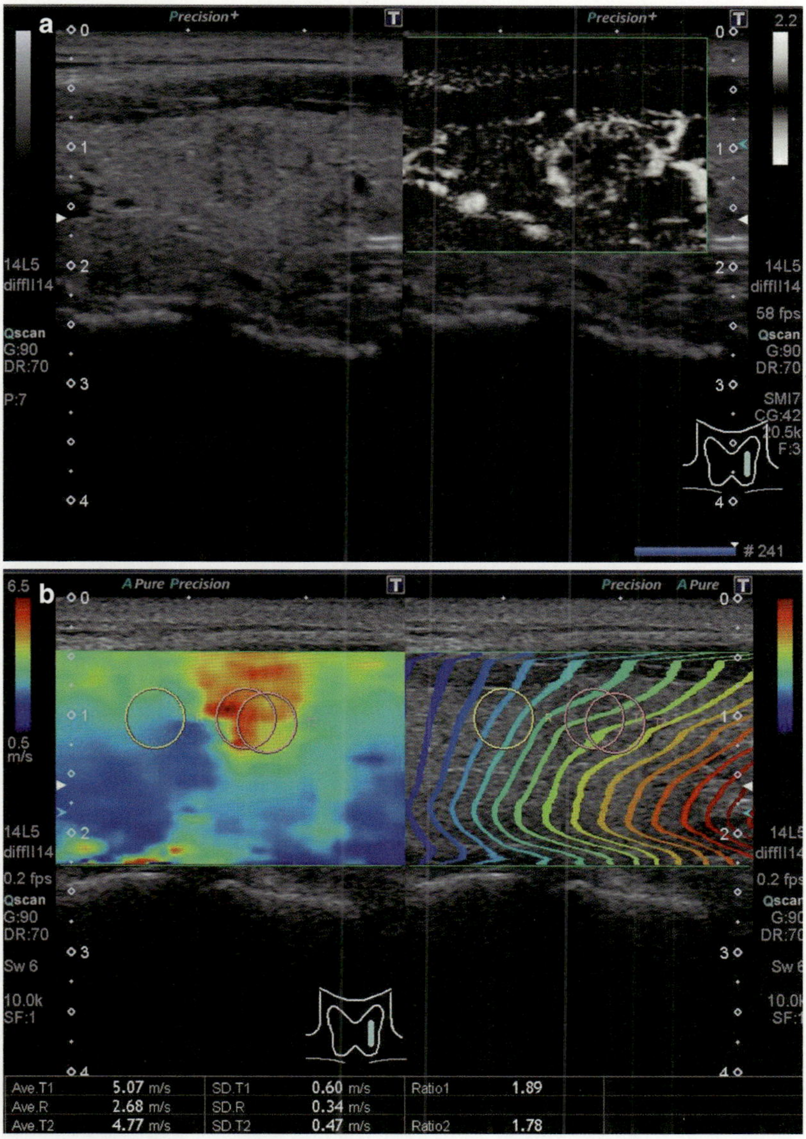

Fig. 7.5 Papillary carcinoma histologically proven. (**a**) Baseline ultrasound shows an isoechoic nodule with a partially continuous halo sign and pattern III at SMI evaluation. (**b**) At shear wave elastography, the lesion appears hard with high elasticity values. It was a carcinoma histologically proven

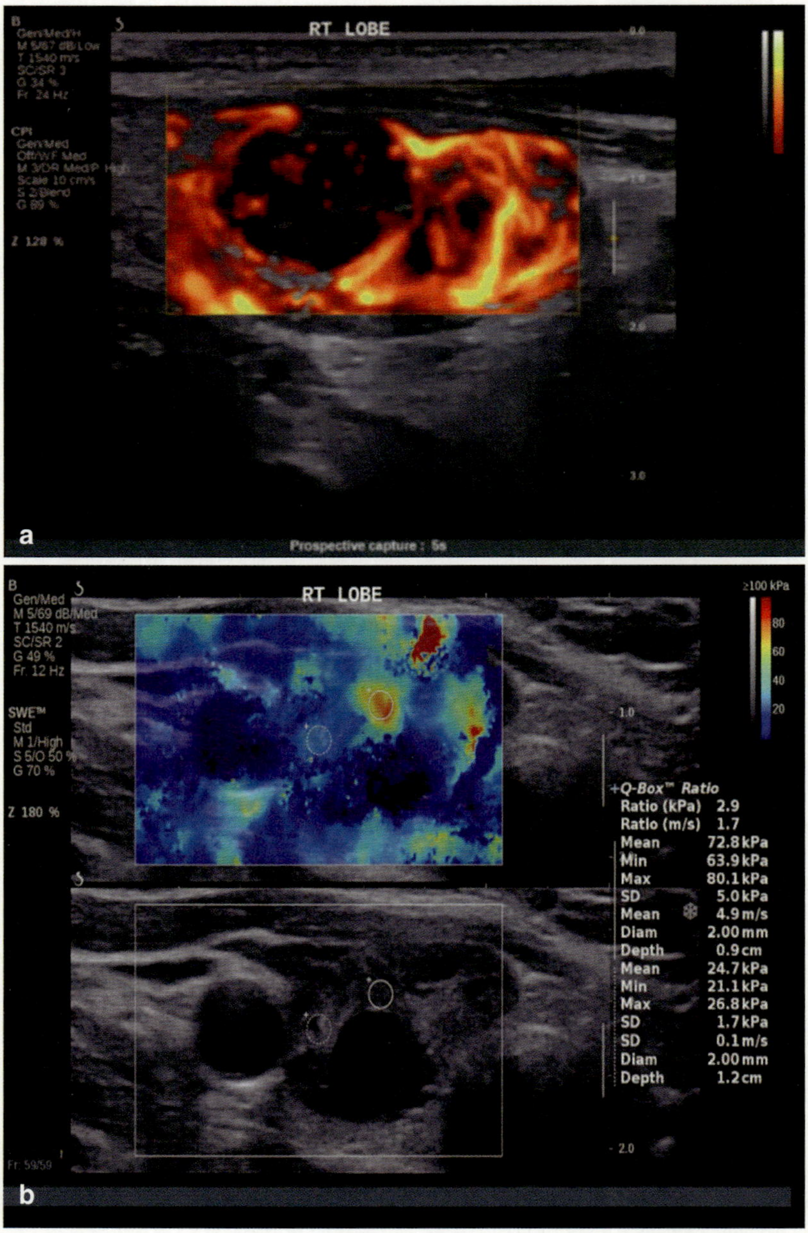

Fig. 7.6 Papillary carcinoma histologically proven. (**a**) Iso-hypoechoic nodule with high peri- and intranodular vascularization (pattern III). (**b**) At SSI the lesion presents mixed stiffness but high elasticity values expressed in m/s and k/Pa

References

1. Bamber J, Cosgrove D, Dietrich CF, et al. EFSUMB guidelines and recommendations on the clinical use of ultrasound elastography. Part 1: basic principles and technology. Ultraschall Med. 2013;34(2):169–84.
2. Shiina T, Nightingale KR, Palmeri ML, et al. WFUMB guidelines and recommendations for clinical use of ultrasound elastography: Part 1: basic principles and terminology. Ultrasound Med Biol. 2015;41(5):1126–47.
3. Remonti LR, Kramer CK, Leitao CB, Pinto LC, Gross JL. Thyroid ultrasound features and risk of carcinoma: a systematic review and meta-analysis of observational studies. Thyroid. 2015;25:538–50.
4. Brander AE, Viikinkoski VP, Nickels JI, Kivisaari LM. Importance of thyroid abnormalities detected at US screening: a 5-year follow-up. Radiology. 2000;215:801–6.
5. Chammas MC, Gerhard R, de Oliveira IR, Widman A, de Barros N, Durazzo M, Ferraz A, Cerri GG. Thyroid nodules: evaluation with power Doppler and duplex Doppler ultrasound. Otolaryngol Head Neck Surg. 2005;132:874–82.
6. Tramalloni J, Leger A, Correas JM, Monpeyssen H, Szwagier-Uzzan C, Helenon O, Moreau JF. Imaging of thyroid nodules. J Radiol. 1999;80:271–7.
7. Reading CC, Charboneau JW, Hay ID, Sebo TJ. Sonography of thyroid nodules: a "classic pattern" diagnostic approach. Ultrasound Q. 2005;21:157–65.
8. Haugen BRM, Alexander EK, Bible KC, Doherty G, Mandel SJ, Nikiforov YE, Pacini F, Randolph G, Sawka A, Schlumberger M, Schuff KG, Sherman SI, Sosa JA, Steward D, Tuttle RMM, Wartofsky L. 2015 American Thyroid Association Management guidelines for adult patients with thyroid nodules and differentiated thyroid cancer. Thyroid. 2015;26(1):1–133.
9. Ferraioli G, Filice C, Castera L, Choi BI, Sporea I, Wilson SR, Cosgrove D, Dietrich CF, Amy D, Bamber JC, Barr R, Chou YH, Ding H, Farrokh A, Friedrich-Rust M, Hall TJ, Nakashima K, Nightingale KR, Palmeri ML, Schafer F, Shiina T, Suzuki S, Kudo M. WFUMB guidelines and recommendations for clinical use of ultrasound elastography: Part 3: liver. Ultrasound Med Biol. 2015;41:1161–79.
10. Tunbridge WM, Evered DC, Hall R, et al. The spectrum of thyroid disease in a community: the Whickham survey. Clin Endocrinol (Oxf). 1977;7(6):481–93.
11. Davies L, Welch HG. Increasing incidence of thyroid cancer in the United States, 1973–2002. JAMA. 2006;295(18):2164–7.
12. Sipos JA. Advances in ultrasound for the diagnosis and management of thyroid cancer. Thyroid. 2009;19:1363–72.
13. Iannuccilli JD, Cronan JJ, Monchik JM. Risk for malignancy of thyroid nodules as assessed by sonographic criteria: the need for biopsy. J Ultrasound Med. 2004;23(11):1455–64.
14. Fish SA, Langer JE, Mandel SJ. Sonographic imaging of thyroid nodules and cervical lymph nodes. Endocrinol Metab Clin North Am. 2008;37(2):401–17.
15. Kim HG, Moon HJ, Kwak JY, Kim EK. Diagnostic accuracy of the ultrasonographic features for subcentimeter thyroid nodules suggested by the revised American Thyroid Association guidelines. Thyroid. 2013;23(12):1583–9.
16. Hoang JK, Lee WK, Lee M, Johnson D, Farrell S. US features of thyroid malignancy: pearls and pitfalls. Radiographics. 2007;27(3):847–60, discussion 861–865.
17. Moon H-G, Jung E-J, Park ST, et al. Role of ultrasonography in predicting malignancy in patients with thyroid nodules. World J Surg. 2007;31(7):1410–6.
18. Horvath E, Majlis S, Rossi R, Franco C, Niedmann JP, Castro A, Dominguez M. An ultrasonogram reporting system for thyroid nodules stratifying cancer risk for clinical management. J Clin Endocrinol Metab. 2009;94:1748–51.
19. Kwak JY, Han KH, Yoon JH, Moon HJ, Son EJ, Park SH, Jung HK, Choi JS, Kim BM, Kim EK. Thyroid imaging reporting and data system for US features of nodules: a step in establishing better stratification of cancer risk. Radiology. 2011;260:892–9.
20. Tee YY, Lowe AJ, Brand CA, Judson RT. Fine-needle aspiration may miss a third of all malignancy in palpable thyroid nodules: a comprehensive literature review. Ann Surg. 2007;246(5):714–20.
21. Peng Y, Wang HH. A meta-analysis of comparing fine-needle aspiration and frozen section for evaluating thyroid nodules. Diagn Cytopathol. 2008;36(12):916–20.
22. Oertel YC, Miyahara-Felipe L, Mendoza MG, Yu K. Value of repeated fine needle aspirations of the thyroid: an analysis of over ten thousand FNAs. Thyroid. 2007;17(11):1061–6.
23. Lyshchik A, Higashi T, Asato R, Tanaka S, Ito J, Mai J, Pellot-Barakat C, Insana M, Brill A, Saga T, Hiraoka M, Togashi K. Thyroid gland tumor diagnosis at US elastography. Radiology. 2005;237:202–11.
24. Ahuja AT. Lupmps and bumps in the head and neck. In: Ahuja AT, Evans R, editors. Practical head and neck ultrasound. London: Greenwich Medical Media Limited; 2000. p. 87–106.
25. Bhatia KS, Rasalkar DD, Lee YP, Wong KT, King AD, Yuen YH, Ahuja AT. Real-time qualitative ultrasound elastography of miscellaneous non-nodal neck masses: applications and limitations. Ultrasound Med Biol. 2010;36:1644–52.
26. Carlsen J, Ewertsen C, Sletting S, Vejborg I, Schäfer FK, Cosgrove D, Bachmann Nielsen M. Ultrasound elastography in breast cancer diagnosis. Ultraschall Med. 2015;36(6):550–62.
27. Cantisani V, Consorti F, Guerrisi A, et al. Prospective comparative evaluation of quantitative-elastosonography (Q-elastography) and contrast-enhanced ultrasound for the evaluation of thyroid nodules: preliminary experience. Eur J Radiol. 2013;82(11):1892–8.
28. Rago T, Vitti P. Potential value of elastosonography in the diagnosis of malignancy in thyroid nodules. Q J Nucl Med Mol Imaging. 2009;53(5):455–64.

29. Ueno E, Itoh A. Diagnosis of breast cancer by elasticity imaging. Eizo Joho Medical. 2004;36(12):2–6.
30. Rubaltelli L, Corradin S, Dorigo A, et al. Differential diagnosis of benign and malignant thyroid nodules at elastosonography. Ultraschall Med. 2009;30(2):175–9.
31. Rago T, Santini F, Scutari M, Pinchera A, Vitti P. Elastography: new developments in ultrasound for predicting malignancy in thyroid nodules. J Clin Endocrinol Metab. 2007;92(8):2917–22.
32. Itoh A, Ueno E, Tohno E, et al. Breast disease: clinical application of US elastography for diagnosis. Radiology. 2006;239(2):341–50.
33. Moon HJ, Sung JM, Kim EK, Yoon JH, Youk JH, Kwak JY. Diagnostic performance of gray-scale US and elastography in solid thyroid nodules. Radiology. 2012;262(3):1002–13.
34. Rago T, Di Coscio G, Basolo F, Scutari M, Elisei R, Berti P, Miccoli P, Romani R, Faviana P, Pinchera A, Vitti P. Combined clinical, thyroid ultrasound and cytological features help to predict thyroid malignancy in follicular and Hupsilonrthle cell thyroid lesions: results from a series of 505 consecutive patients. Clin Endocrinol (Oxf). 2007;66:13–20.
35. Rago T, Vitti P. Role of thyroid ultrasound in the diagnostic evaluation of thyroid nodules. Best Pract Res Clin Endocrinol Metab. 2008;22:913–28.
36. Ning CP, Jiang SQ, Zhang T, Sun LT, Liu YJ, Tian JW. The value of strain ratio in differential diagnosis of thyroid solid nodules. Eur J Radiol. 2012;81(2):286–91.
37. Park SH, Kim SJ, Kim EK, Kim MJ, Son EJ, Kwak JY. Interobserver agreement in assessing the sonographic and elastographic features of malignant thyroid nodules. AJR Am J Roentgenol. 2009;193(5):W416–23.
38. Kim JK, Baek JH, Lee JH, et al. Ultrasound elastography for thyroid nodules: a reliable study? Ultrasound Med Biol. 2012;38(9):1508–13.
39. Chong Y, Shin JH, Ko ES, Han BK. Ultrasonographic elastography of thyroid nodules: is adding strain ratio to colour mapping better? Clin Radiol. 2013;68:1241–6.
40. Vorländer C, Wolff J, Saalabian S, Lienenlüke RH, Wahl RA. Real-time ultrasound elastography – a noninvasive diagnostic procedure for evaluating dominant thyroid nodules. Langenbecks Arch Surg. 2010;395(7):865–71.
41. Ding J, Cheng HD, Huang J, Zhang Y, Liu J. An improved quantitative measurement for thyroid cancer detection based on elastography. Eur J Radiol. 2012;81(4):800–5.
42. Dudea SM, Botar-Jid C. Ultrasound elastography in thyroid disease. Med Ultrasound. 2015;17(1):74–96.
43. Cakir B, Aydin C, Korukluoğlu B, et al. Diagnostic value of elastosonographically determined strain index in the differential diagnosis of benign and malignant thyroid nodules. Endocrine. 2011;39(1):89–98.
44. Ciledag N, Arda K, Aribas BK, Aktas E, Köse SK. The utility of ultrasound elastography and MicroPure imaging in the differentiation of benign and malignant thyroid nodules. AJR Am J Roentgenol. 2012;198(3):W244–9.
45. Xing P, Wu L, Zhang C, Li S, Liu C, Wu C. Differentiation of benign from malignant thyroid lesions: calculation of the strain ratio on thyroid sonoelastography. J Ultrasound Med. 2011;30(5):663–9.
46. Cantisani V, D'Andrea V, Biancari F, Medvedyeva O, Di Segni M, Olive M, Patrizi G, Redler A, De Antoni EE, Masciangelo R, Frezzotti F, Ricci P. Prospective evaluation of multiparametric ultrasound and quantitative elastosonography in the differential diagnosis of benign and malignant thyroid nodules: preliminary experience. Eur J Radiol. 2012;81:2678–83.
47. Cantisani V, Grazhdani H, Drakonaki E, D'Andrea V, Di Segni M, Kaleshi E, Calliada F, Catalano C, Redler A, Brunese L, Drudi FM, Fumarola A, Carbotta G, Frattaroli F, Di Leo N, Ciccariello M, Caratozzolo M, D'Ambrosio F. Strain US elastography for the characterization of thyroid nodules: advantages and limitation. Int J Endocrinol. 2015;2015:908575.
48. Ding J, Cheng H, Ning C, Huang J, Zhang Y. Quantitative measurement for thyroid cancer characterization based on elastography. J Ultrasound Med. 2011;30:1259–66.
49. Kagoya R, Monobe H, Tojima H. Utility of elastography for differential diagnosis of benign and malignant thyroid nodules. Otolaryngol Head Neck Surg. 2010;143:230–4.
50. Aydin R, Elmali M, Polat AV, Danaci M, Akpolat I. Comparison of muscle-to-nodule and parenchyma-to-nodule strain ratios in the differentiation of benign and malignant thyroid nodules: which one should we use? Eur J Radiol. 2014;83:e131–6.
51. Lim DJ, Luo S, Kim MH, Ko SH, Kim Y. Interobserver agreement and intraobserver reproducibility in thyroid ultrasound elastography. AJR Am J Roentgenol. 2012;198(4):896–901.
52. Dighe M, Bae U, Richardson ML, Dubinsky TJ, Minoshima S, Kim Y. Differential diagnosis of thyroid nodules with US elastography using carotid artery pulsation. Radiology. 2008;248(2):662–9.
53. Luo S, Kim EH, Dighe M, Kim Y. Screening of thyroid nodules by ultrasound elastography using diastolic strain variation. Conf Proc IEEE Eng Med Biol Soc. 2009;2009:4420–3.
54. Dighe M, Kim J, Luo S, Kim Y. Utility of the ultrasound elastographic systolic thyroid stiffness index in reducing fine-needle aspirations. J Ultrasound Med. 2010;29(4):565–74.
55. Dighe M, Luo S, Cuevas C, Kim Y. Efficacy of thyroid ultrasound elastography in differential diagnosis of small thyroid nodules. Eur J Radiol. 2013;82(6):e274–80.
56. Luo S, Lim DJ, Kim Y. Objective ultrasound elastography scoring of thyroid nodules using spatiotemporal strain information. Med Phys. 2012;39(3):1182–9.
57. Cantisani V, Lodise P, Grazhdani H, Mancuso E, Maggini E, Di Rocco G, D'Ambrosio F, Calliada F, Redler A, Ricci P, Catalano C. Ultrasound elastography in the evaluation of thyroid pathology. Current status. Eur J Radiol. 2014;83:420–8.

58. Shuzhen C. Comparison analysis between conventional ultrasonography and ultrasound elastography of thyroid nodules. Eur J Radiol. 2012;81:1806–11.
59. Barr RG, Lackey AE. The utility of the "bull's-eye" artifact on breast elasticity imaging in reducing breast lesion biopsy rate. Ultrasound Q. 2011;27(3):151–5.
60. Tranquart F, Bleuzen A, Pierre-Renoult P, Chabrolle C, Sam Giao M, Lecomte P. Elastosonography of thyroid lesions. J Radiol. 2008;89:35–9.
61. Wang HL, Zhang S, Xin XJ, Zhao LH, Li CX, Mu JL, Wei XQ. Application of real-time ultrasound elastography in diagnosing benign and malignant thyroid solid nodules. Cancer Biol Med. 2012;9:124–7.
62. Merino S, Arrazola J, Cárdenas A, et al. Utility and interobserver agreement of ultrasound elastography in the detection of malignant thyroid nodules in clinical care. AJNR Am J Neuroradiol. 2011;32(11):2142–8.
63. Wang Y, Dan HJ, Dan HY, Li T, Hu B. Differential diagnosis of small single solid thyroid nodules using real-time ultrasound elastography. J Int Med Res. 2010;38(2):466–72.
64. Bhatia KS, Rasalkar DP, Lee YP, et al. Cystic change in thyroid nodules: a confounding factor for real-time qualitative thyroid ultrasound elastography. Clin Radiol. 2011;66(9):799–807.
65. Garra BS. Elastography: current status, future prospects, and making it work for you. Ultrasound Q. 2011;27(3):177–86.
66. Barr RG. Breast elastography. New York: Thieme; 2014.
67. Liu BX, Xie XY, Liang JY, et al. Shear wave elastography versus real-time elastography on evaluation thyroid nodules: a preliminary study. Eur J Radiol. 2014;83(7):1135–43.
68. Sporea I, Sirli R, Bota S, Vlad M, Popescu A, Zosin I. ARFI elastography for the evaluation of diffuse thyroid gland pathology: preliminary results. World J Radiol. 2012;4(4):174–8.
69. Park AY, Son EJ, Han K, Youk JH, Kim JA, Park CS. Shear wave elastography of thyroid nodules for the prediction of malignancy in a large scale study. Eur J Radiol. 2015;84(3):407–12.
70. Veyrieres JB, Albarel F, Lombard JV, et al. A threshold value in Shear Wave elastography to rule out malignant thyroid nodules: a reality? Eur J Radiol. 2012;81(12):3965–72.
71. Friedrich-Rust M, Romenski O, Meyer G, Dauth N, Holzer K, Grunwald F, Kriener S, Herrmann E, Zeuzem S, Bojunga J. Acoustic Radiation Force Impulse-Imaging for the evaluation of the thyroid gland: a limited patient feasibility study. Ultrasonics. 2012;52:69–74.
72. Fukuhara T, Matsuda E, Endo Y, Takenobu M, Izawa S, Fujiwara K, Kitano H. Correlation between quantitative shear wave elastography and pathologic structures of thyroid lesions. Ultrasound Med Biol. 2015;41:2326–32.
73. Bhatia KS, Tong CS, Cho CC, Yuen EH, Lee YY, Ahuja AT. Shear wave elastography of thyroid nodules in routine clinical practice: preliminary observations and utility for detecting malignancy. Eur Radiol. 2012;22(11):2397–406.
74. Sebag F, Vaillant-Lombard J, Berbis J, et al. Shear wave elastography: a new ultrasound imaging mode for the differential diagnosis of benign and malignant thyroid nodules. J Clin Endocrinol Metab. 2010;95(12):5281–8.
75. Slapa RZ, Piwowonski A, Jakubowski WS, et al. Shear wave elastography may add a new dimension to ultrasound evaluation of thyroid nodules: case series with comparative evaluation. J Thyroid Res. 2012;2012:657147.
76. Grazhdani H, Cantisani V, Lodise P, Di Rocco G, Proietto MC, Fioravanti E, Rubini A, Redler A. Prospective evaluation of acoustic radiation force impulse technology in the differentiation of thyroid nodules: accuracy and interobserver variability assessment. J Ultrasound. 2014;17:13–20.
77. Magri F, Chytiris S, Capelli V, et al. Shear wave elastography in the diagnosis of thyroid nodules: feasibility in the case of coexistent chronic autoimmune Hashimoto's thyroiditis. Clin Endocrinol (Oxf). 2012;76(1):137–41.
78. Gu J, Du L, Bai M, et al. Preliminary study on the diagnostic value of acoustic radiation force impulse technology for differentiating between benign and malignant thyroid nodules. J Ultrasound Med. 2012;31(5):763–71.
79. Zhan J, Jin JM, Diao XH, Chen Y. Acoustic radiation force impulse imaging (ARFI) for differentiation of benign and malignant thyroid nodules-A meta-analysis. Eur J Radiol. 2015;84:2181–6.
80. Lin P, Chen M, Liu B, Wang S, Li X. Diagnostic performance of shear wave elastography in the identification of malignant thyroid nodules: a meta-analysis. Eur Radiol. 2014;24:2729–38.
81. Zhang YF, Xu HX, He Y, Liu C, Guo LH, Liu LN, Xu JM. Virtual touch tissue quantification of acoustic radiation force impulse: a new ultrasound elastic imaging in the diagnosis of thyroid nodules. PLoS One. 2012;7:e49094.
82. Rago T, Scutari M, Santini F, et al. Real-time elastosonography: useful tool for refining the presurgical diagnosis in thyroid nodules with indeterminate or nondiagnostic cytology. J Clin Endocrinol Metab. 2010;95(12):5274–80.
83. Xu JM, Xu HX, Xu XH, Liu C, Zhang YF, Guo LH, Liu LN, Zhang J. Solid hypo-echoic thyroid nodules on ultrasound: the diagnostic value of acoustic radiation force impulse elastography. Ultrasound Med Biol. 2014;40:2020–30.
84. Bojunga J, Dauth N, Berner C, et al. Acoustic radiation force impulse imaging for differentiation of thyroid nodules. PLoS One. 2012;7(8):e42735.
85. Tatar IG, Kurt A, Yilmaz KB, Akinci M, Kulacoglu H, Hekimoglu B. The learning curve of real time elastosonography: a preliminary study conducted for the assessment of malignancy risk in thyroid nodules. Med Ultrason. 2013;15:278–84.
86. Hegedüs L. Can elastography stretch our understanding of thyroid histomorphology? J Clin Endocrinol Metab. 2010;95(12):5213–5.

8 Carotid Artery

Dirk-André Clevert

Stroke is the third leading cause of death after ischaemic heart disease and cancer [1]. Atherosclerosis may affect the intracranial vessels themselves; 88 % of patients with amaurosis fugax or hemispheric transient ischemic attacks have atherosclerotic disease at the carotid bifurcation [2].

Approximately 25–50 % of all strokes are caused by an unstable carotid artery plaque and about 80 % of all strokes are ischaemic [3, 4].

A reliable differentiation of a high-grade stenosis, pseudo-occlusion or occlusion in preoperative diagnostics is relevant for the therapy of internal carotid artery (ICA) stenoses [5–11].

The results of the "North American Symptomatic Carotid Endarterectomy Trial" (NASCET) and the "European Carotid Surgery Trial" (ECST) [12, 13] have shown that symptomatic patients with high-grade (70–90 %) stenoses of the internal carotid artery (ICA) do profit from carotid endarterectomy (CEA). In the guidelines of the American Heart Association and the Executive Committee for the Asymptomatic Carotid Atherosclerosis Study [14, 15], CEA is also recommended as the method of choice for the treatment of asymptomatic patients with high-grade stenoses of the ICA.

However, whilst surgical endarterectomy or stenting treatment of a carotid artery stenosis can significantly reduce stroke risk, 3–9 % of patients undergoing interventional treatment are expected to suffer stroke or death as a complication from such a treatment. Patient that undergoes carotid stenting has a higher risk for major complications than patients with carotid endarterectomy [15].

A well-established non-invasive method of assessment of carotid diseases is colour and spectral Doppler ultrasound for the primary examination of the extracranial carotid arterial systems [17, 18]. Doppler ultrasound however has some limitations and does not always provide a full diagnostic assessment in the differentiation of critical stenosis from complete occlusion when the Duplex ultrasound study is suboptimal [19–26].

At the moment there are only a limited papers published regarding the use of tissue strain analytics measurement in vascular disease [26–29].

D.-A. Clevert
Department of Clinical Radiology,
Interdisciplinary Ultrasound-Center,
University of Munich-Grosshadern Campus,
Marchioninistr. 15, 81377 Munich, Germany
e-mail: Dirk.Clevert@med.uni-muenchen.de

D.-A. Clevert et al. (eds.), *Atlas of Elastosonography*, DOI 10.1007/978-3-319-44201-3_8

8.1 Image Gallery

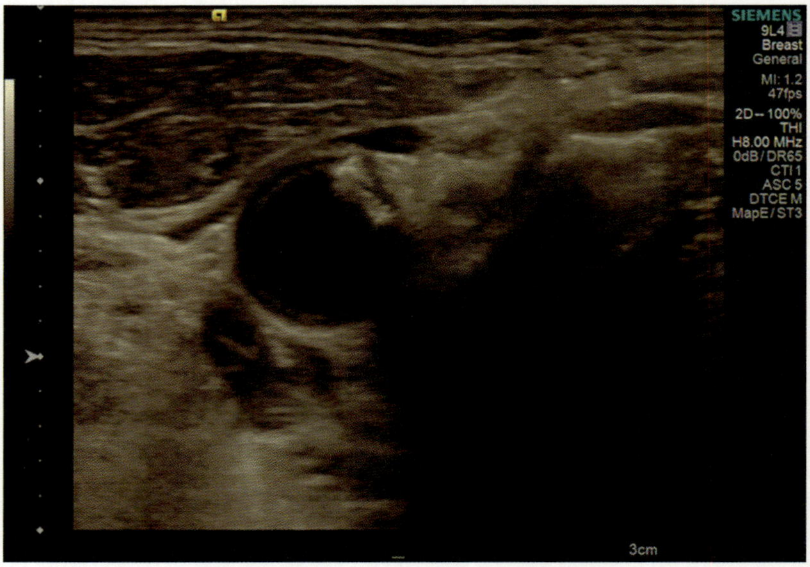

Fig. 8.1 68-year-old male patient with recent ischaemic neurological symptoms, B-scan shows a hard plaque of the common carotid artery (CCA)

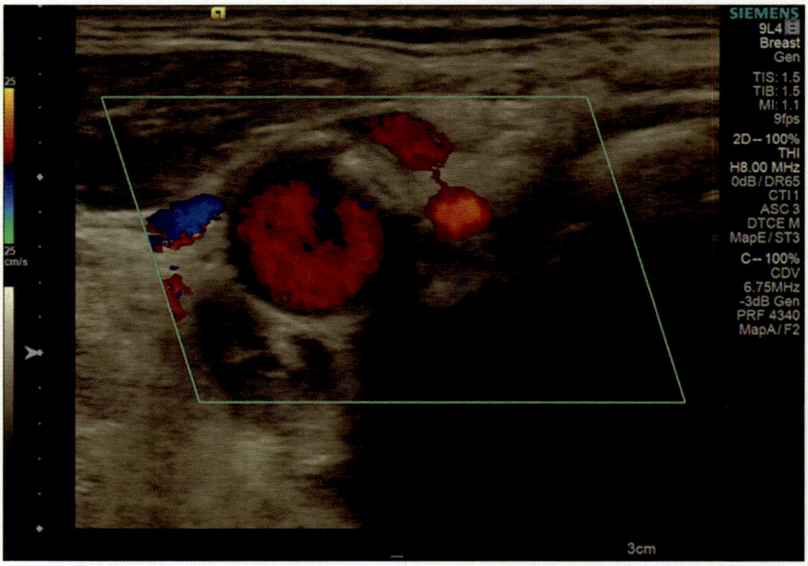

Fig. 8.2 Duplex ultrasonography depicted no high-degree stenosis of the CCA

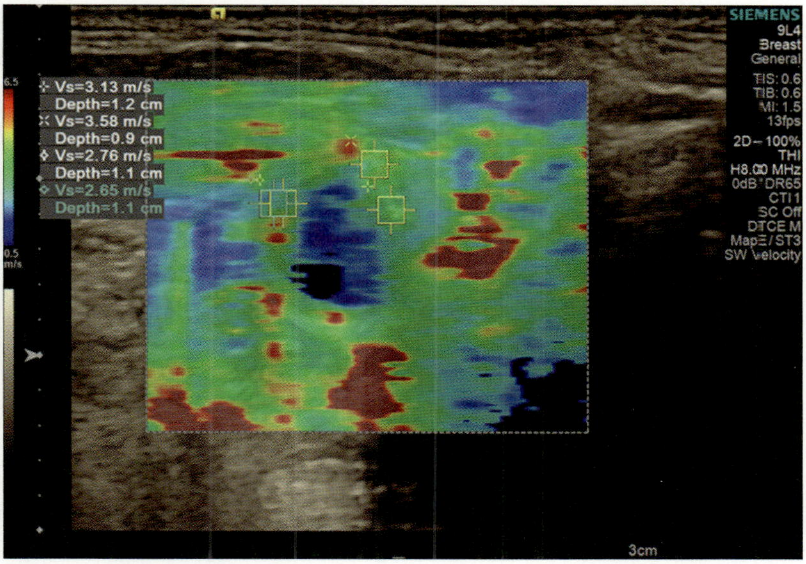

Fig. 8.3 VTIQ velocity colour overlay displayed relative shear wave velocities according to the adjacent colour spectrum, *red areas* corresponding to higher values and *blue areas* corresponding to lower values. Shear wave velocity was measured in the plaque between $v = 3.13$ and 3.58 m/s

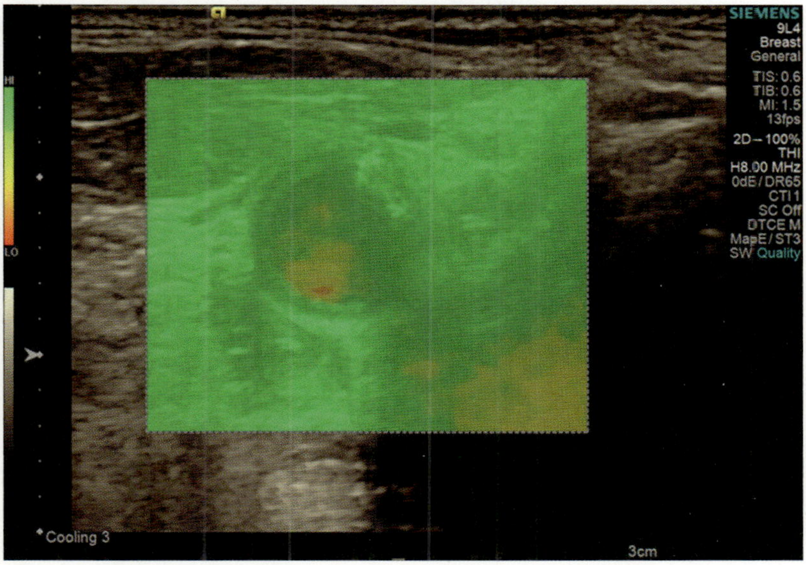

Fig. 8.4 Same patient as Fig. 8.3. The low-quality shear wave signal area representing the fluid parts of the carotid artery in *dark yellow*, the background tissue provides a high-quality signal as indicated by *green area* in the shear wave quality display in the same image

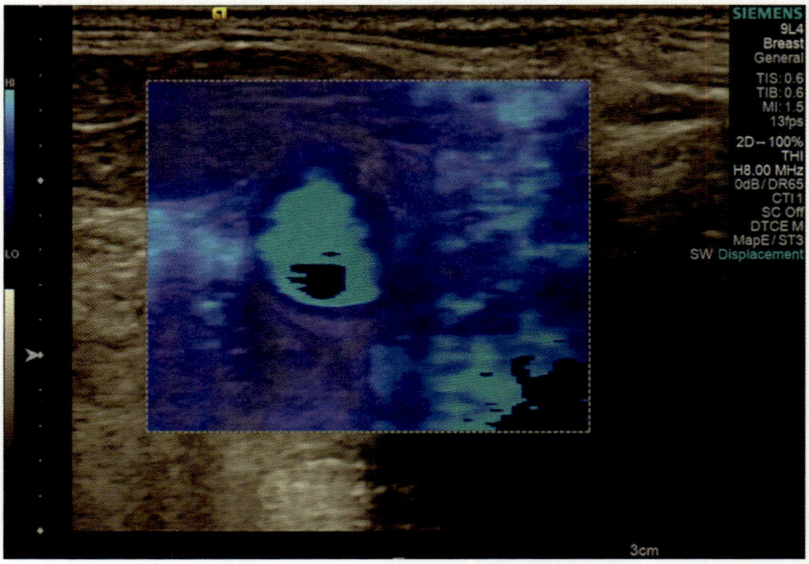

Fig. 8.5 Same lesion as Figs. 8.3 and 8.4. VTIQ displacement mode showed a low deformation of the plaque displayed as *dark blue*

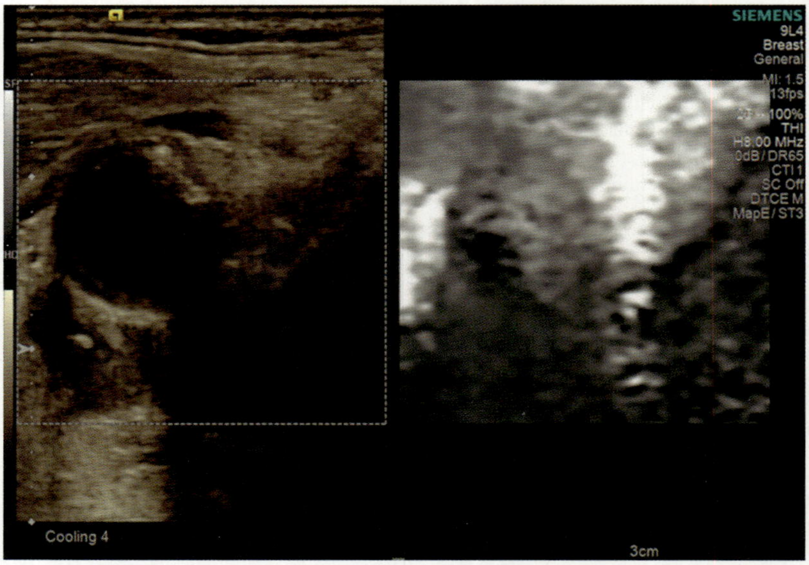

Fig. 8.6 In VTI mode elastography, the plaque appears in *dark grey* as an indicator for stiff tissue

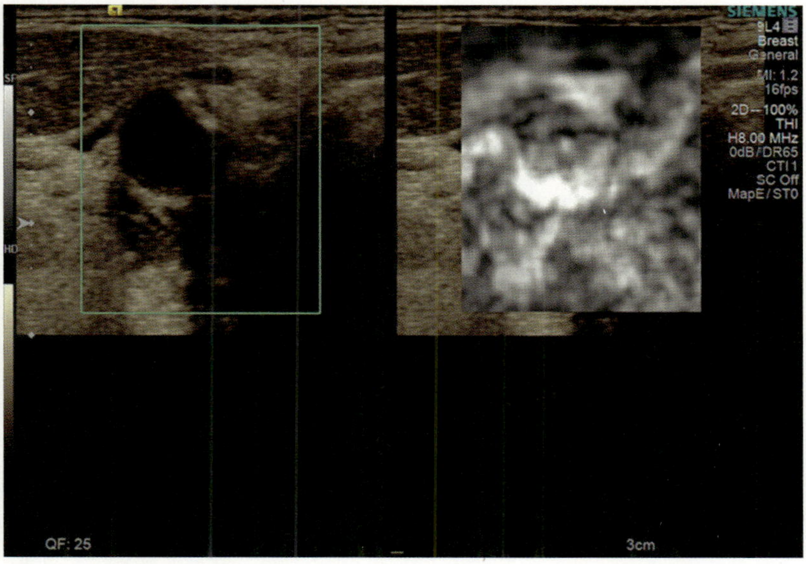

Fig. 8.7 In sonoelastography, the plaque appears in *dark grey* as an indicator for a stiff tissue and confirmed the finding from Fig. 8.6

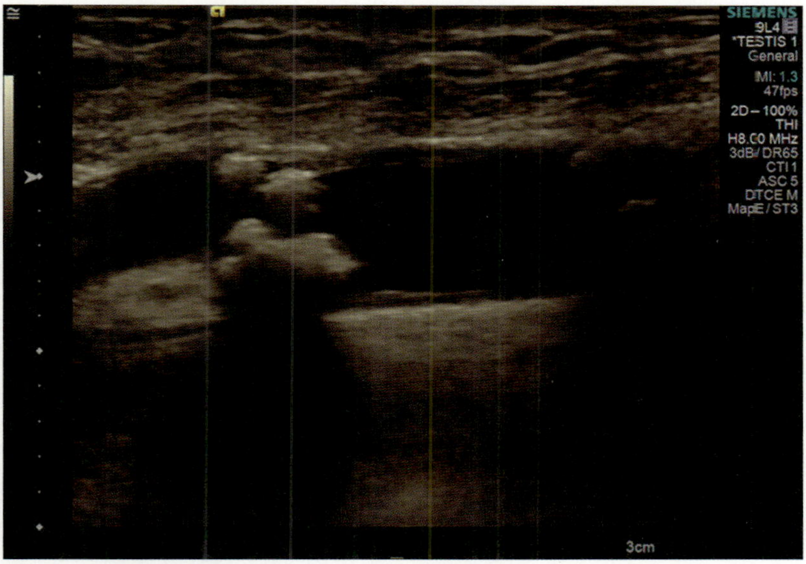

Fig. 8.8 75-year-old male patient with recent ischaemic neurological symptoms. B-scan shows a high-degree internal carotid artery (ICA) stenosis with hard plaques on both sides of the vessel

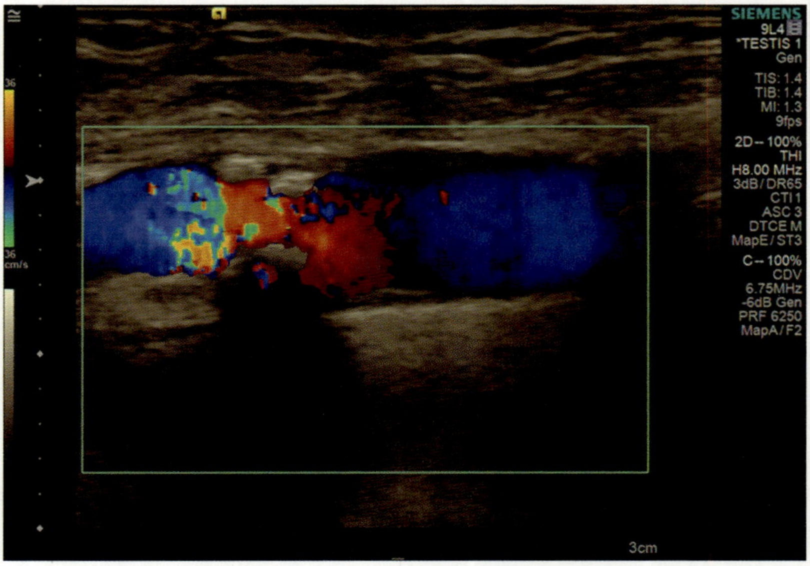

Fig. 8.9 Duplex ultrasonography depicted a high-degree stenosis of the ICA with overwriting artefacts of the vessel wall

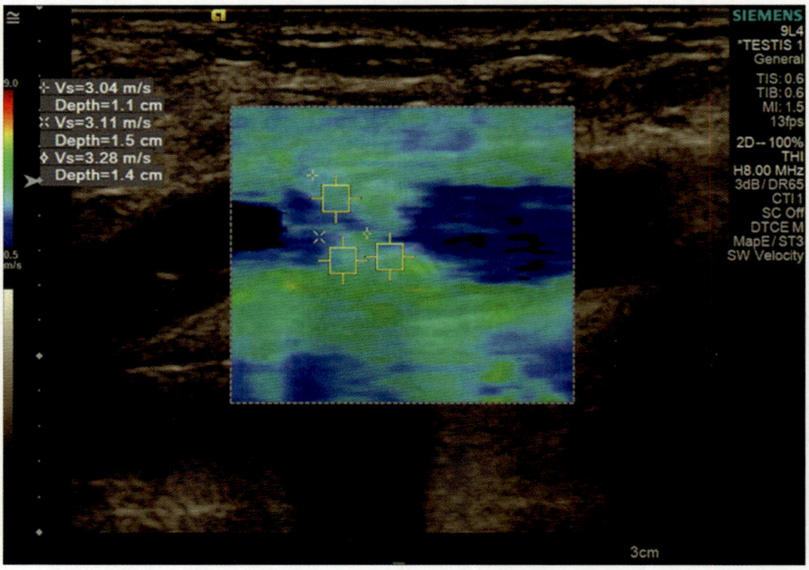

Fig. 8.10 VTIQ velocity colour overlay displayed relative shear wave velocities according to the adjacent colour spectrum, *red areas* corresponding to higher values and *blue areas* corresponding to lower values. Shear wave velocity was measured in the plaques on both vessel walls between $v = 3.04$ and 3.28 m/s

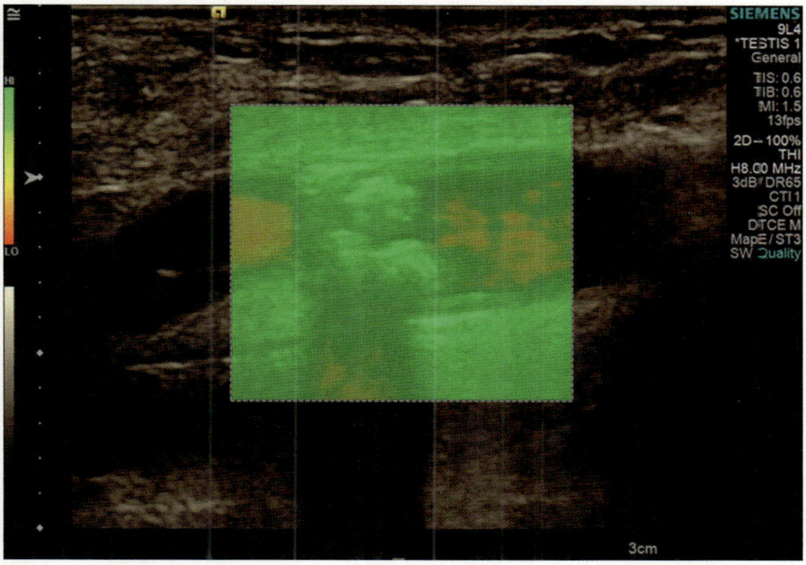

Fig. 8.11 Same lesion as Fig. 8.10. The low-quality shear wave signal area representing the fluid parts of the vessel coded in *yellow*, the background tissue and the plaques provide a high-quality signal as indicated by *green area* in the shear wave quality display

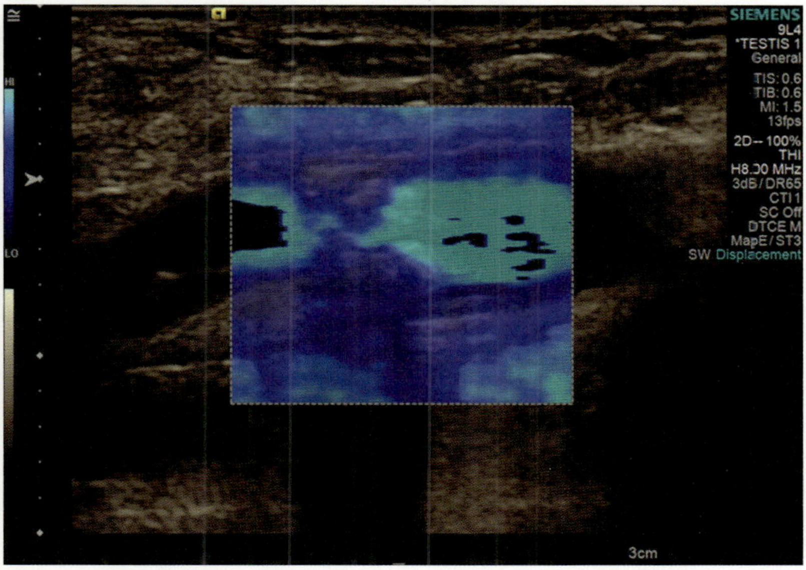

Fig. 8.12 Same lesion as Figs. 8.10 and 8.11. VTIQ displacement mode showed a low deformation of the plaques displayed as *dark blue* and depicted the residual lumen of the high-degree stenosis

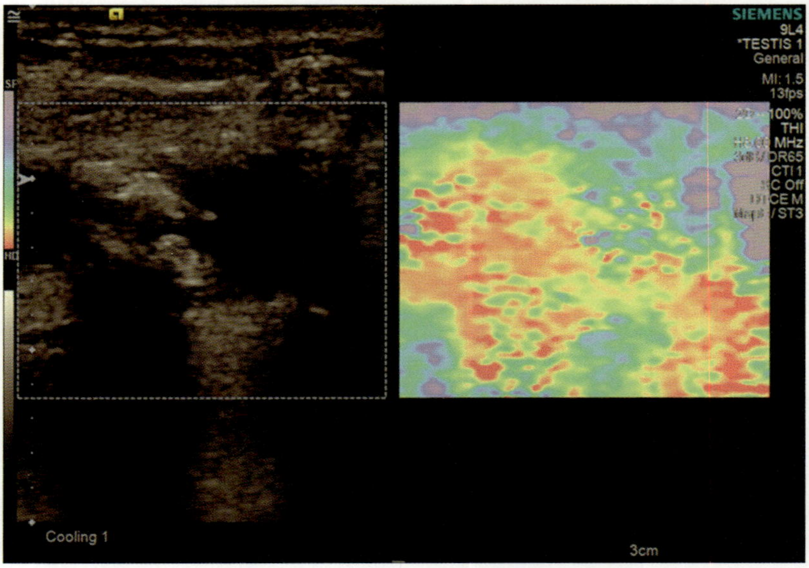

Fig. 8.13 In VTI mode elastography, the plaques appear in *red*, as an indicator for stiff tissue

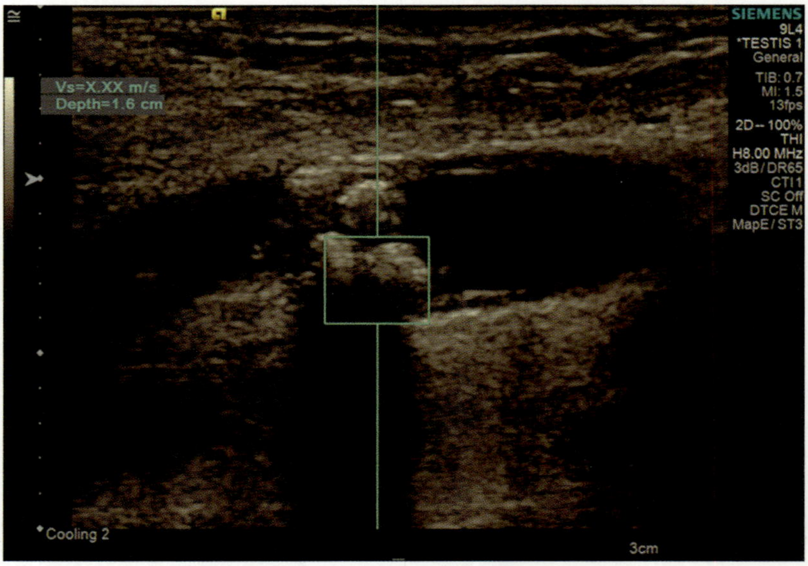

Fig. 8.14 In VTQ mode, the shear wave velocity could not be measured in the plaque $v = XXX$ m/s

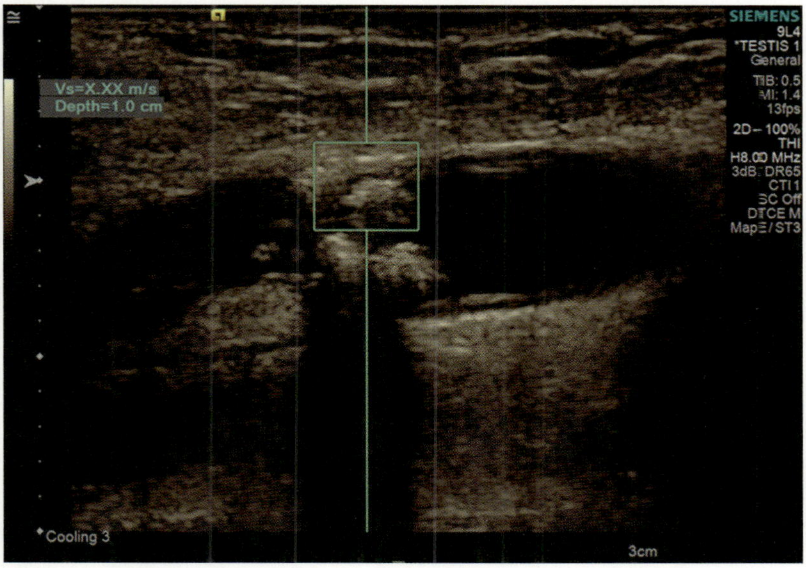

Fig. 8.15 In VTQ mode, the shear wave velocity was measured in the ventral carotid wall; no velocity could be measured *v* = XXX m/s

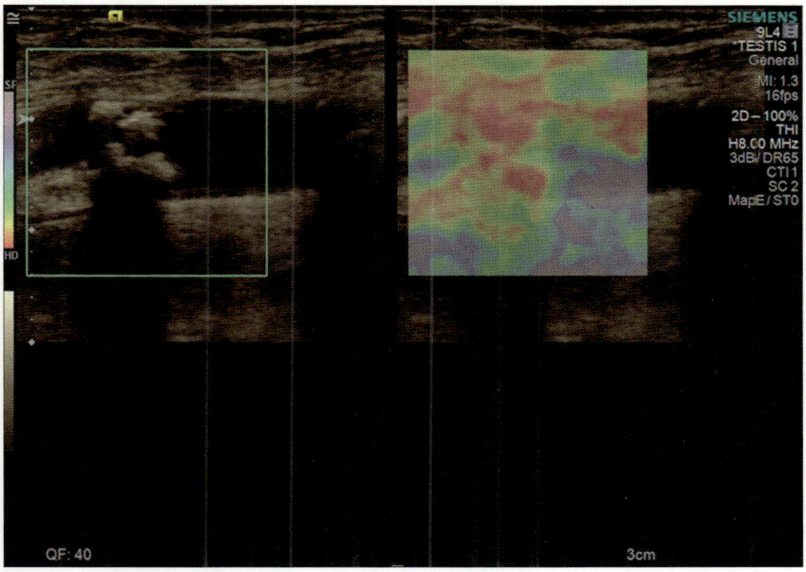

Fig. 8.16 In sonoelastography, the plaques appear in *dark red* as an indicator for a very stiff tissue. The borders of the plaques are displayed well in this technique

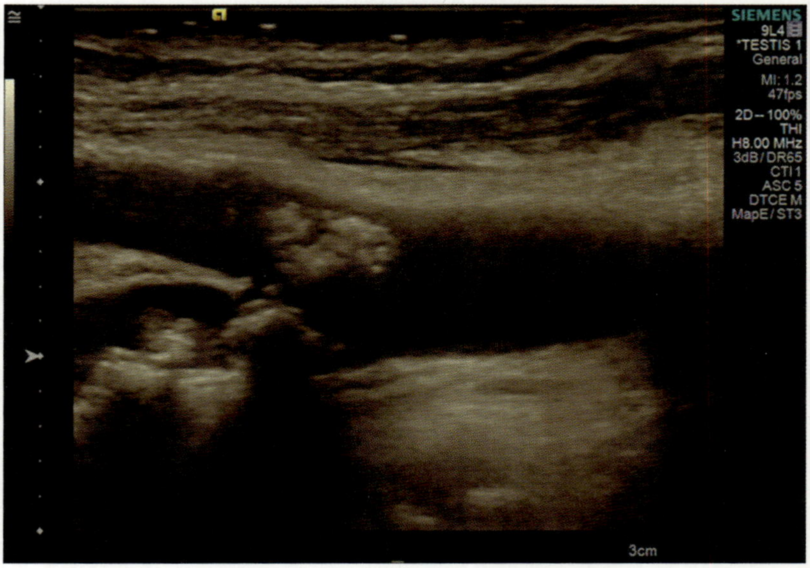

Fig. 8.17 67-year-old woman patient with ischaemic neurological symptoms. B-scan shows a high-degree internal carotid artery (ICA) and external carotid artery (ECA) stenosis with hard plaques on both vessel walls

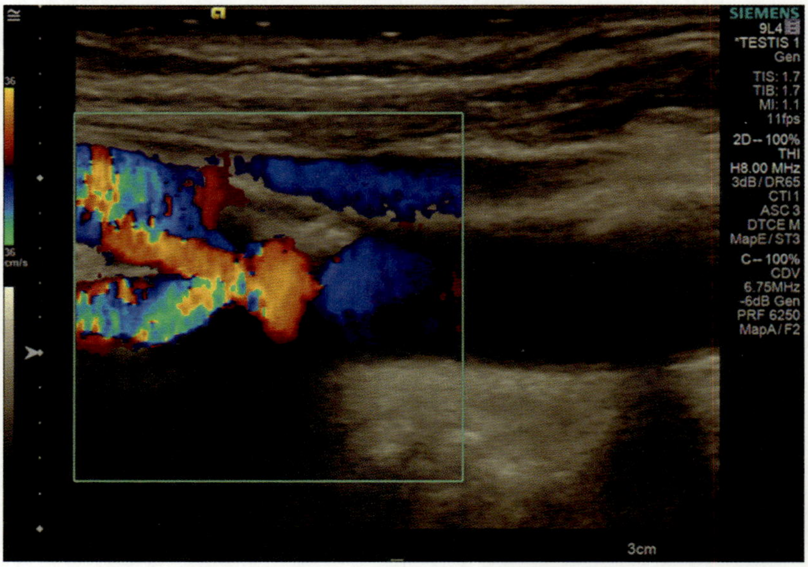

Fig. 8.18 Duplex ultrasonography depicted a high-degree stenosis of the internal carotid artery (*ICA*) and external carotid artery (*ECA*) stenosis with hard plaques

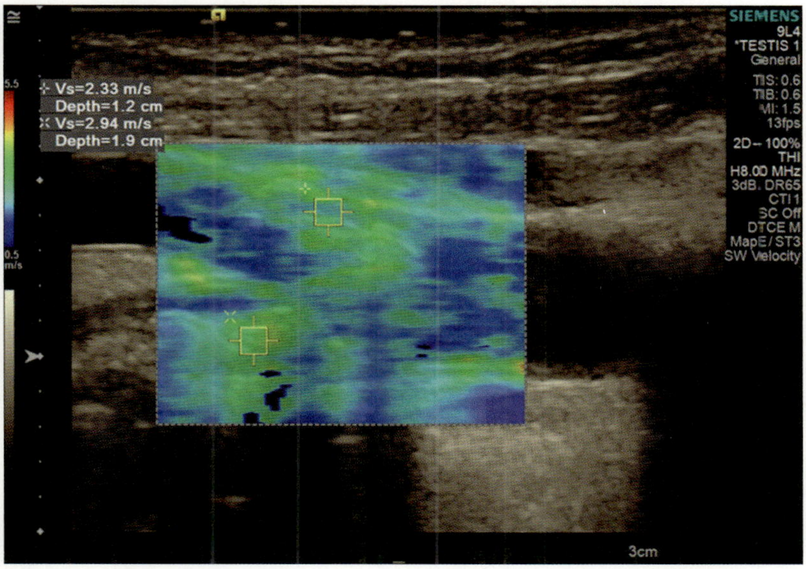

Fig. 8.19 VTIQ velocity colour overlay displayed relative shear wave velocities according to the adjacent colour spectrum, *red areas* corresponding to higher values and *blue areas* corresponding to lower values. Shear wave velocity was measured in the plaques between $v = 2.33$ and 2.94 m/s

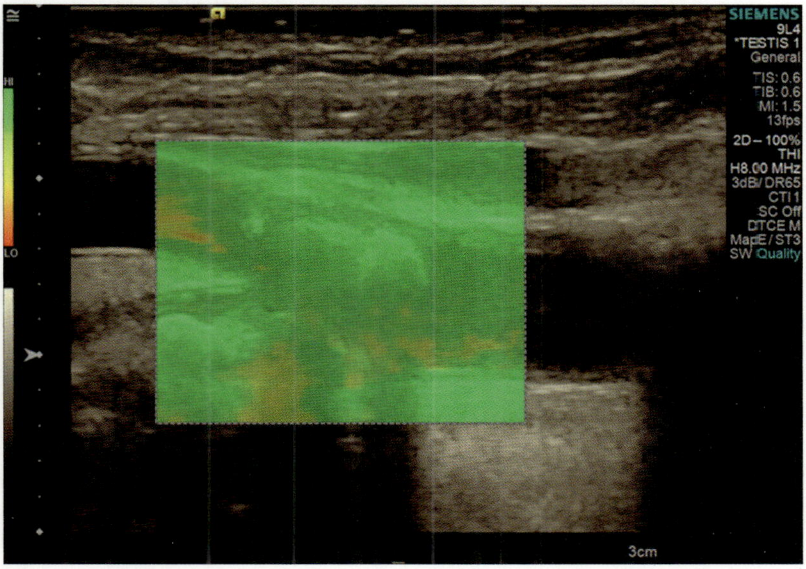

Fig. 8.20 Same lesion as Fig. 8.19. Most of the plaques are coloured in *green*, as an indicator for a high quality of generated shear waves

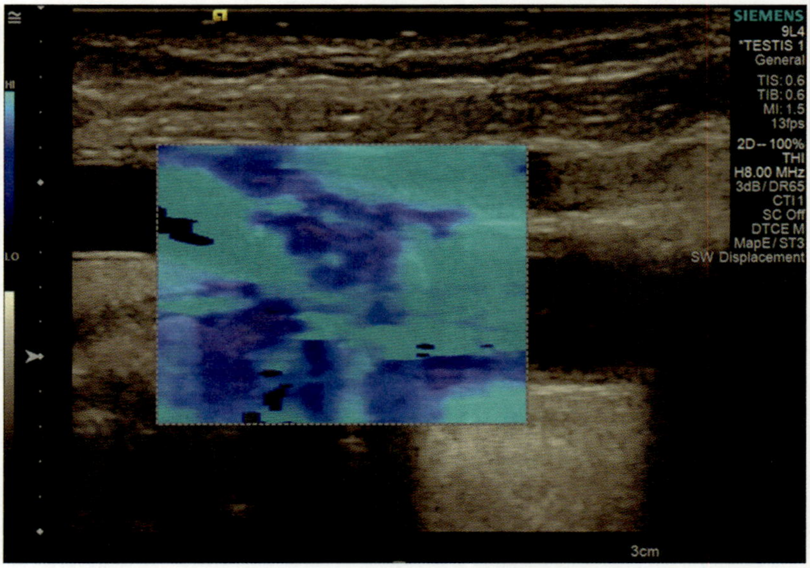

Fig. 8.21 Same lesion as Figs. 8.19 and 8.20. VTIQ displacement mode showed a low deformation of the plaques displayed as *dark blue*

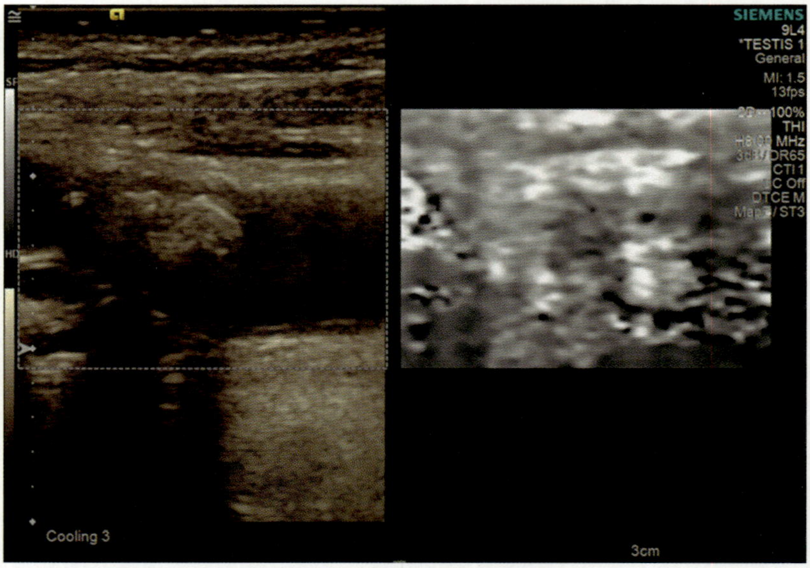

Fig. 8.22 In VTI mode elastography, the plaques appear in *dark grey*, as an indicator for stiff tissue

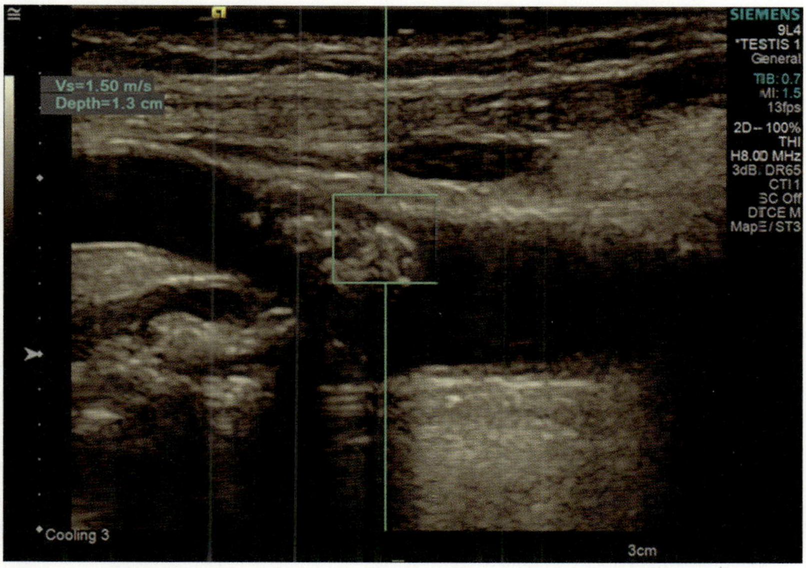

Fig. 8.23 In VTQ mode, the shear wave velocity was measured in the ventral carotid plaque with a velocity of $v = 1.50$ m/s

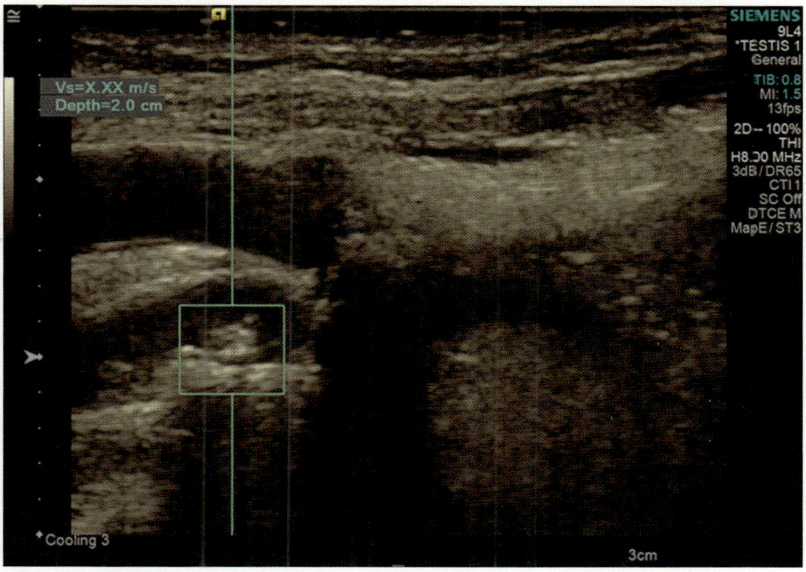

Fig. 8.24 In VTQ mode, no velocity could be measured in the dorsal carotid plaque $v = \text{XXX}$ m/s

References

1. World Health Organization (WHO). The atlas of heart disease and stroke. http://www.who.int/cardiovascular_diseases/en/cvd_atlas_16_death_from_stroke.pdf.
2. Eisenberg RL, Nemzek WR, Moore WS, et al. Relationship of transient ischemic attack and angiographically demonstrable lesions of carotid artery. Stroke. 1977;8:483–6.
3. Adams HP, Bendixen BH, Kapelle LJ, et al. Classification of subtype of acute ischemic stroke. Definitions for use in a multicenter clinical trial. TOAST. Trial of ORG 10172 in acute stroke treatment. Stroke. 1993;24(1):35e41.
4. Hermus L, van Dam GM, Zeebregts CJ. Advanced carotid plaque imaging. Eur J Vasc Endovasc Surg. 2010;39:125e133.
5. North American Symptomatic Carotid Endarterectomy Trial Collaborators. Beneficial effect of carotid endarterectomy in symptomatic patients with high-grade stenosis. N Engl J Med. 1991;325:445–52.
6. European Carotid Surgery Trialists Collaborative Group. Risk of stroke in the distribution of an asymptomatic carotid artery. Lancet. 1995;345:445–53.
7. Hetzel A, Eckenweber B, Trummer B, et al. Colour-coded duplex sonography of preocclusive carotid stenoses. Eur J Ultrasound. 1998;8:183–91.
8. Mead GE, Lewis SC, Wardlaw JM. Variability in Doppler ultrasound influences referral of patients for carotid surgery. Eur J Ultrasound. 2000;12:137–43.
9. Schminke U, Motsch L, Hilker L, et al. Three-dimensional ultrasound observation of carotid artery plaque ulceration. Stroke. 2000;31:1651–5.
10. Fürst G, Saleh A, Wenserski F, et al. Reliability and validity of noninvasive imaging of internal carotid artery pseudo-occlusion. Stroke. 1999;30:1444–9.
11. Polak JF. Carotid ultrasound. Radiol Clin North Am. 2001;39:569–89.
12. Saloner D. Determinants of image appearance in contrast – enhanced magnetic resonance angiography. A review. Invest Radiol. 1998;33:488–95.
13. Krinsky GA, Kaminer E, Lee VS, et al. The effects of apnea on timing examinations for optimization of gadolinium – enhanced MRA of the thoracic aorta and arch vessels. J Comput Assist Tomogr. 1998;22:677–81.
14. Executive Committee for the Asymptomatic Carotid Artherosclerosis Study. Endarterectomy for asymptomatic carotid artery stenosis. J Am Med Assoc. 1995;273:1421–8.
15. Moore WS, Barnett HJM, Beebe H. Guidelines for carotid endarterectomy. Circulation. 1995;91:556–79.
16. van der Vaart MG, Meerwaldt R, Reijnen MM, et al. Endarterectomy or carotid artery stenting: the quest continues. Am J Surg. 2008;195(2):259–69.
17. Sidhu PS, Allan PL. The extended role of carotid artery ultrasound. Clin Radiol. 1997;52:643–53.
18. Sidhu PS, Allan PL. Ultrasound assessment of internal carotid artery stenosis. Clin Radiol. 1997;52:654–8.
19. Sidhu PS, Allan PL, Cattin F, et al. Diagnostic efficacy of SonoVue, a second generation contrast agent, in the assessment of extracranial carotid or peripheral arteries using colour and spectral Doppler ultrasound: a multicentre study. Br J Radiol. 2006;79:44–51.
20. Clevert DA, Paprottka P, Sommer WH, Helck A, Reiser MF, Zengel P. The role of contrast-enhanced ultrasound in imaging carotid arterial diseases. Semin Ultrasound CT MR. 2013;34(3):204–12.
21. Clevert DA, Sommer WH, Helck A, Reiser M. Duplex and contrast enhanced ultrasound (CEUS) in evaluation of in-stent restenosis after carotid stenting. Clin Hemorheol Microcirc. 2011;48(1):199–208.
22. Clevert DA, Sommer WH, Helck A, Saam T, Reiser M. Improved carotid atherosclerotic plaques imaging with contrast-enhanced ultrasound (CEUS). Clin Hemorheol Microcirc. 2011;48(1):141–8.
23. Clevert DA, Sommer WH, Zengel P, Helck A, Reiser M. Imaging of carotid arterial diseases with contrast-enhanced ultrasound (CEUS). Eur J Radiol. 2011;80(1):68–76.
24. Finkenzeller T, Tacke J, Clevert DA, Jung W, Kubale R, Schreyer A, Feuerbach S, Jung EM. Quantification of extracranial ICA stenoses with vessel ultrasound by CCDS and B-flow in comparison to 64-slice multidector CTA, contrast-enhanced MRA and DSA. Ultraschall Med. 2008;29(3):294–301.
25. Clevert DA, Johnson T, Jung EM, Clevert DA, Flach PM, Strautz TI, Ritter G, Gallegos MT, Kubale R, Becker C, Reiser M. Color Doppler, power Doppler and B-flow ultrasound in the assessment of ICA stenosis: comparison with 64-MD-CT angiography. Eur Radiol. 2007;17(8):2149–59.
26. Clevert DA, Johnson T, Michaely H, Jung EM, Flach PM, Strautz TI, Clevert DA, Reiser M, Schoenberg SO. High-grade stenoses of the internal carotid artery: comparison of high-resolution contrast enhanced 3D MRA, duplex sonography and power Doppler imaging. Eur J Radiol. 2006;60(3):379–86.
27. Widman E, Maksuti E, Amador C, Urban MW, Caidahl K, Larsson M. Shear wave elastography quantifies stiffness in Ex vivo porcine artery with stiffened arterial region. Ultrasound Med Biol. 2016;42(10):2423–35.
28. Widman E, Maksuti E, Larsson D, Urban MW, Bjällmark A, Larsson M. Shear wave elastography plaque characterization with mechanical testing validation: a phantom study. Phys Med Biol. 2015;60(8):3151–74.
29. Ramnarine KV, Garrard JW, Dexter K, Nduwayo S, Panerai RB, Robinson TG. Shear wave elastography assessment of carotid plaque stiffness: in vitro reproducibility study. Ultrasound Med Biol. 2014;40(1):200–9.

Testis

9

Dirk-André Clevert

Ultrasound is a sensitive and accurate technique for the evaluation of testicular abnormalities and is widely accepted as the first-line imaging technique and gold standard for many common and uncommon testicular diseases although it does not provide a histological diagnosis [1–3].

Due to the continuous development of modern ultrasonography such as high-frequency transducers, colour Doppler and real-time elastography, ultrasonography is considered the imaging modality of choice in small parts and scrotal disorders [4–7].

Real-time elastography, also known as strain elastography, was introduced over 20 years ago, enabling non-invasive assessment of the mechanical properties of tissue and imaging the elasticity of biological tissue [8–10].

Real-time elastography has already demonstrated promising value in the detection and differentiation of nodules in the breast, prostate, thyroid gland, and lymph nodes [11–13]. However, there are only a few studies in the literature concerning the efficacy of real-time tissue elastography for scrotal mass evaluation [14–16].

During the use of free-hand real-time elastography, the operator-induced mechanical waves provide only qualitative or semi-quantitative results. Due to this fact, the use of this technique can be subject to a degree of variability.

D.-A. Clevert
Department of Clinical Radiology, Interdisciplinary Ultrasound-Center, University of Munich-Grosshadern Campus, Marchioninistr. 15, 81377 Munich, Germany
e-mail: Dirk.Clevert@med.uni-muenchen.de

The use of less operator-dependent imaging techniques is one of the goals of improving diagnostic performance.

Virtual Touch imaging quantification (VTIQ, Siemens, Erlangen Germany) is a new imaging modality that measures tissue stiffness in real time [7]. It was previously used for the assessment of breast diseases [17–19].

VTIQ, as opposed to free-hand strain elastography, employs automatically generated acoustic radiation force impulses (ARFI) to induce shear waves within the targeted area [17].

The VTIQ technique does not rely on the investigator's ability to apply appropriate mechanical pressure to the tissue. It also overcomes the limitations of traditional strain elastography by offering quantitative information about the examined structures, such as shear wave propagation speed values measured in m/s, and also displays them on a two-dimensional colour-coded map.

Studies performed on the testes have resulted in standard values for healthy testicular tissue showing that the stiffness of healthy tissue varies from pathological tissue, and these studies have presented ARFI as a reliable method of evaluation [20–23]. The higher the shear wave velocity measured, the stiffer the tissue under investigation.

However, since shear waves do not result in a deformation in fluid, we could not obtain any measurements in testicular cysts and thus could confirm the similar findings of Barr and Trottmann et al. [24, 25].

D.-A. Clevert et al. (eds.), *Atlas of Elastosonography*, DOI 10.1007/978-3-319-44201-3_9

9.1 Image Gallery

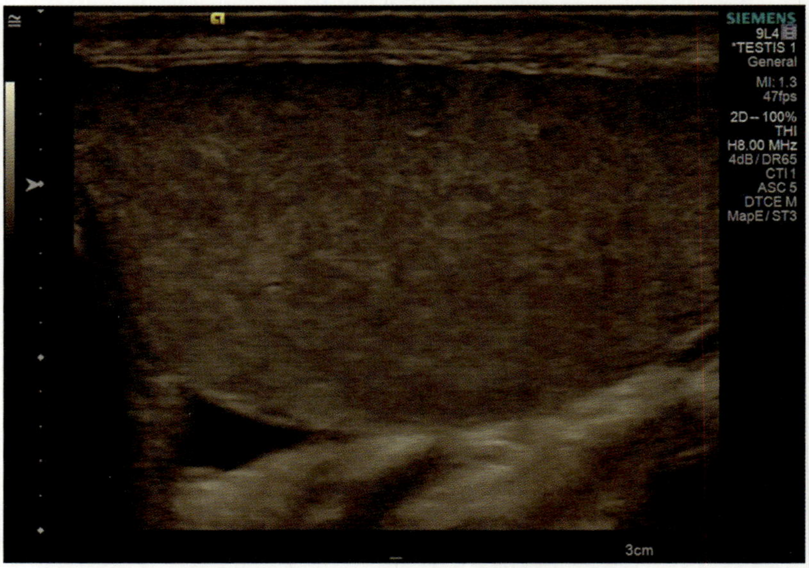

Fig. 9.1 B-mode ultrasound demonstrates normal testicular tissue

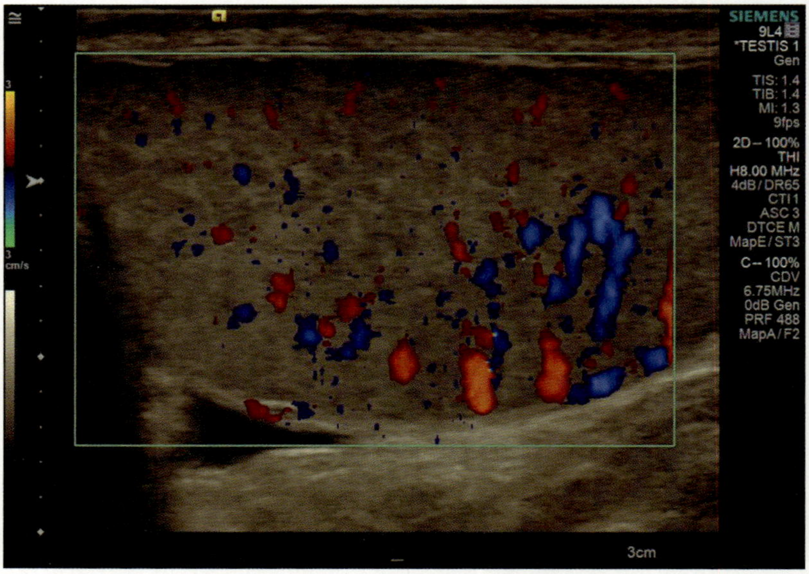

Fig. 9.2 Colour Doppler ultrasound demonstrates internal vascularity of the normal testicular tissue

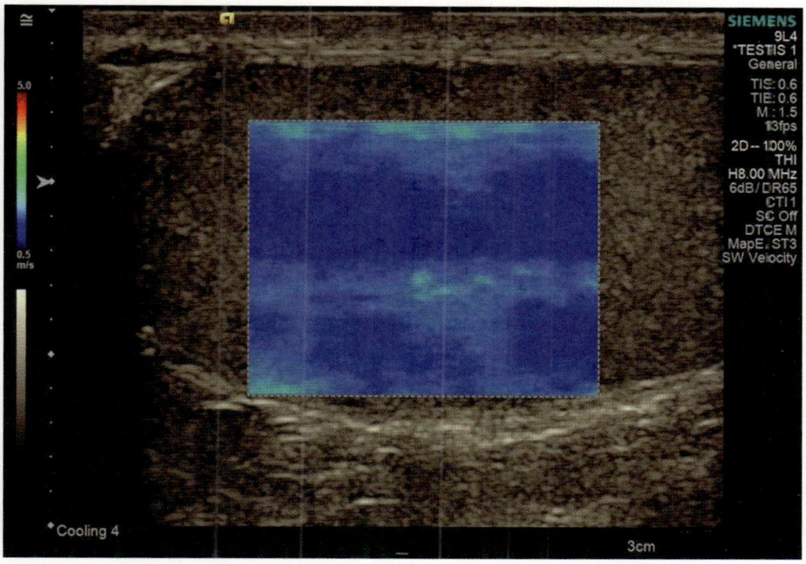

Fig. 9.3 VTIQ velocity colour overlay displays relative shear wave velocities (*SWV*) according to the adjacent colour spectrum, *red areas* corresponding to higher SWV values and *blue areas* corresponding to lower values

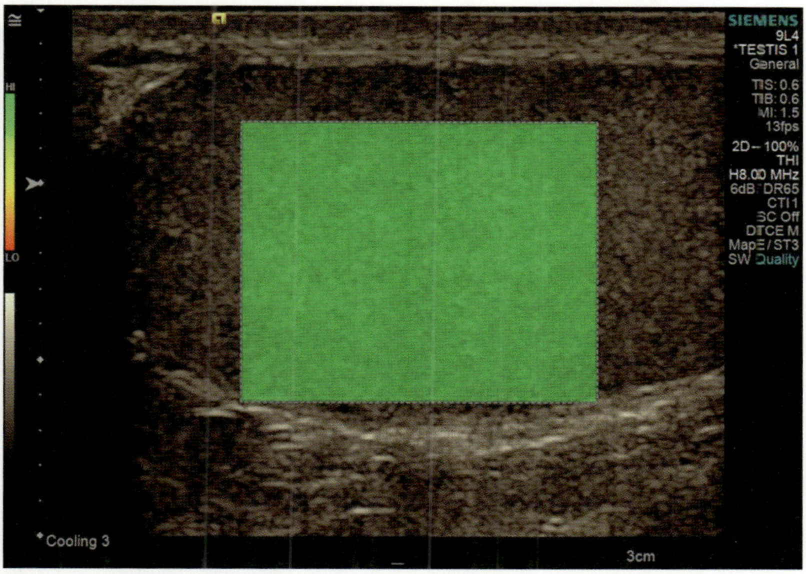

Fig. 9.4 Same lesion as Figs. 9.1, 9.2, and 9.3. Using the VTIQ quality map, the entire testis is coloured *green*, which is an indicator of high-quality generated shear waves

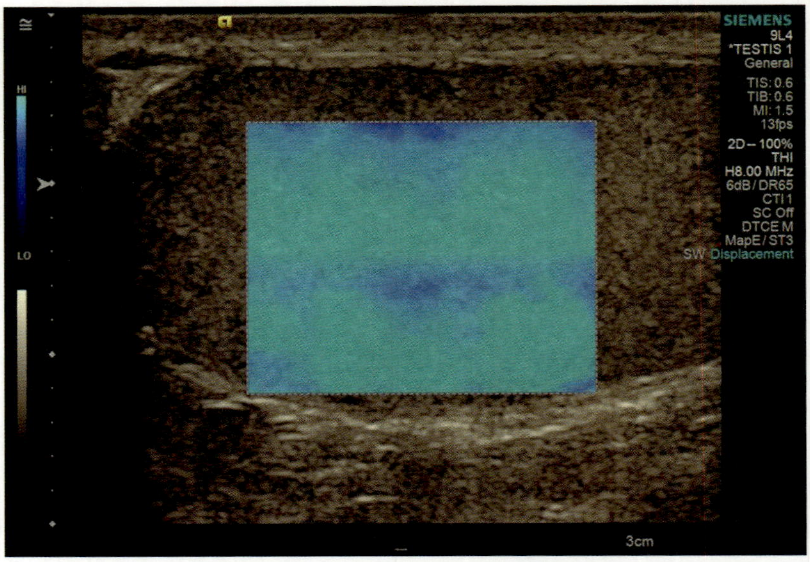

Fig. 9.5 Same lesion as Figs. 9.1, 9.2, 9.3, and 9.4. VTIQ displacement mode shows normal deformation of the testis displayed as *bright blue*

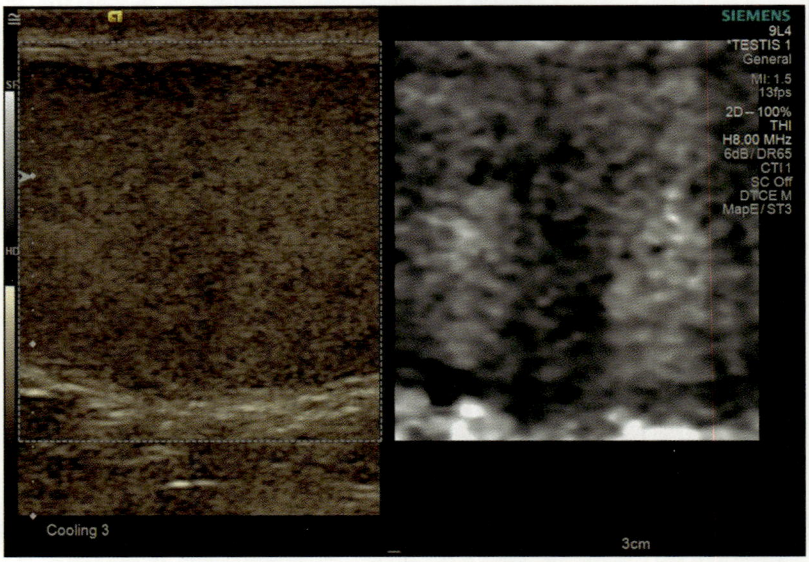

Fig. 9.6 In VTI elastography mode, the testicular tissue appears *grey*, indicating an intermediate stiffness of the tissue

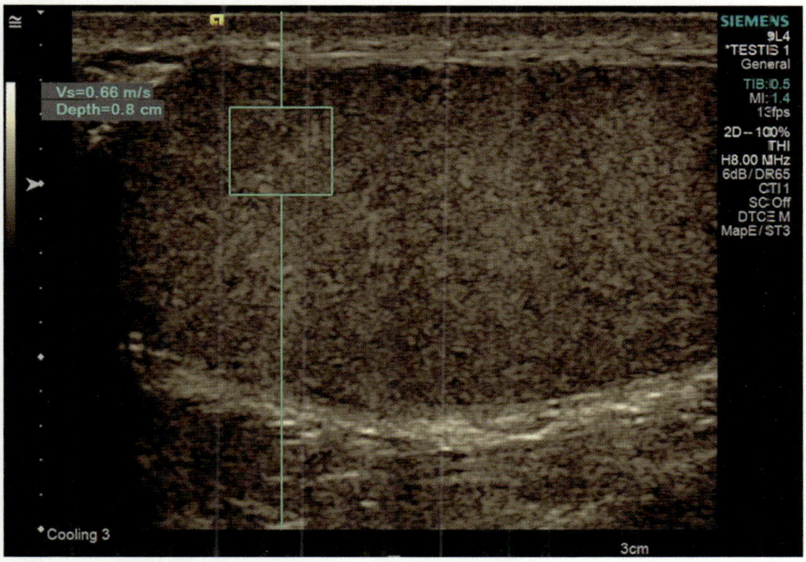

Fig. 9.7 In VTQ mode, the shear wave velocity in the upper pole of the normal testicular tissue was measured with a velocity of $v = 0.66$ m/s

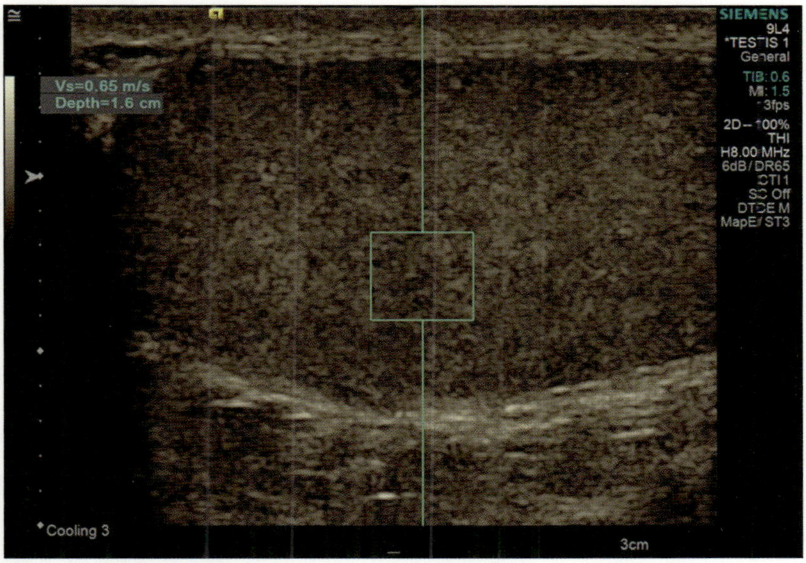

Fig. 9.8 In VTQ mode, the shear wave velocity was measured in the middle of the normal testicular tissue with a velocity of $v = 0.65$ m/s

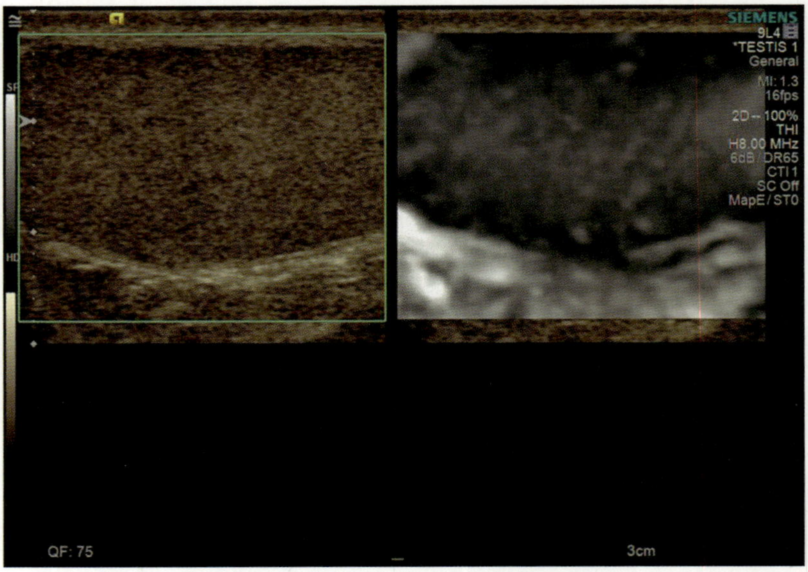

Fig. 9.9 Strain elastogram image shows a homogenous *grey colour*, as indicating normal testicular tissue. The testis has the same size in the strain elastogram mode in comparison to the B-mode

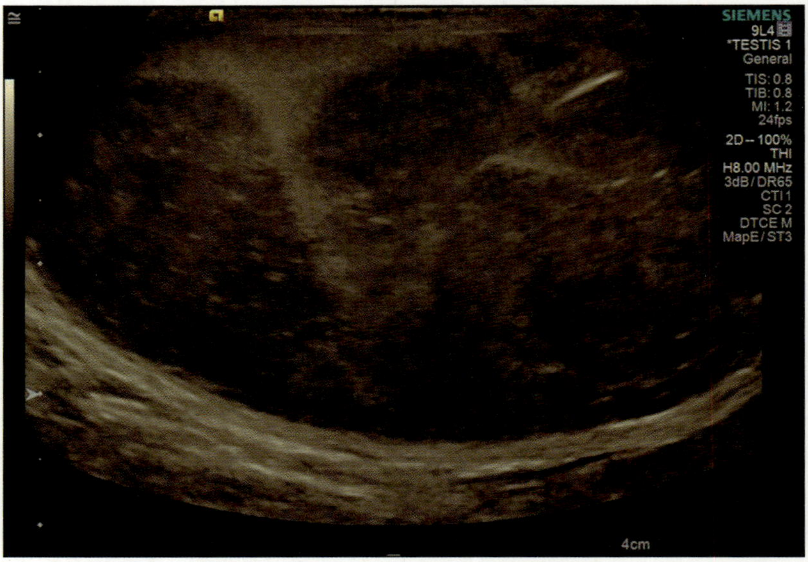

Fig. 9.10 Ultrasound images of a 35-year-old man. B-mode ultrasound demonstrates a huge testicular lesion measuring 55 mm, with uniform low reflectivity. The surgically proven histological diagnosis was a seminoma

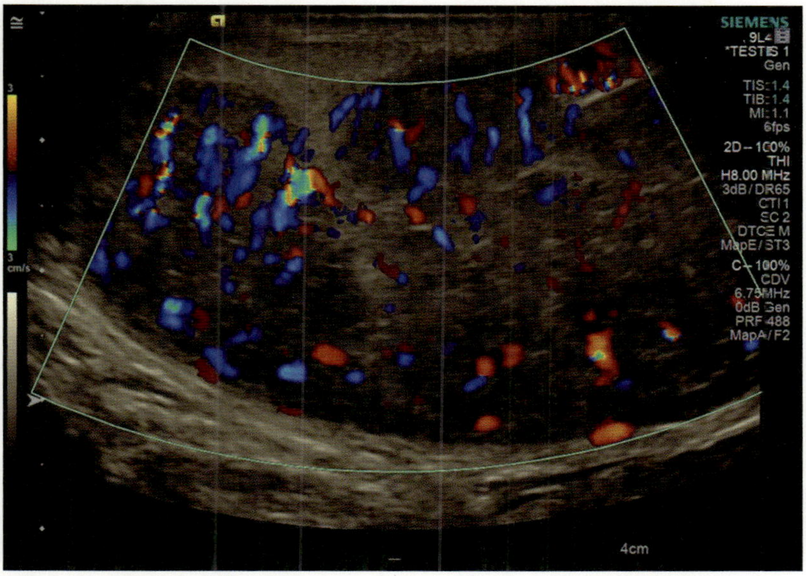

Fig. 9.11 Colour Doppler ultrasound demonstrates a high vascularity within the tumour

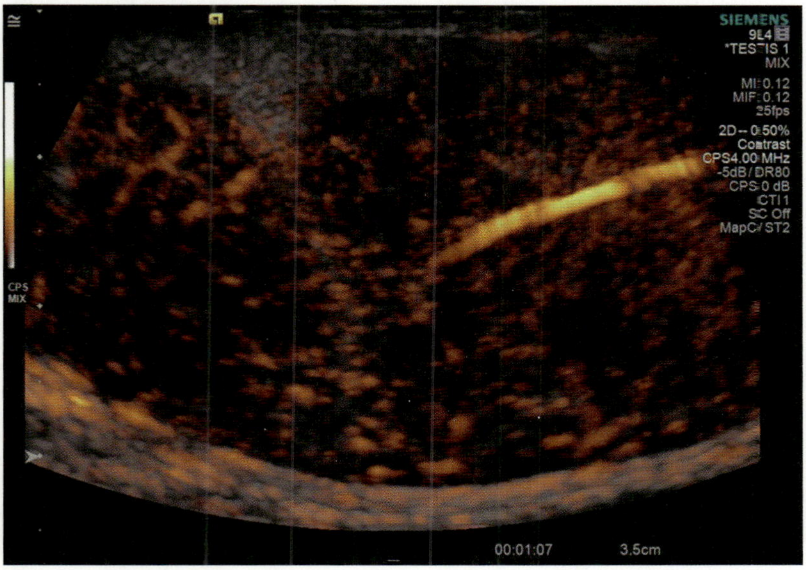

Fig. 9.12 Contrast-enhanced ultrasound confirmed the finding of colour Doppler ultrasound with a high vascularity within the tumour in comparison to the surrounding tissue

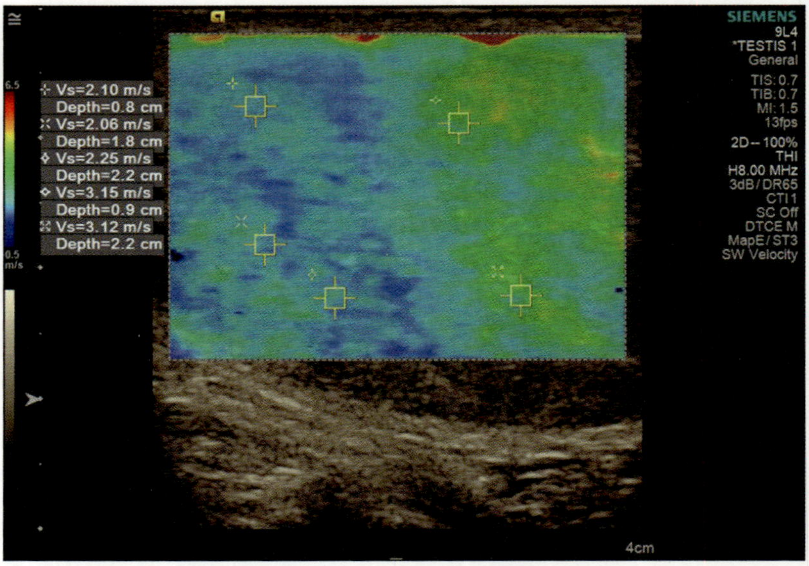

Fig. 9.13 VTIQ velocity colour overlay displayed relative shear wave velocities according to the adjacent colour spectrum, *red areas* corresponding to higher values (stiffer tissue) and *blue areas* corresponding to lower values (softer tissue). Shear wave velocity (*SWV*) was measured in the lesion between $v = 2.06–3.15$ m/s

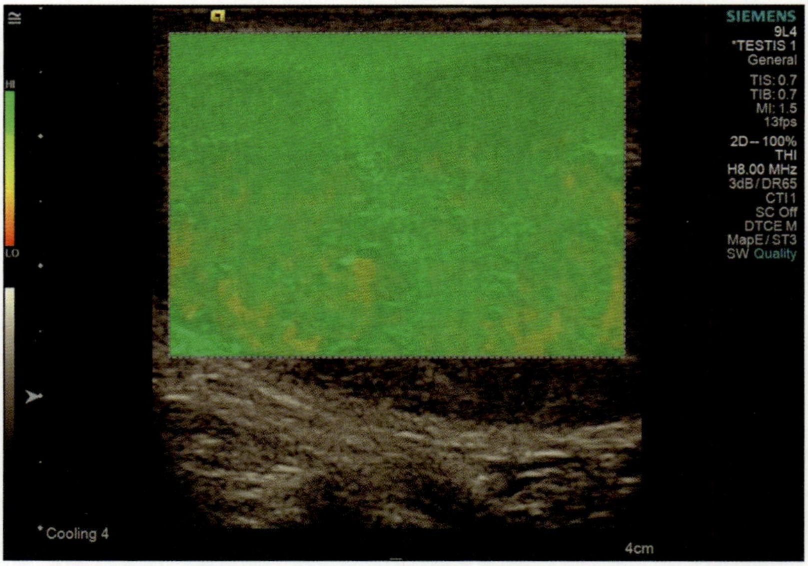

Fig. 9.14 Same lesion as Fig. 9.12. Using the VTIQ quality map, most of the testis and the lesion are coloured *green*, indicating a high quality of generated shear waves

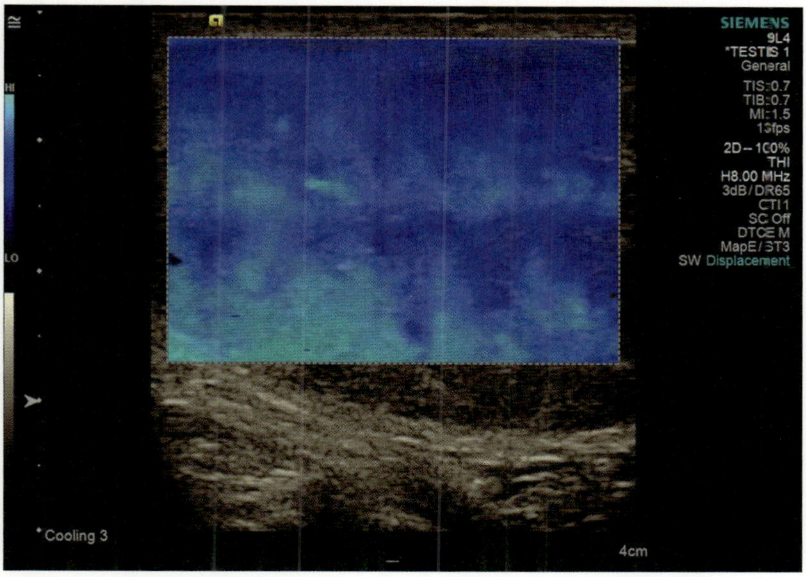

Fig. 9.15 Same lesion as Figs. 9.13 and 9.14. The *dark blue* VTIQ displacement mode indicates reduced deformation of the tumour tissue

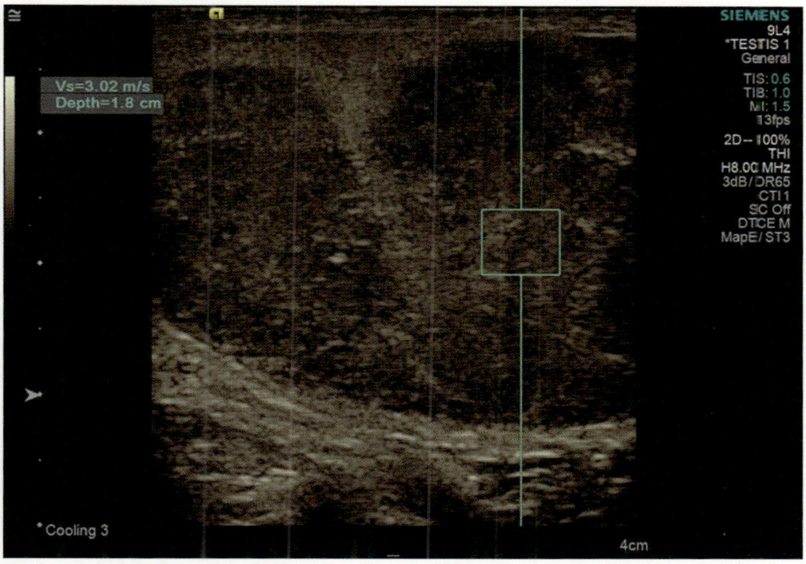

Fig. 9.16 In VTQ mode, the shear wave velocity was measured on the right side of the tumour tissue with a velocity of $v = 3.02$ m/s

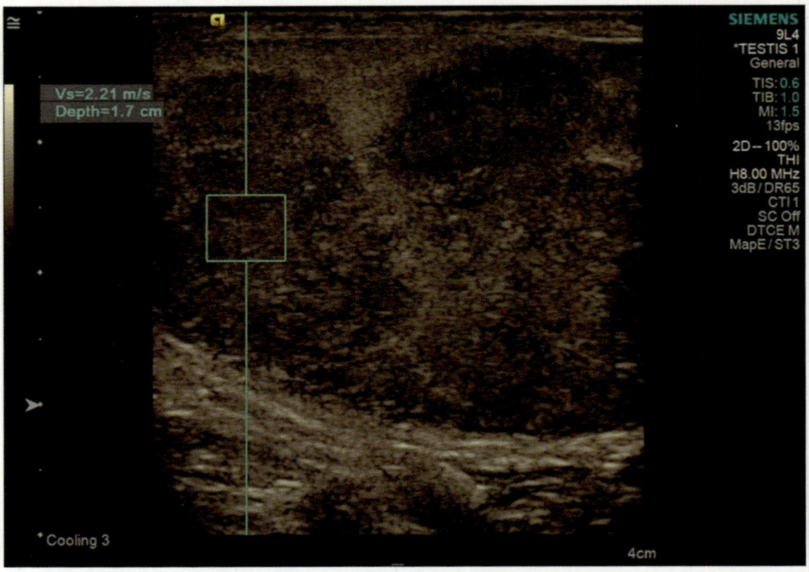

Fig. 9.17 In VTQ mode, the shear wave velocity was measured on the left side of the tumour tissue with a velocity of $v = 2.21$ m/s

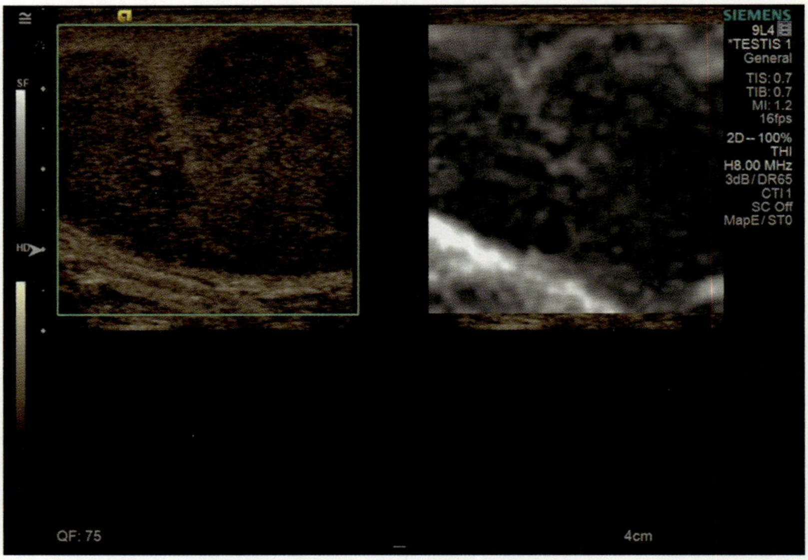

Fig. 9.18 In the strain elastogram, the lesion appears *dark grey*, an indicator of stiff tissue. The border of the lesions is displayed well in this technique

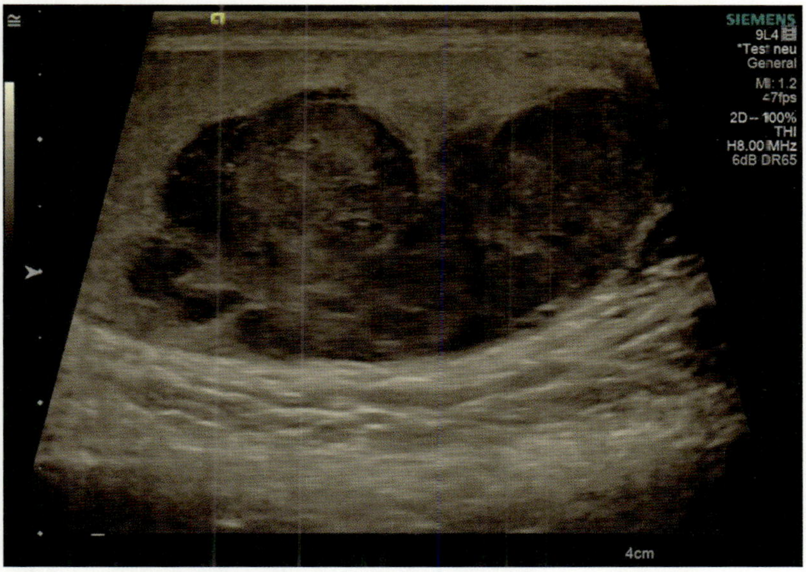

Fig. 9.19 Ultrasound images of a 27-year-old man. B-mode ultrasound demonstrates a hypoechoic lesion. The surgically proven histological diagnosis was a seminoma

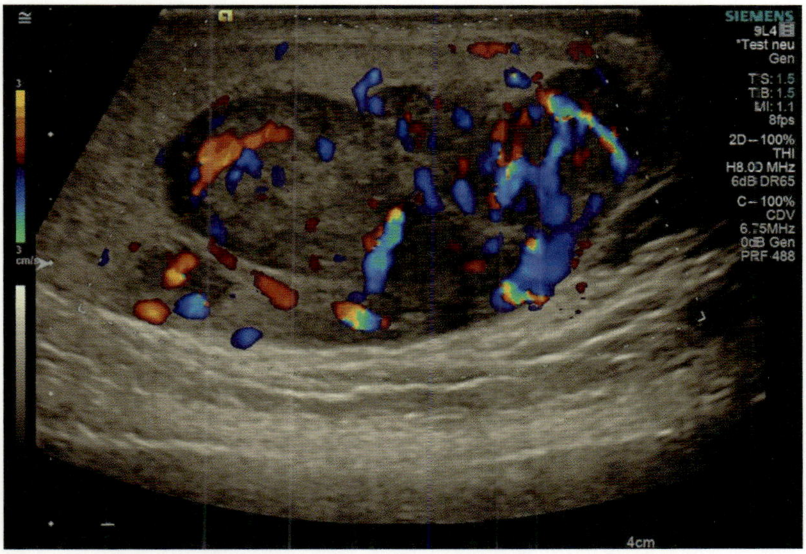

Fig. 9.20 Colour Doppler ultrasound demonstrates a high vascularity within the tumour

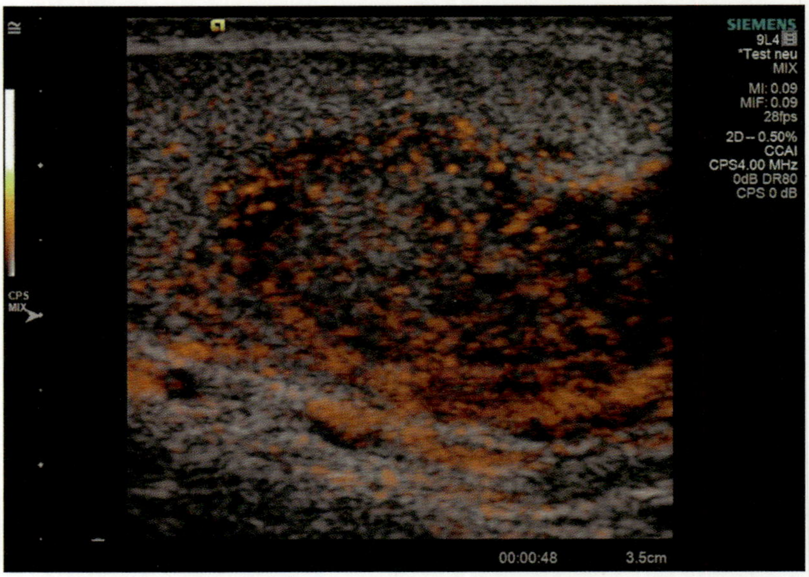

Fig. 9.21 Contrast-enhanced ultrasound confirmed the finding of colour Doppler ultrasound with a high vascularity within the tumour in comparison to the surrounding tissue

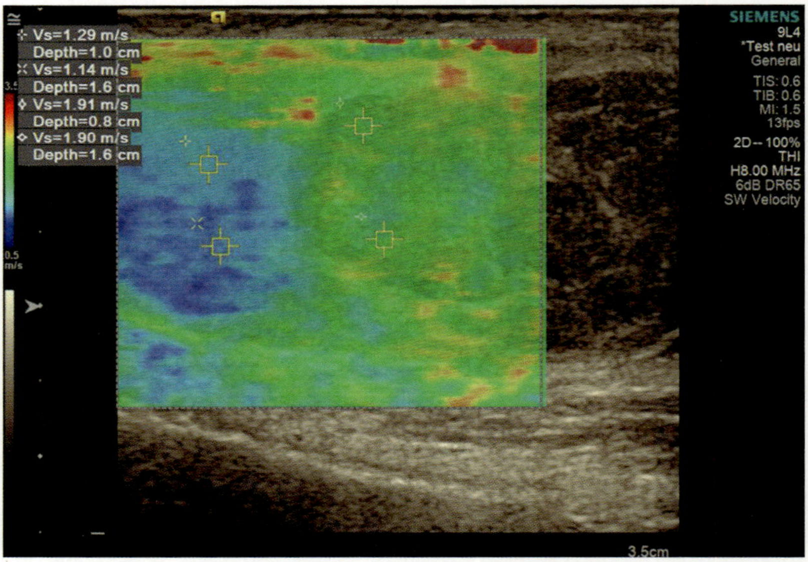

Fig. 9.22 VTIQ velocity colour overlay displayed relative shear wave velocities according to the adjacent colour spectrum, *red areas* corresponding to higher values and *blue areas* corresponding to lower values. Shear wave velocity was measured in the lesion $v = 1.90$–1.91 m/s and in the surrounding tissue level between $v = 1.14$–1.29 m/s

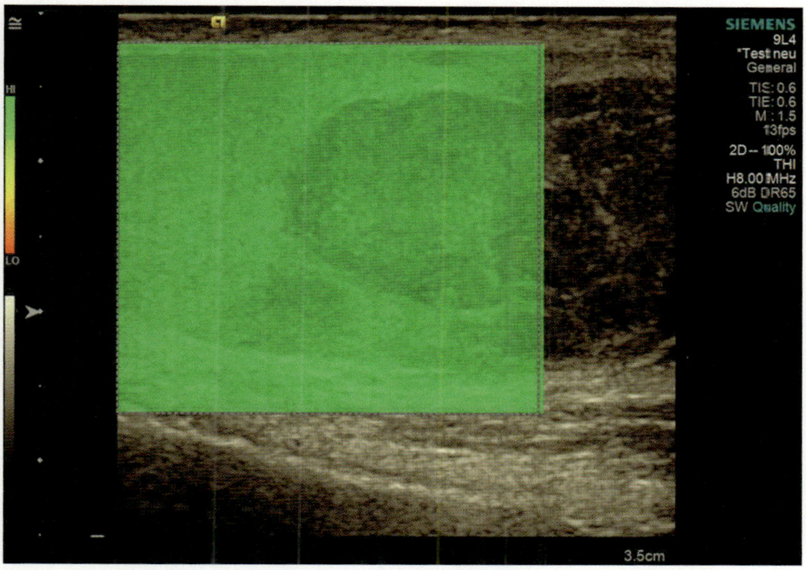

Fig. 9.23 Same lesion as Fig. 9.22. Using the VTIQ quality map, the entire testicular tissue and the lesion are coloured *green*, indicating a high quality of generated shear waves

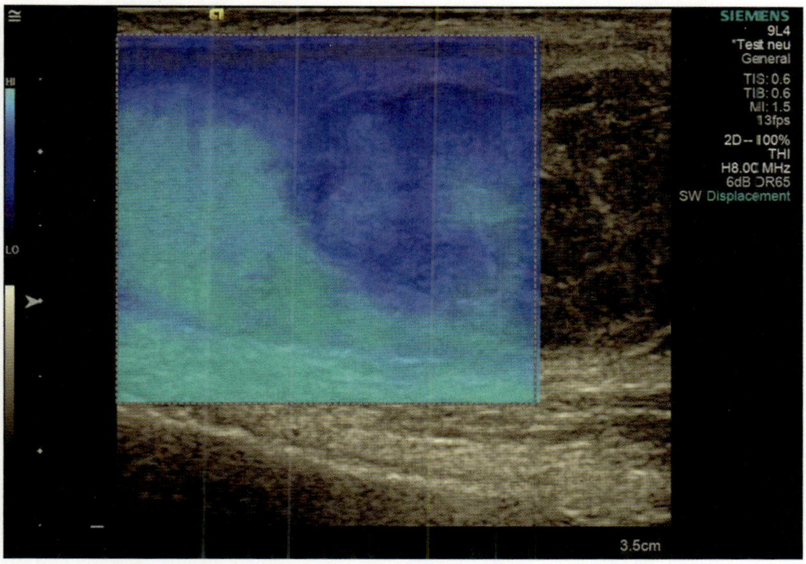

Fig. 9.24 Same lesion as Figs. 9.22 and 9.23. VTIQ displacement mode showed as *dark blue* within the tumour, indicating a low deformation of the tumour tissue in comparison to good displacement of the surrounding tissue as displayed in *bright blue*

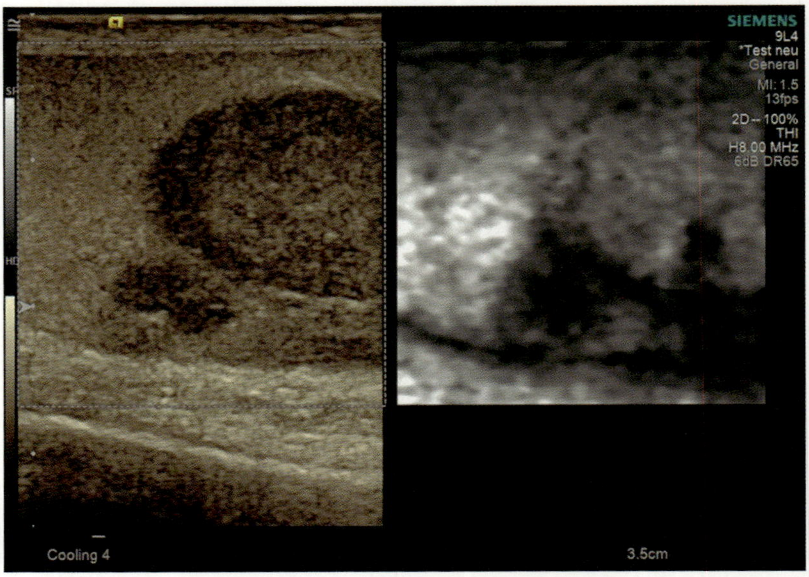

Fig. 9.25 In VTI elastography mode, the tumour appears *dark grey* indicative of a stiff lesion in comparison to the *light grey* display of the normal surrounding tissue

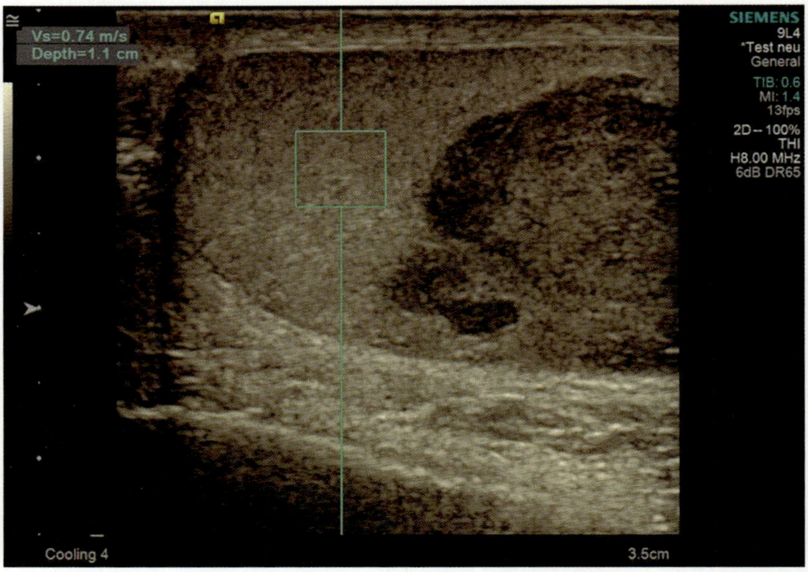

Fig. 9.26 In VTQ mode, the shear wave velocity was measured in the normal tissue with a velocity of $v = 0.74$ m/s

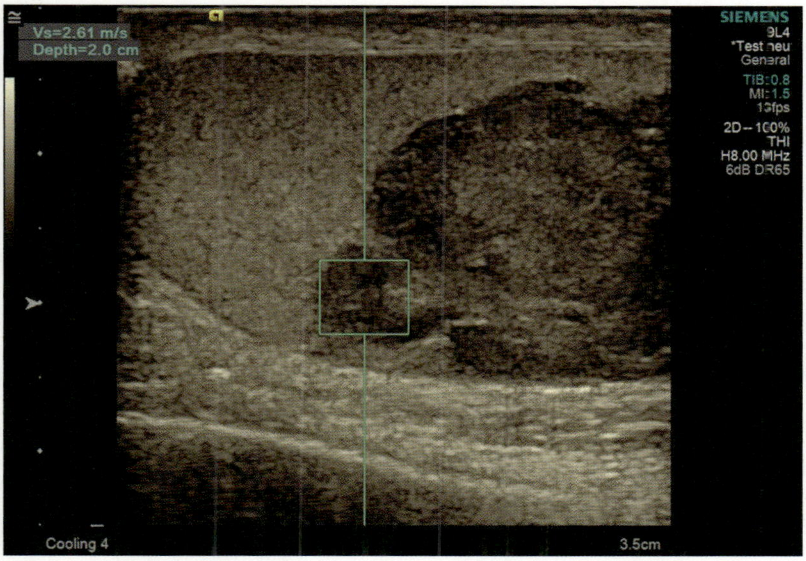

Fig. 9.27 In VTQ mode, the shear wave velocity was measured in the tumour tissue with a velocity of $v = 2.61$ m/s

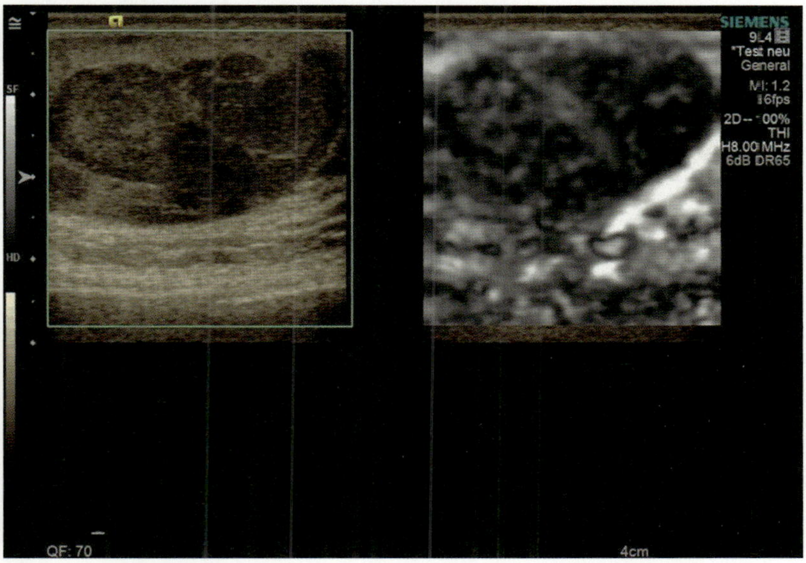

Fig. 9.28 In the strain elastogram, the lesion appears in *dark grey*, an indicator of very stiff tissue. The border of the lesions is displayed well in this technique

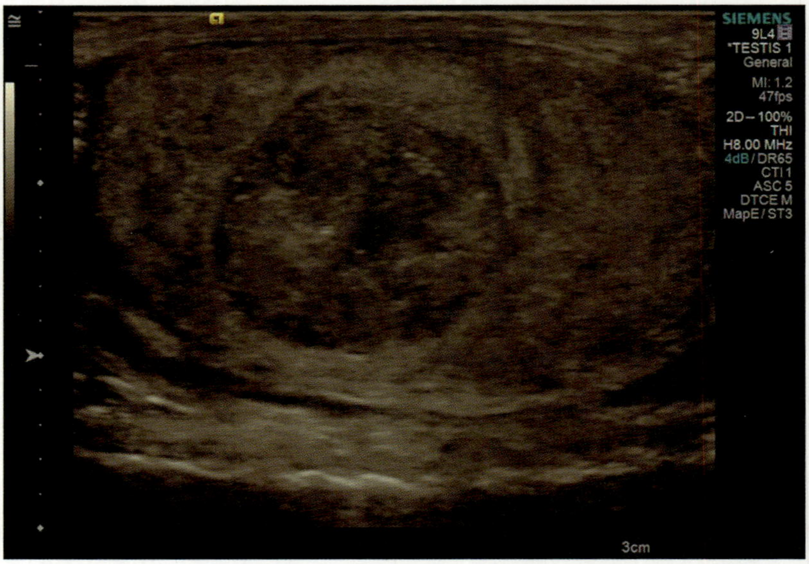

Fig. 9.29 Ultrasound images of a 47-year-old man. B-mode ultrasound demonstrates a hypoechoic lesion which was stable for more than 3 years. The diagnosis was a haemorrhagic cyst. The surgically proven histological diagnosis was that of a seminoma

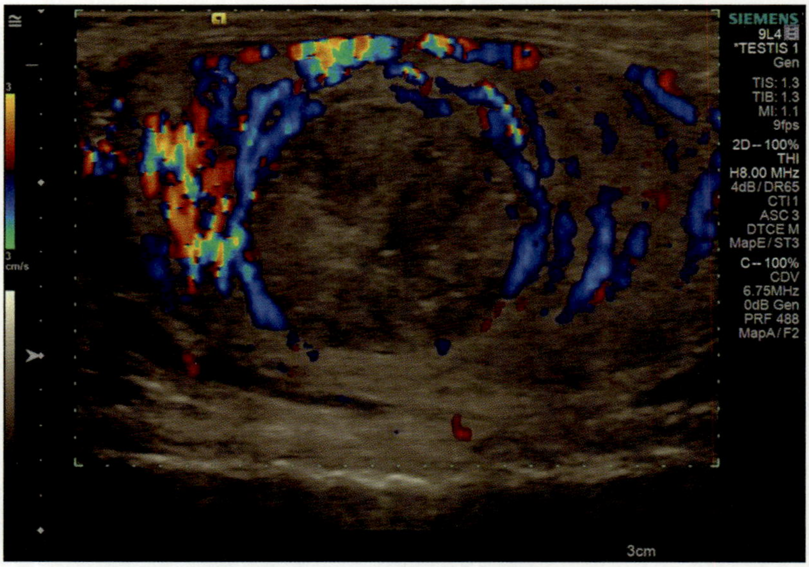

Fig. 9.30 Colour Doppler sonography indicates no vascularity of the lesion

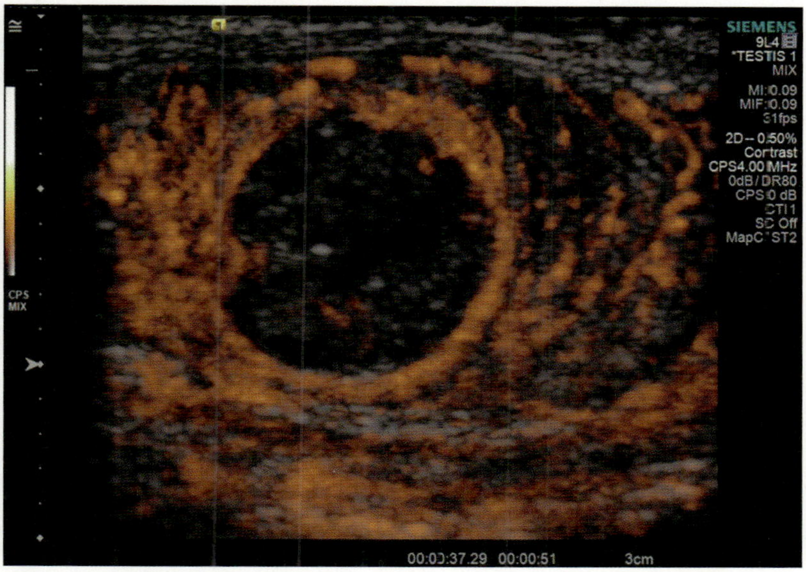

Fig. 9.31 Contrast-enhanced ultrasound confirmed a marginal contrast uptake in the tumour, which is not consistent with a haemorrhagic cyst

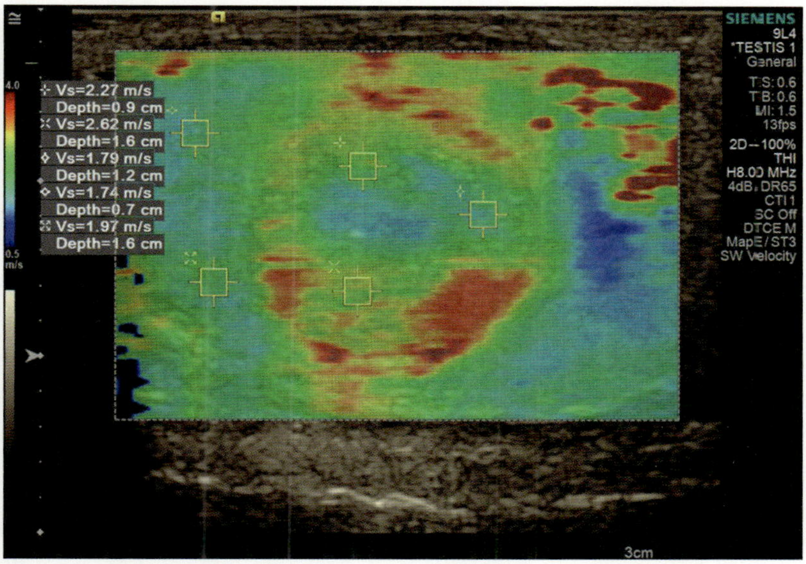

Fig. 9.32 VTIQ velocity colour overlay displays relative shear wave velocities according to the adjacent colour spectrum, *red areas* corresponding to higher values and *blue areas* corresponding to lower values. Shear wave velocity was measured in the lesion $v = 1.79$–2.62 m/s and in the surrounding tissue level between $v = 1.74$–1.97 m/s

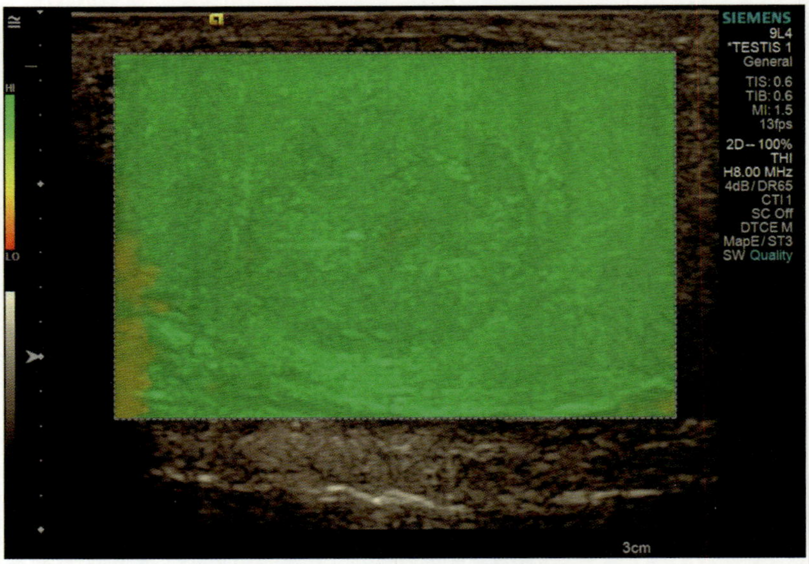

Fig. 9.33 Same lesion as Fig. 9.32. Using the VTIQ quality map, the entire testicular tissue and the lesion are coloured *green*, indicating high-quality shear waves

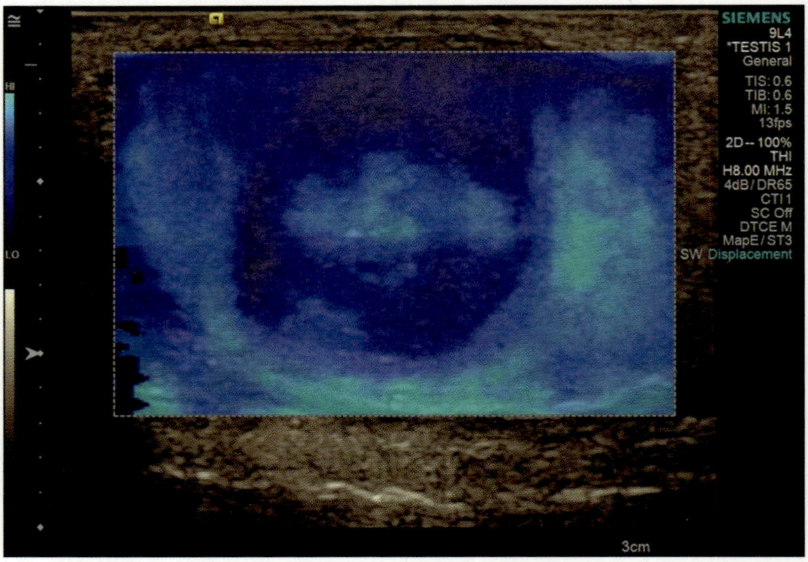

Fig. 9.34 Same lesion as Figs. 9.32 and 9.33. VTIQ displacement mode showed a low deformation of the tumour border displayed as *dark blue* in comparison to good displacement inside the tumour and the surrounding tissue displayed in *bright blue*

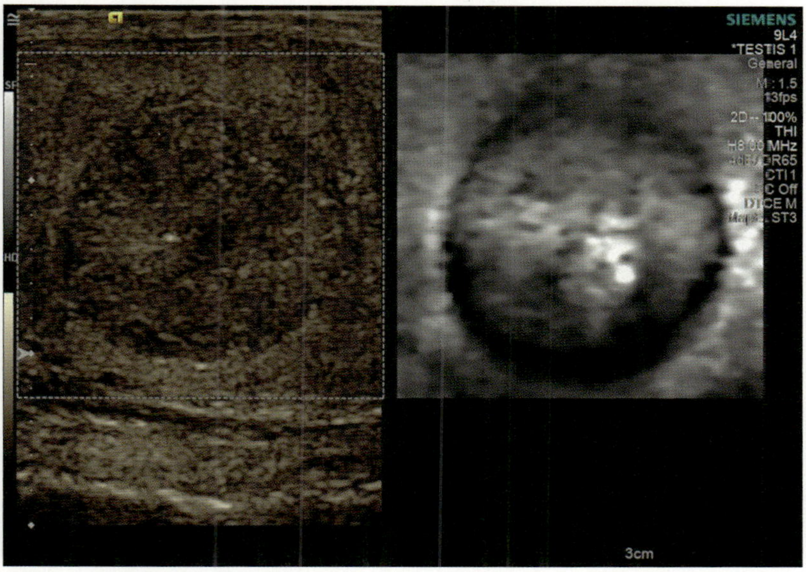

Fig. 9.35 In VTI elastography mode, the periphery of the tumour tissue appears *dark grey*, whereas the centre of the tumour appears *bright grey/white*

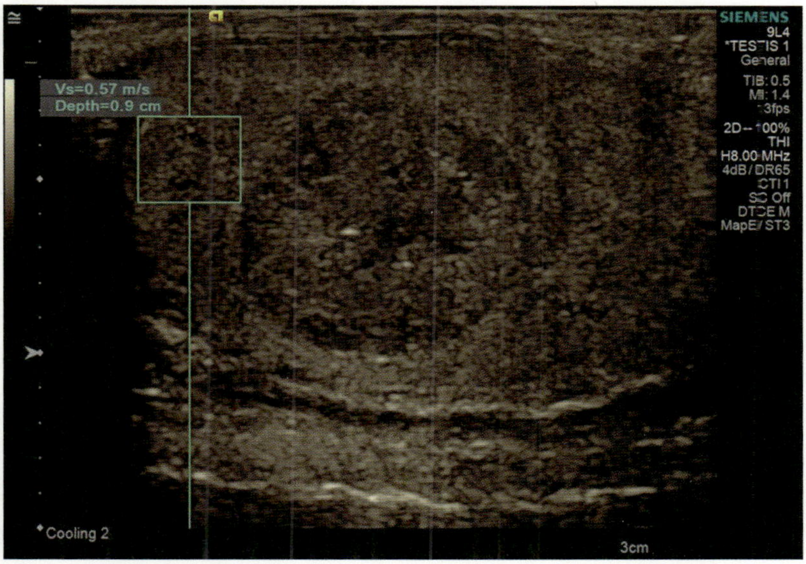

Fig. 9.36 In VTQ mode, the shear wave velocity was measured in the normal tissue with a velocity of $v=0.57$ m/s

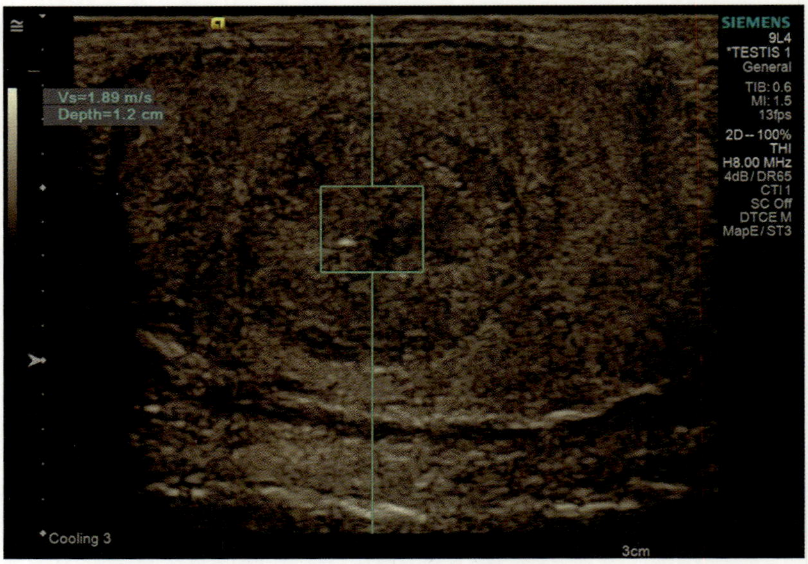

Fig. 9.37 In VTQ mode, the shear wave velocity was measured in the tumour tissue with a velocity of $v = 1.89$ m/s

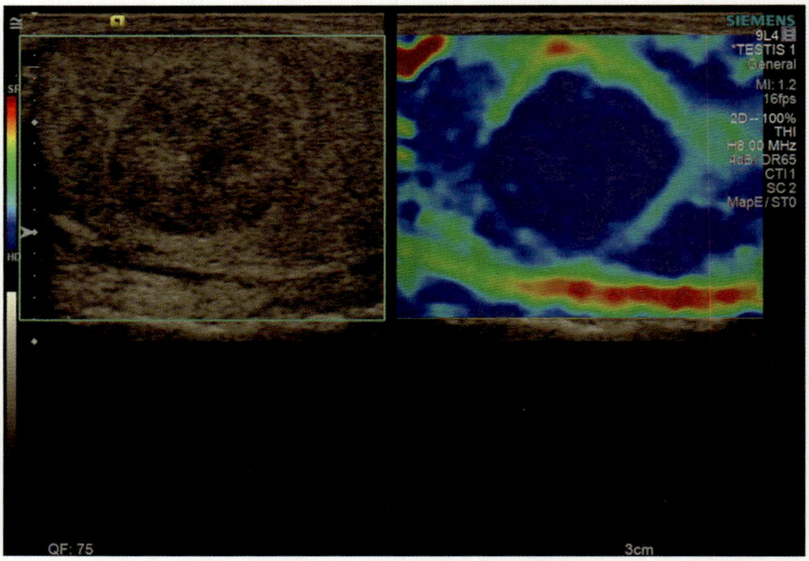

Fig. 9.38 In the strain elastogram, the lesion appears in *dark blue* indicating stiff tissue. The border of the lesions is displayed well in this technique

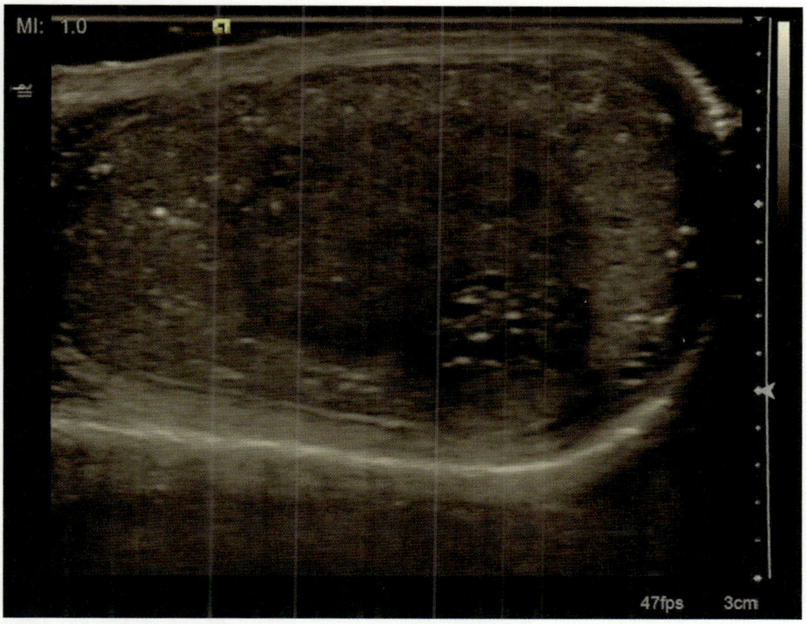

Fig. 9.39 Ultrasound images of a 41-year-old man. B-mode ultrasound demonstrates a hypoechoic lesion. The surgically proven histological diagnosis was a teratoma

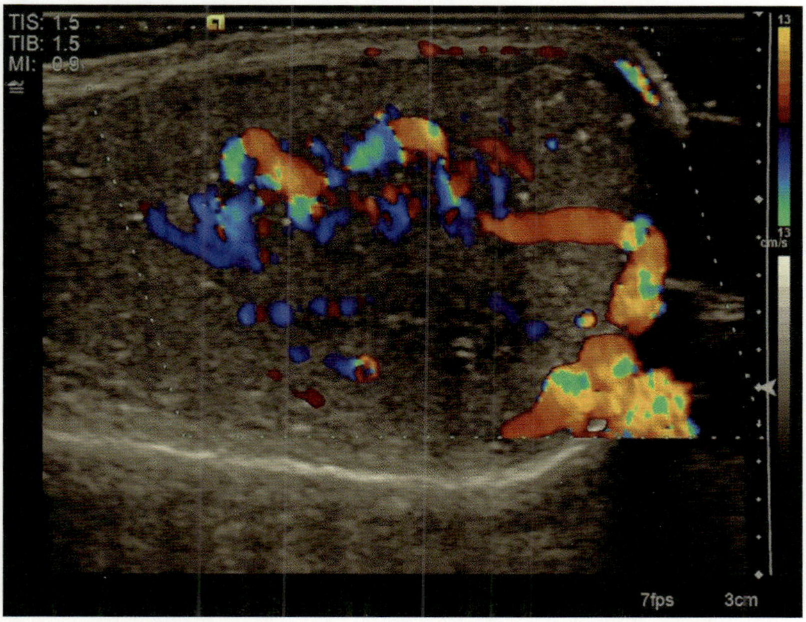

Fig. 9.40 Colour Doppler ultrasound demonstrates a high vascularity within the tumour

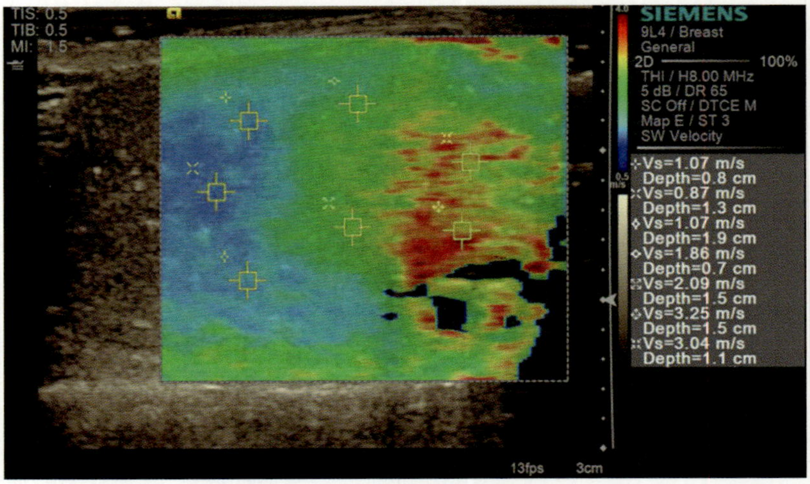

Fig. 9.41 VTIQ velocity colour overlay displays relative shear wave velocities according to the adjacent colour spectrum, *red areas* corresponding to higher values and *blue areas* corresponding to lower values. Shear wave velocity was measured in the lesion $v = 1.86$–3.25 m/s and in the surrounding tissue level between $v = 0.87$–1.07 m/s

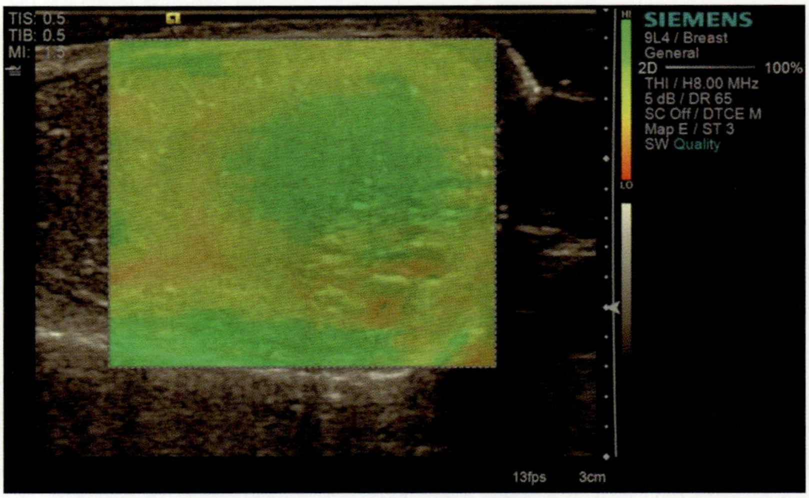

Fig. 9.42 Same lesion as Fig. 9.41. Using the VTIQ quality map, most of the testicular tumour is coloured *green*, indicating the generated shear waves are of good quality. Most of the normal testicular tissue is coloured in *yellow*, as an indicator for a moderate quality of generated shear waves

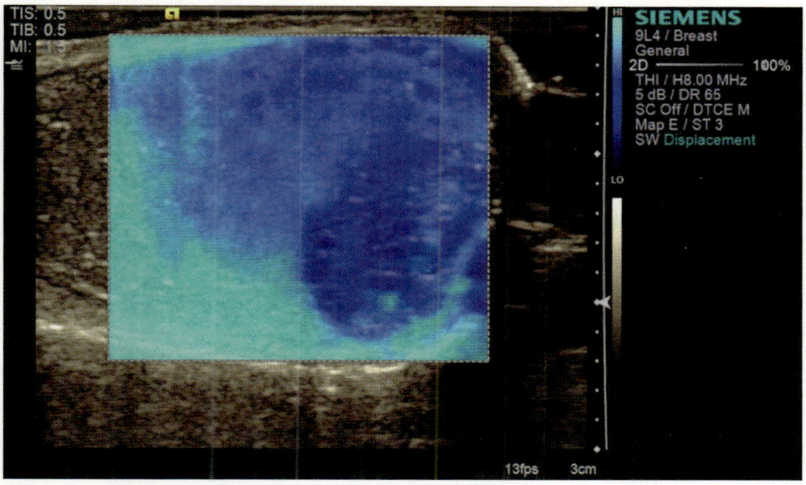

Fig. 9.43 Same lesion as Figs. 9.41 and 9.42. VTIQ displacement mode showed a low deformation of the tumour border displayed as *dark blue* in comparison to good displacement of the normal testicular tissue displayed in *bright blue*

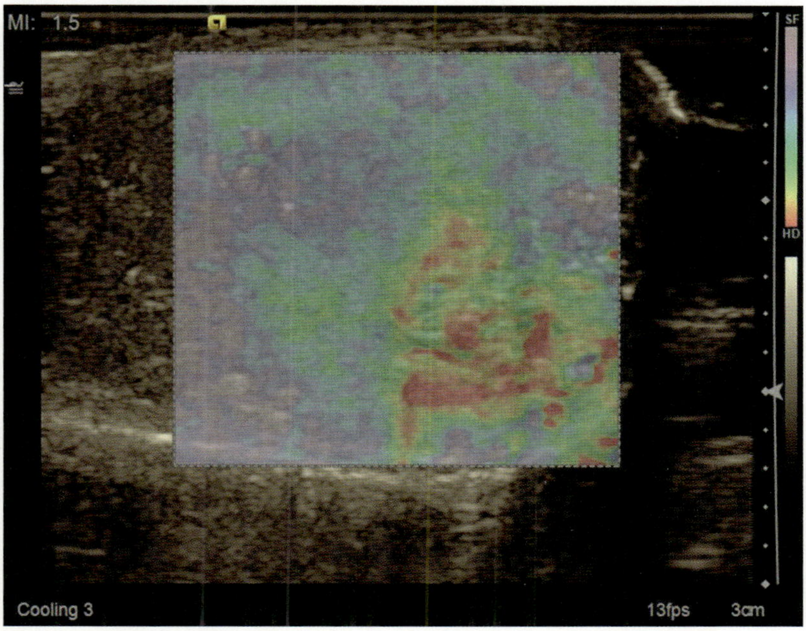

Fig. 9.44 In VTI elastography mode, the periphery of the tumour tissue is displayed in *red* and *green*, indicating stiffer tissue in the lesion in comparison to the surrounding tissue

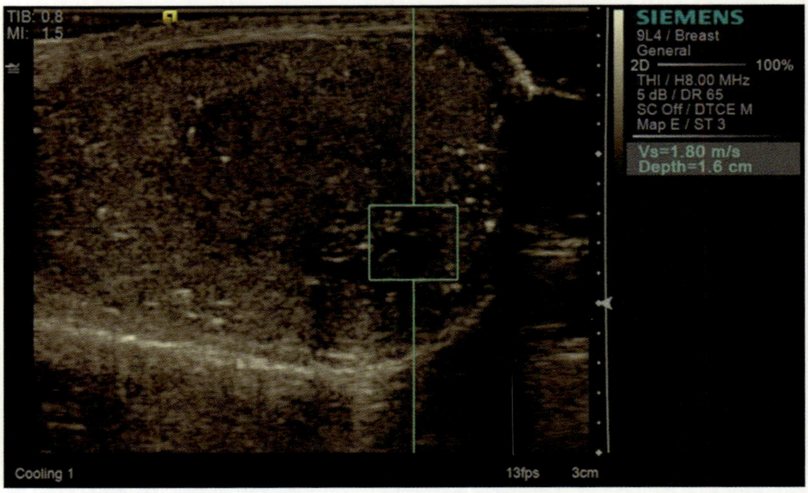

Fig. 9.45 In VTQ mode, the shear wave velocity was measured in the tumour tissue with a velocity of $v = 1.80$ m/s

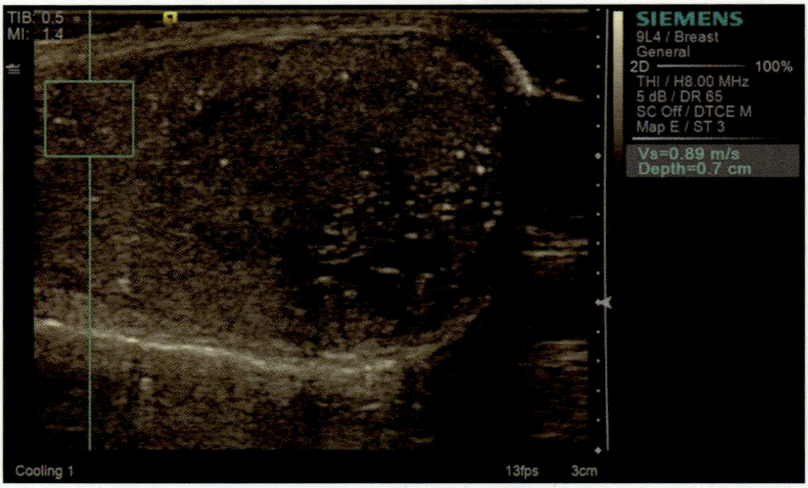

Fig. 9.46 In VTQ mode, the shear wave velocity was measured in the normal tissue with a velocity of $v = 0.89$ m/s

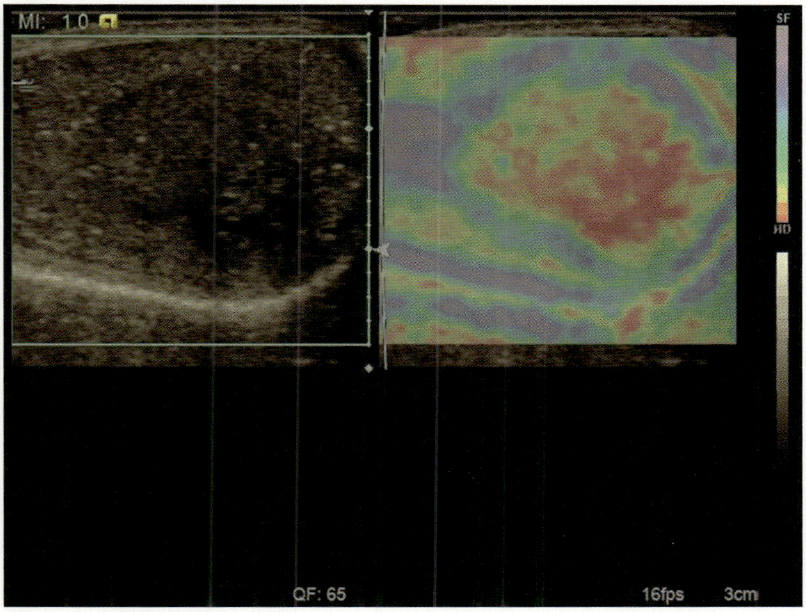

Fig. 9.47 In the strain elastogram, the lesion appears *red* indicative of very stiff tissue. The border of the lesions is well displayed using this technique

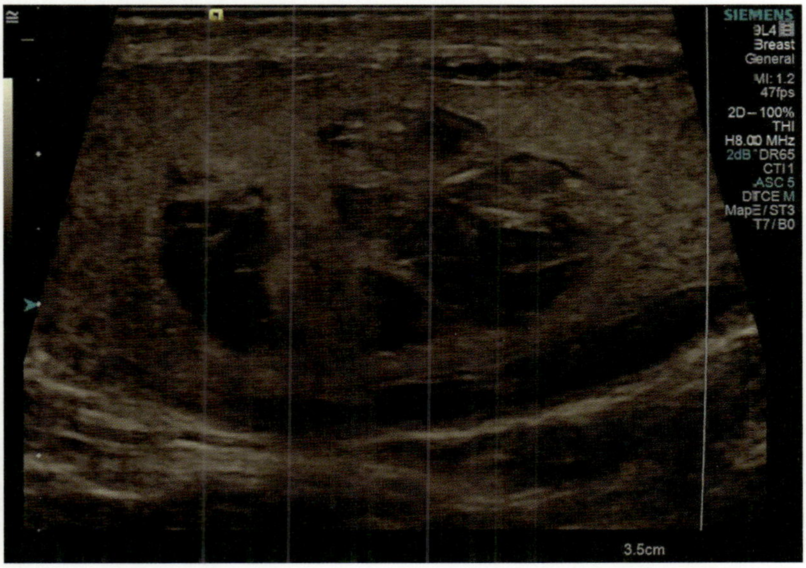

Fig. 9.48 Ultrasound images of a 37-year-old man following a soccer trauma. B-mode ultrasound demonstrates a hypoechoic lesion confirming the haematoma

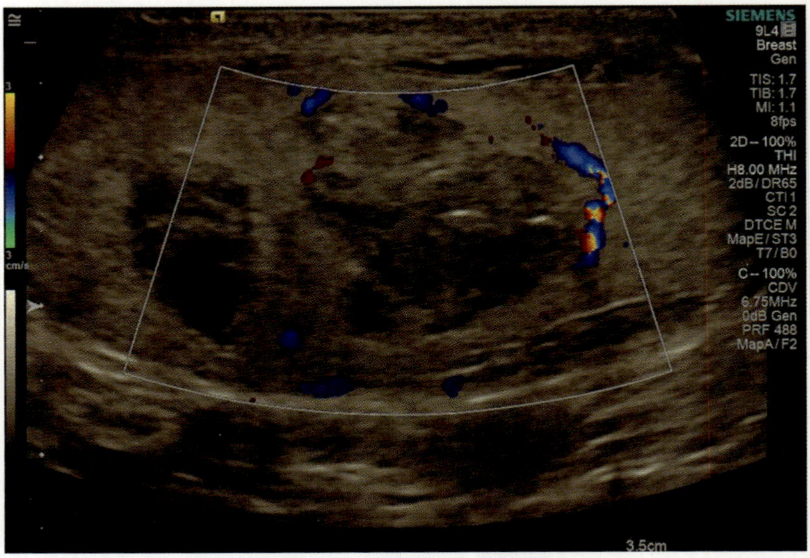

Fig. 9.49 Colour Doppler ultrasound demonstrates no vascularity within the haematoma

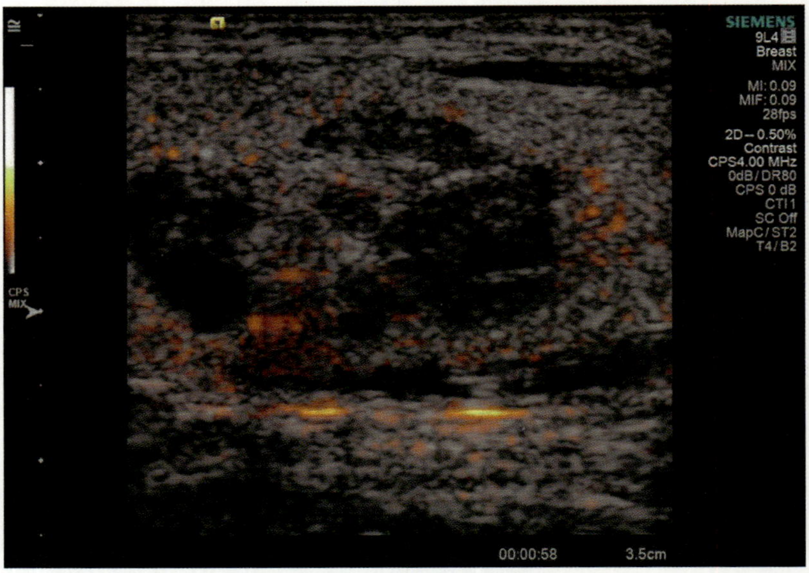

Fig. 9.50 Contrast-enhanced ultrasound confirmed no contrast uptake in the haematoma, indicating no active bleeding

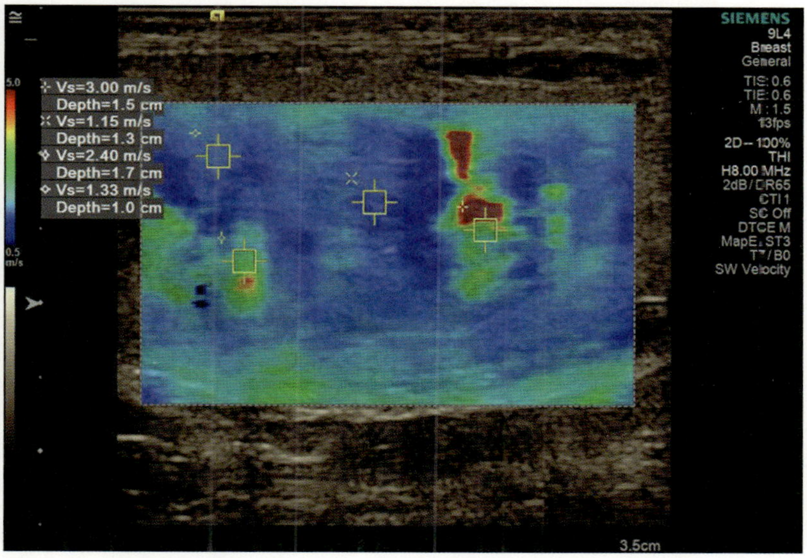

Fig. 9.51 VTIQ velocity colour overlay displayed relative shear wave velocities according to the adjacent colour spectrum, *red areas* corresponding to higher values and *blue areas* corresponding to lower values. Shear wave velocity was measured in the haematoma $v = 1.33$–3.00 m/s and in the surrounding tissue level between $v = 1.15$ m/s

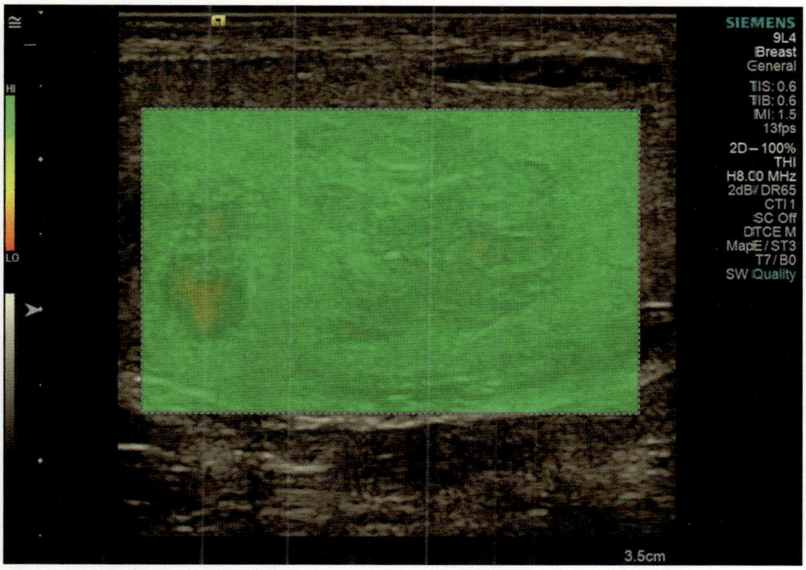

Fig. 9.52 Same lesion as Fig. 9.51. Using the VTIQ quality map, most of the testicular haematoma and the surrounding tissue is coloured *green*, an indicator of the good quality of the generated shear waves

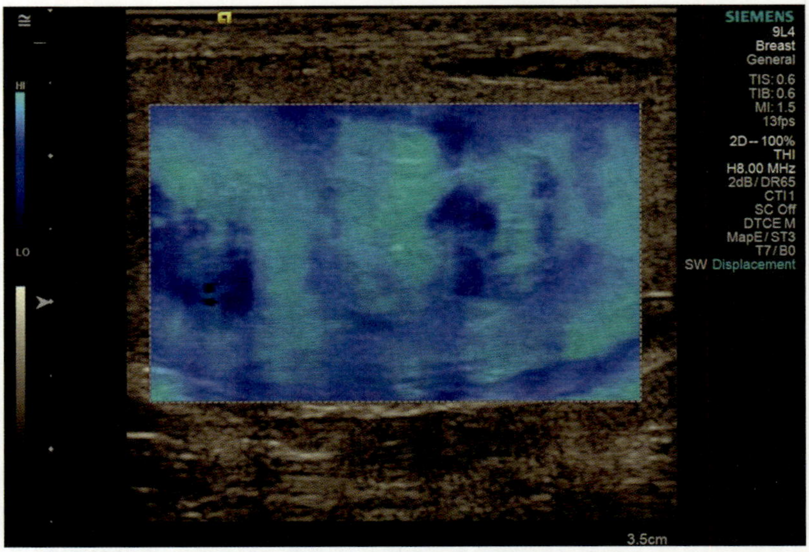

Fig. 9.53 Same lesion as Figs. 9.51 and 9.52. VTIQ displacement mode showed a low deformation of part of the haematoma displayed as *dark blue* in comparison to good displacement of the normal testicular tissue displayed in *bright blue*

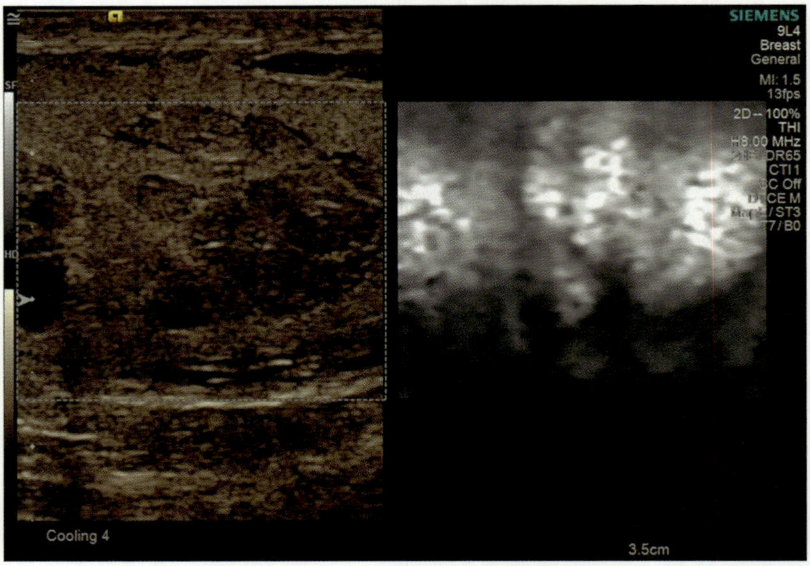

Fig. 9.54 In VTI elastography mode, the tissue in the periphery of the haematoma appears *dark grey*, indicative of stiffer tissue in this region in comparison to the surrounding tissue

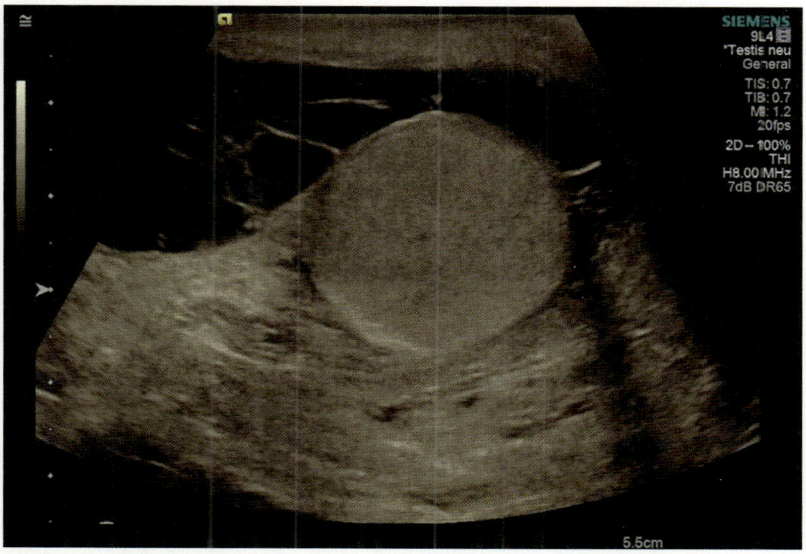

Fig. 9.55 Ultrasound images of a 57-year-old man. B-mode ultrasound demonstrates a hydrocele

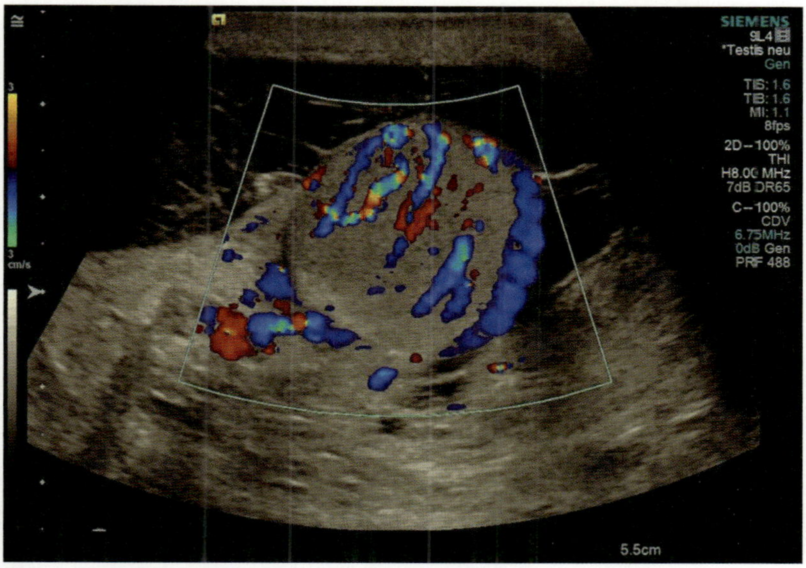

Fig. 9.56 Colour Doppler ultrasound demonstrates normal vascularity within the testicular tissue

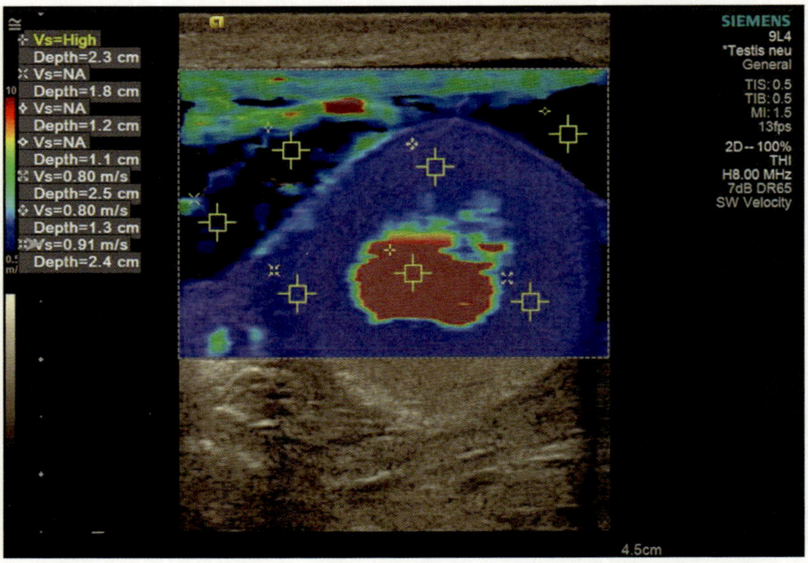

Fig. 9.57 VTIQ velocity colour overlay displayed relative shear wave velocities according to the adjacent colour spectrum, *red areas* corresponding to higher values and *blue areas* corresponding to lower values. Shear wave velocity was measured in the normal testicular tissue $v = 0.80–0.91$ m/s; shear wave velocity could not be measured in the surrounding fluid. At the centre of the testis is actually a reflection artefact, caused by the round geometry of the testis, and shear waves reflecting off the lateral edges of the testis appear, which are interpreted as higher velocity

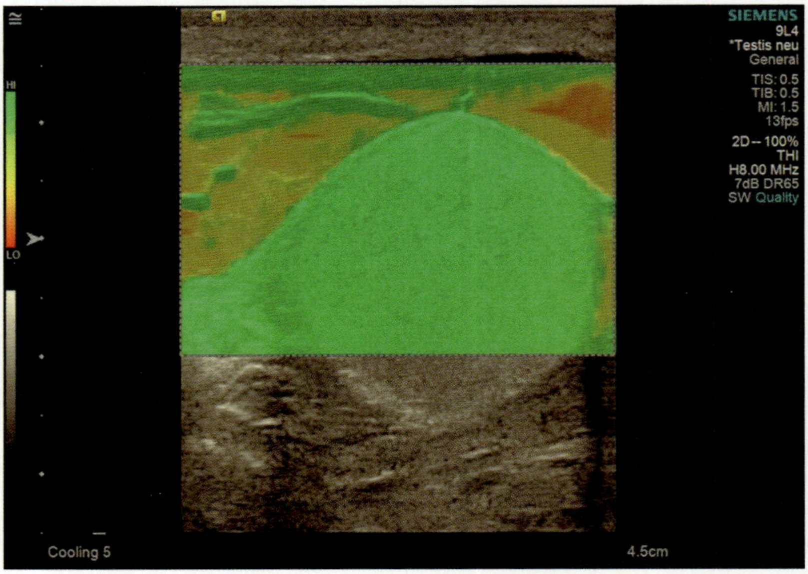

Fig. 9.58 Same lesion as Fig. 9.57. Using the VTIQ quality map, the shear wave signals from the fluid parts of the hydrocele are coded in *dark yellow* indicating poor quality or no shear waves generated, whereas the shear waves generated by the background tissue and the normal testicular tissue are of a high quality as indicated by their *green colour* coding

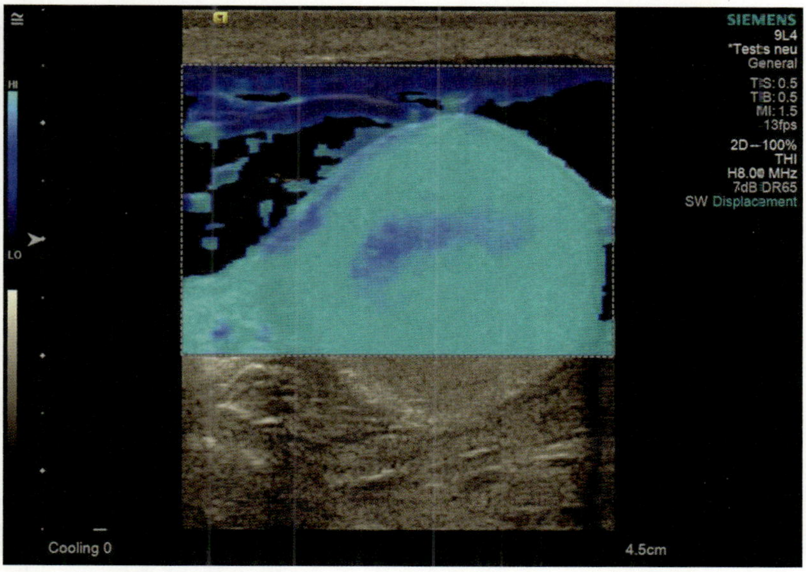

Fig. 9.59 Same lesion as Figs. 9.57 and 9.58. VTIQ displacement mode showed a high deformation of the normal testicular tissue displayed as *bright blue* in comparison to no displacement of the fluid parts of the hydrocele

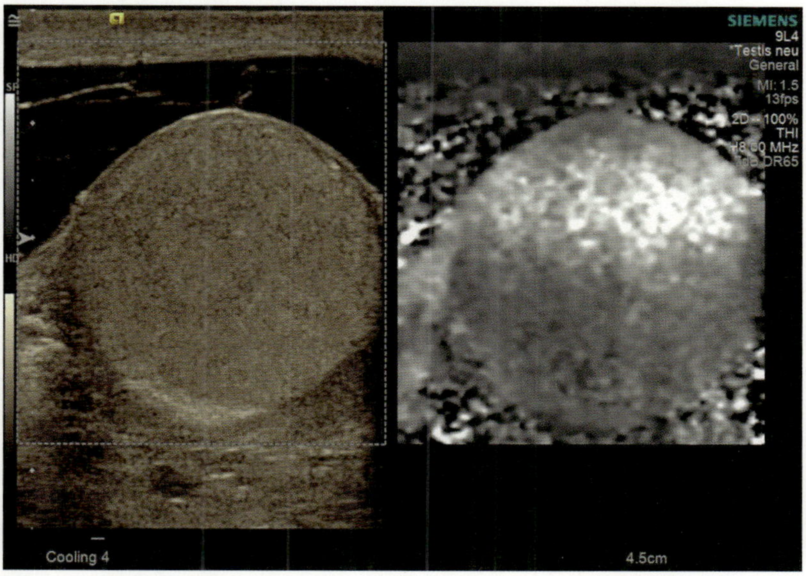

Fig. 9.60 In VTI elastography mode, the normal testicular tissue appears *bright grey*, indicating soft tissue in comparison to the fluid parts of the hydrocele which are displayed as a patchy mosaic indicative of artefact

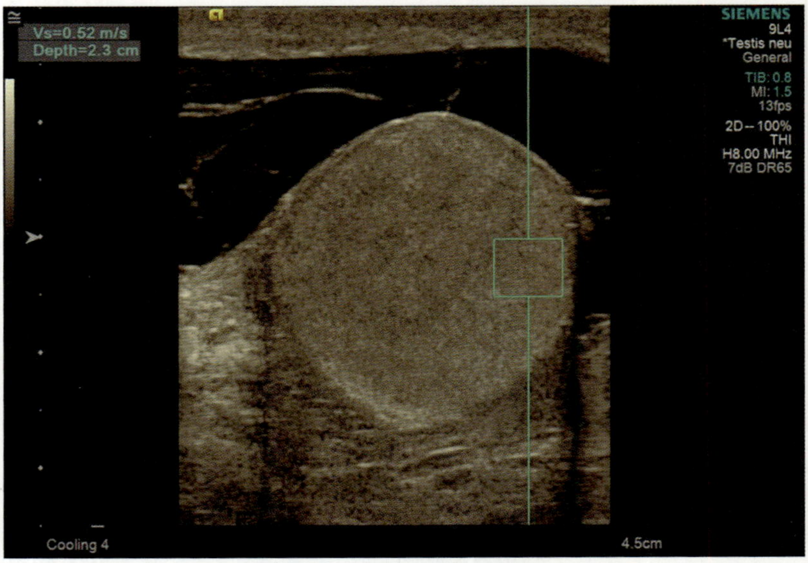

Fig. 9.61 In VTQ mode, the shear wave velocity was measured in the normal tissue with a velocity of $v = 0.52$ m/s

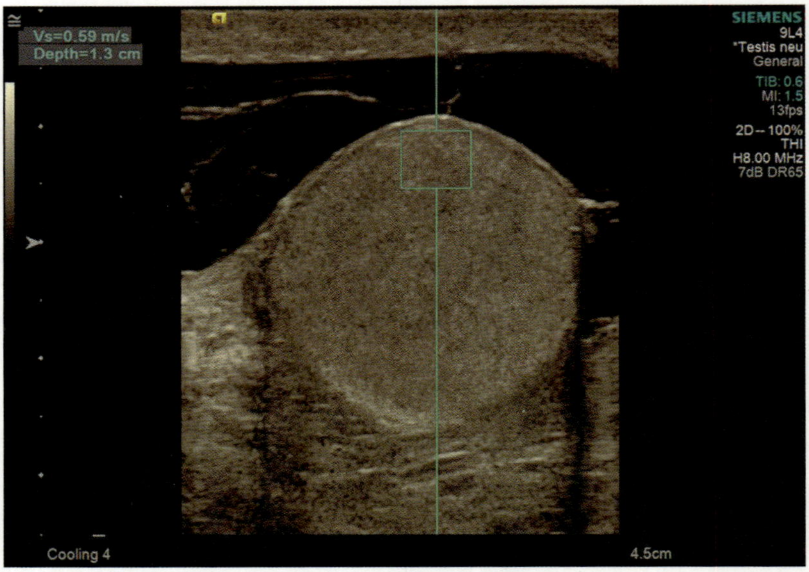

Fig. 9.62 In VTQ mode, the shear wave velocity was measured in the normal tissue with a velocity of $v = 0.59$ m/s

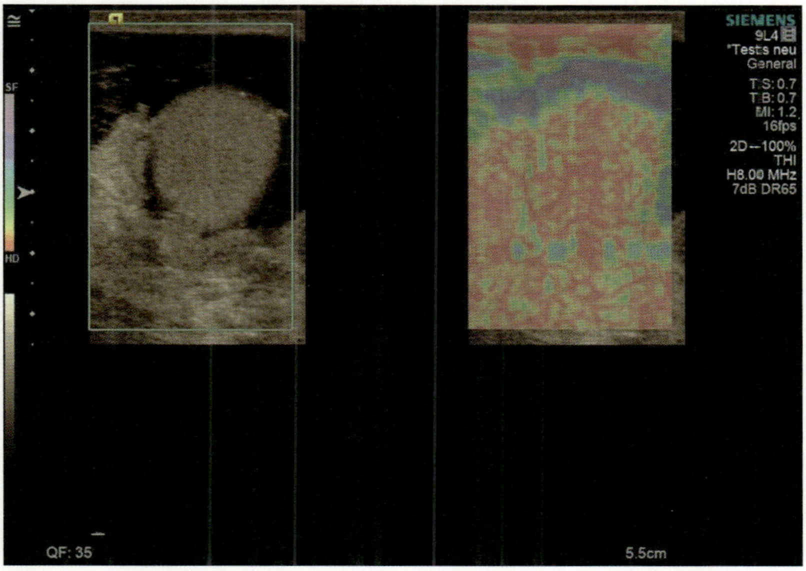

Fig. 9.63 In the strain elastogram, the lesion appears *red* indicating stiff tissue. The border of the lesions is displayed well in this technique

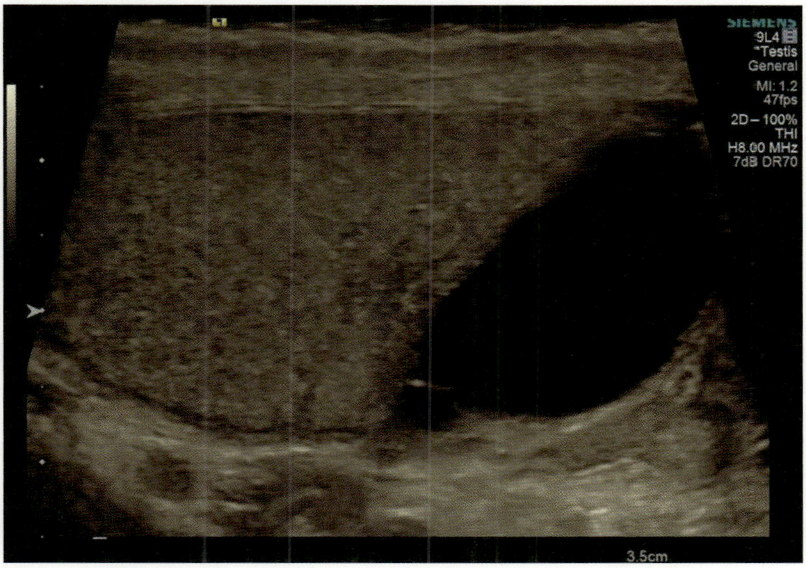

Fig. 9.64 A 20-mm anechoic cystic lesion with a thin wall is noted in the testicular periphery

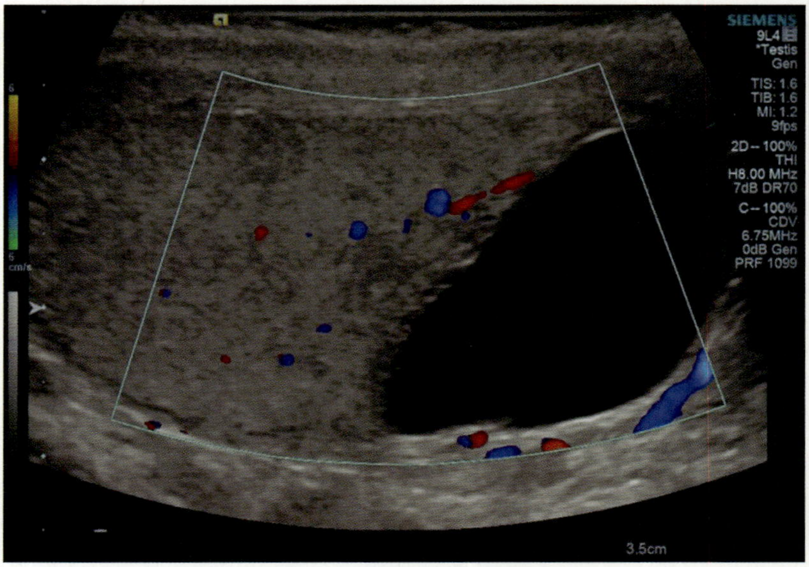

Fig. 9.65 No internal colour Doppler signal is demonstrated within the cyst

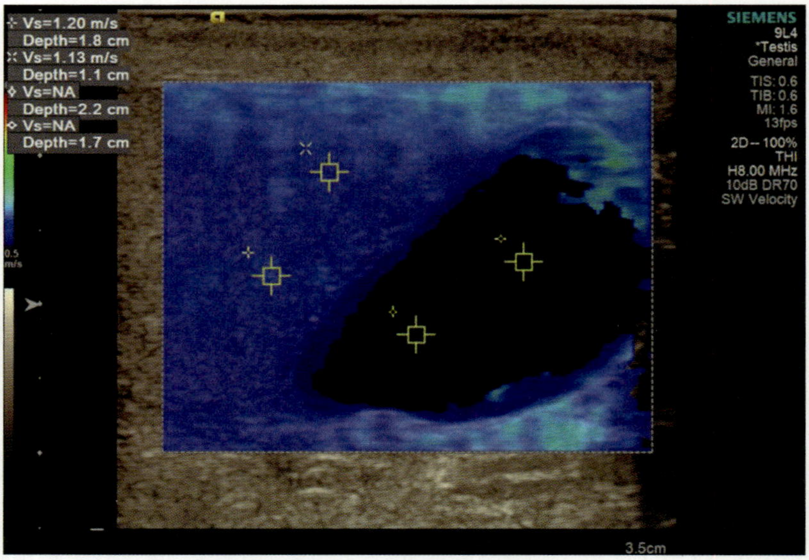

Fig. 9.66 VTIQ velocity colour overlay displayed relative shear wave velocities according to the adjacent colour spectrum. Shear wave velocity could not be measured in the lesion. Shear wave velocity in the surrounding tissue level between $v = 1.13$–1.20 m/s at the operator defined regions of interest

Fig. 9.67 Same lesion as Fig. 9.66. The shear waves from the cystic lesion are displayed in *dark yellow* and *red* indicating poor quality or no shear waves generated, whereas the background tissue generates high-quality shear waves as indicated by the *green colour* coding of that area

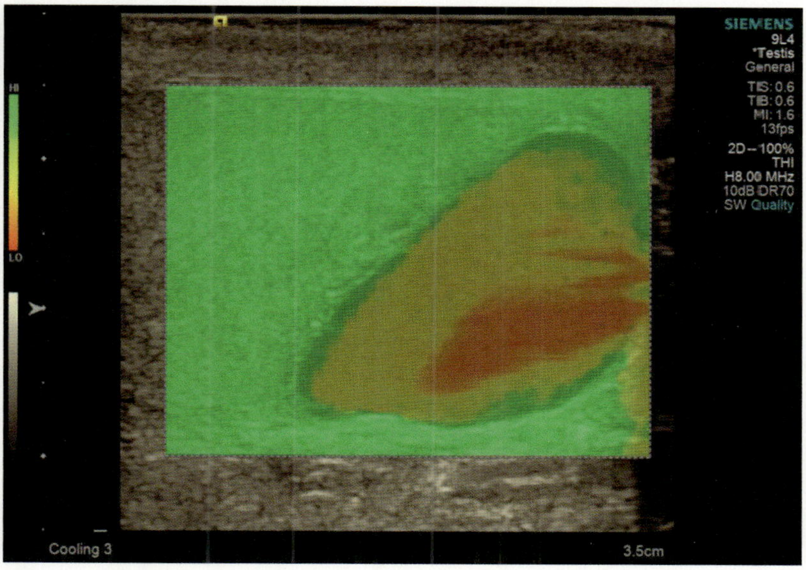

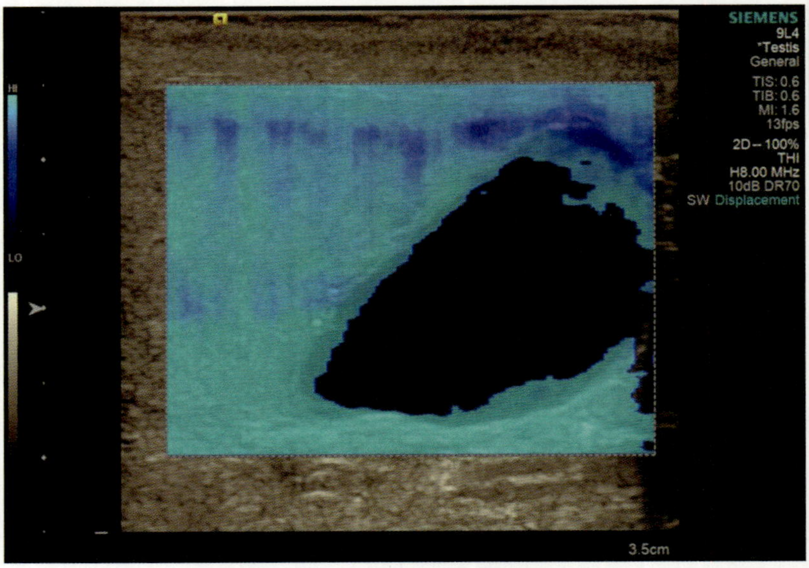

Fig. 9.68 Same lesion as Figs. 9.66, 9.67. VTIQ displacement mode showed an area of no signal in the cystic lesion, indicated that the acoustic push pulse does not deform fluid material, in contrast to the *light blue colour* of the surrounding tissue indicative of good tissue deformation

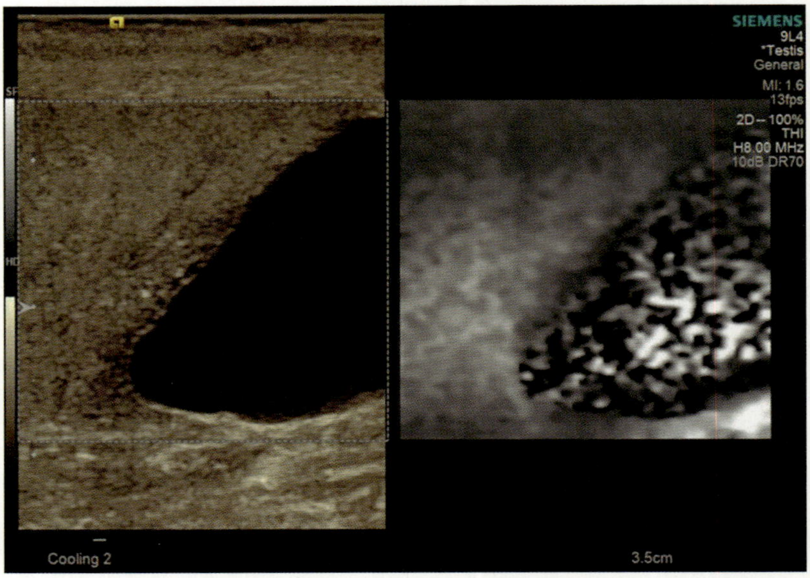

Fig. 9.69 In VTI elastography mode, the cyst appears as a patchy mosaic indicative of artefact; the peripheral tissue is displayed as *bright grey* indicating soft tissue

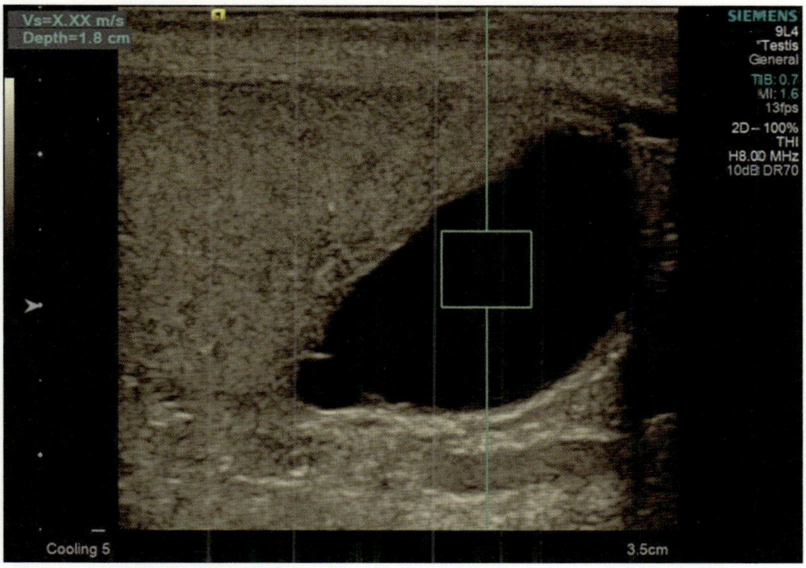

Fig. 9.70 In VTQ mode, the shear wave reading was measured in the cyst as $v = XXX$ m/s indicating no shear wave velocity could be measured

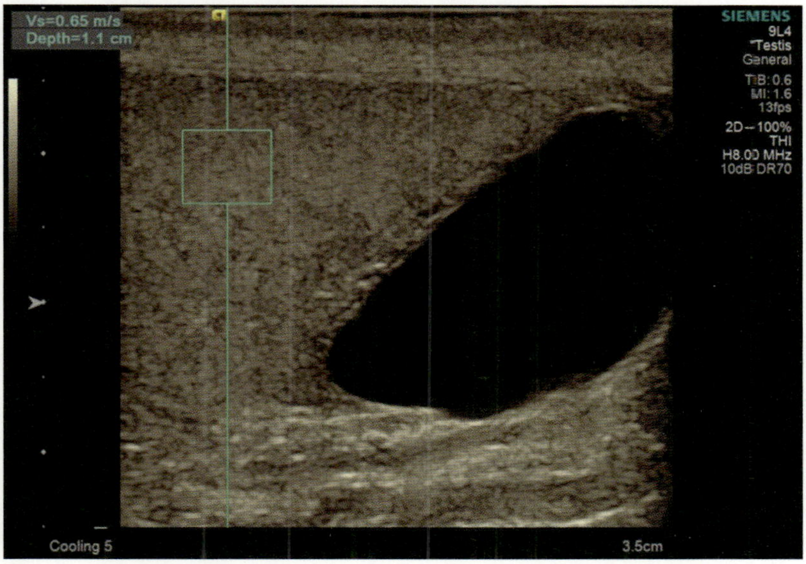

Fig. 9.71 In VTQ mode, the shear wave velocity was measured in the normal tissue with a velocity of $v = 0.65$ m/s

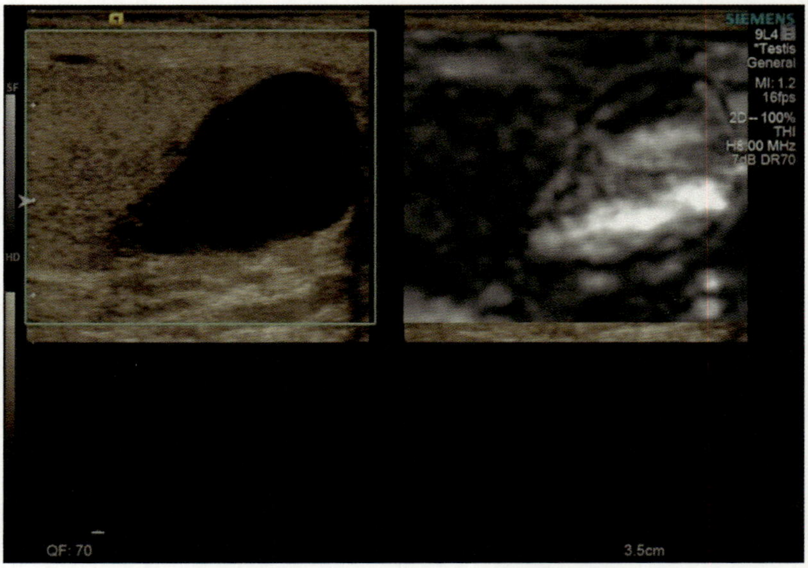

Fig. 9.72 In the strain elastogram, the cyst appears as a ring-shaped area with a *white* (soft) central portion, typical elastographic appearance of a cyst. The surrounding normal tissue is *light grey*, indicating soft tissue

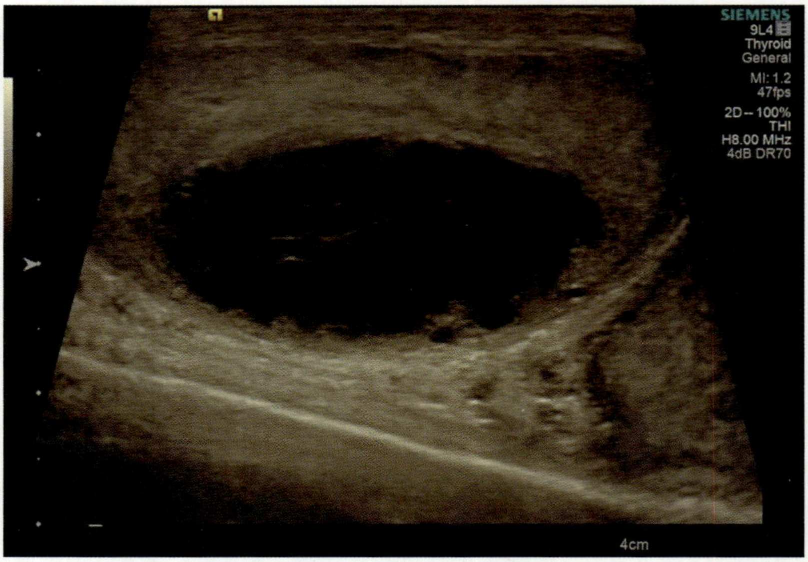

Fig. 9.73 A 35-year-old man with testicular pain. A 30-mm hypoechoic lesion is noted in the centre of the testis

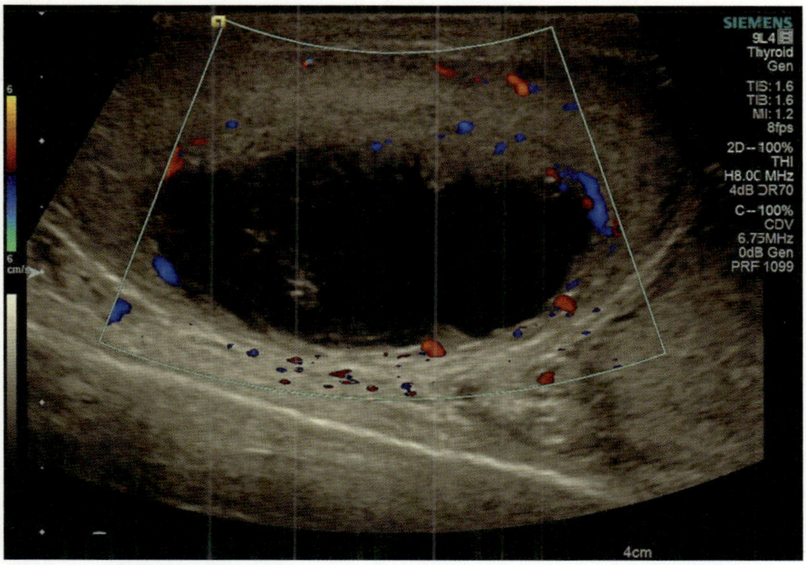

Fig. 9.74 No colour Doppler signal is demonstrated within the lesion

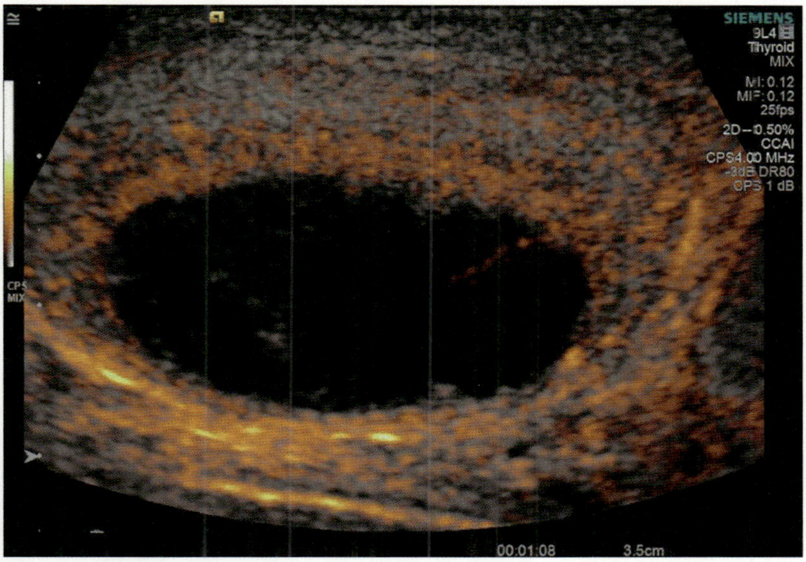

Fig. 9.75 Contrast-enhanced ultrasound confirmed no central contrast uptake of the lesion, but the peripheral uptake seen is consistent with that of an abscess

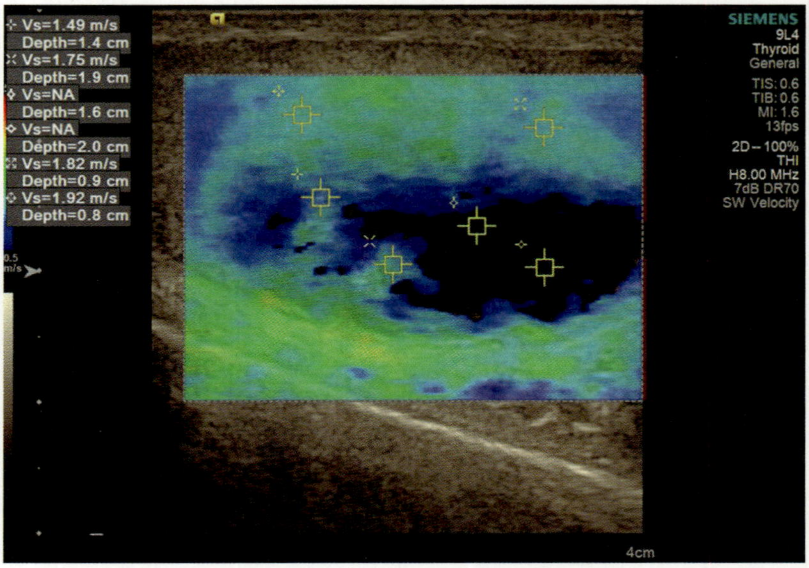

Fig. 9.76 VTIQ velocity colour overlay displayed relative shear wave velocities according to the adjacent colour spectrum, *red areas* corresponding to higher values and *blue areas* corresponding to lower values. Shear wave velocity was measured in the abscess $v = 1.75$–1.92 m/s and in the surrounding tissue level between $v = 1.49$ m/s. In part of the abscess, no VTIQ measurement could be calculated (NA)

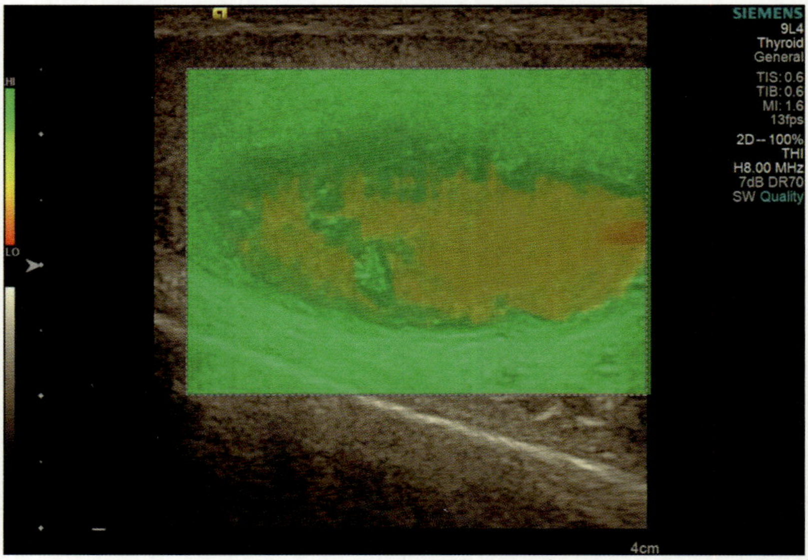

Fig. 9.77 Same lesion as Fig. 9.76. The colour display in the majority of the abscess is *orange* indicating the low quality of the shear waves generated in this region, whereas the background tissue is shown as *green*, indicating the high quality of the generated shear waves

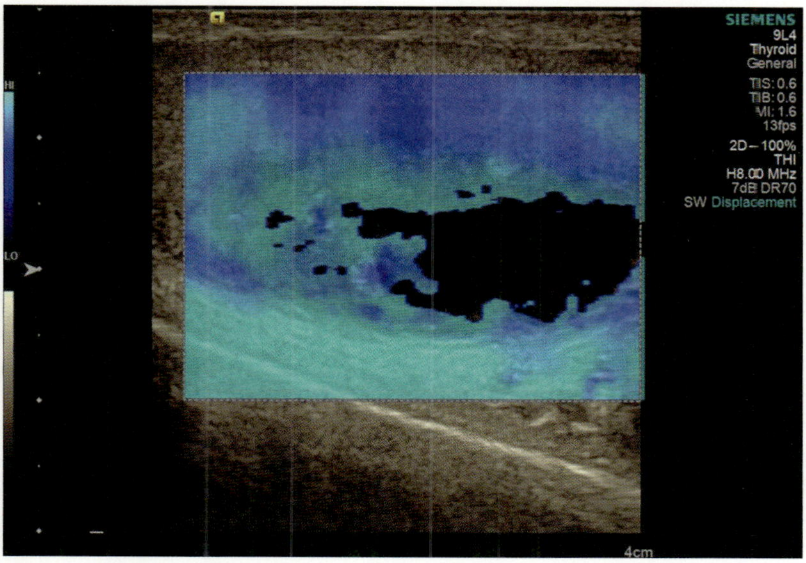

Fig. 9.78 Same lesion as Figs. 9.76 and 9.77. VTIQ displacement mode shows an area of *black* in part of the abscess indicating that there is no deformation in this region, compared with the mid to *light blue* displayed in the surrounding area showing mild to good tissue deformation

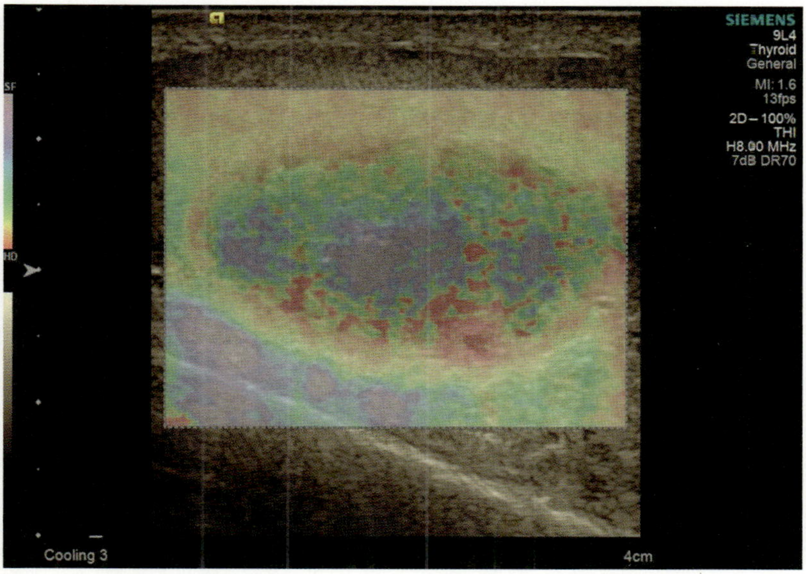

Fig. 9.79 In VTI mode elastography, the abscess appears in a patchy mosaic as an indicator for artefacts, the peripheral tissue in *red* an indicator for the capsule of the abscess

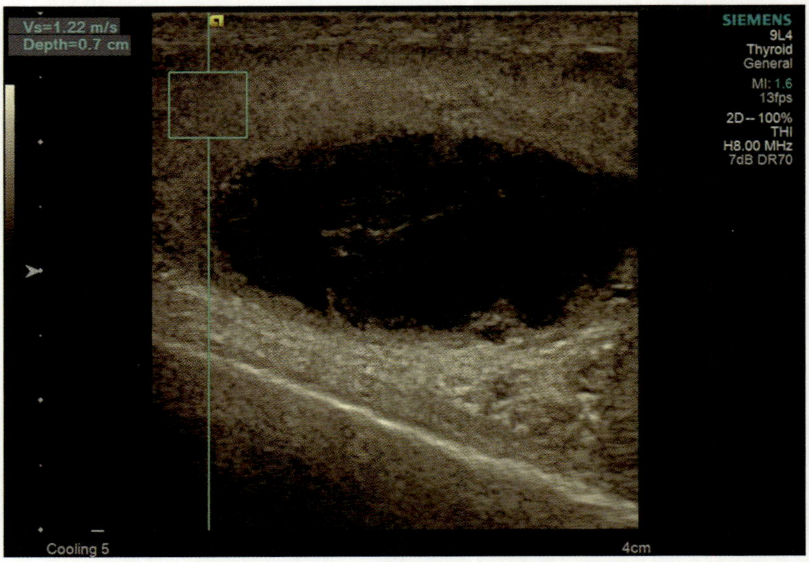

Fig. 9.80 In VTQ mode, the shear wave velocity was measured in the normal tissue, a velocity could be measured $v = 1.22$ m/s

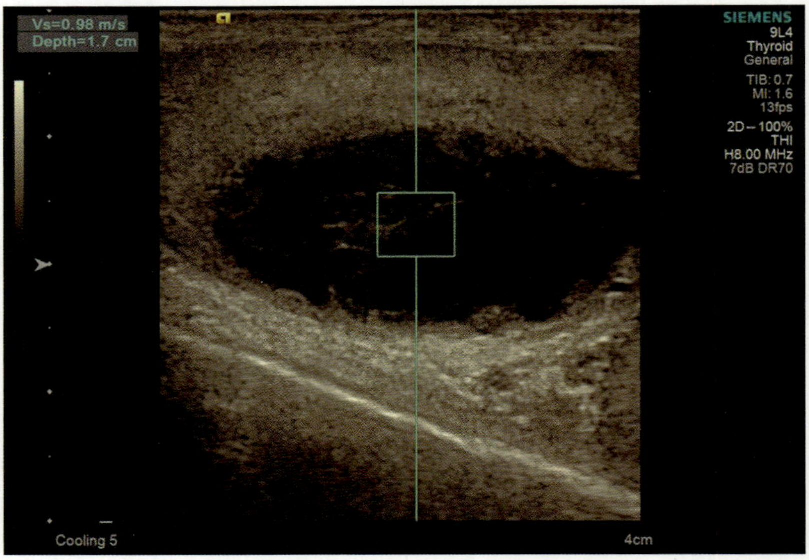

Fig. 9.81 In VTQ mode, the shear wave velocity was measured in the abscess with a velocity that could be measured $v = 0.98$ m/s

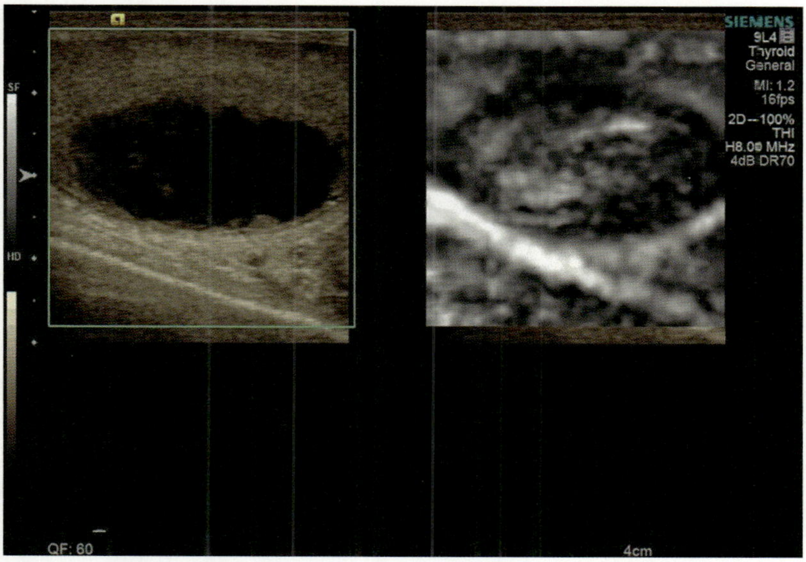

Fig. 9.82 In sonoelastography, the abscess appears in patchy mosaic pattern as an indicator for an intermediate stiffness tissue. The border of the abscess is displayed in *black* in this technique

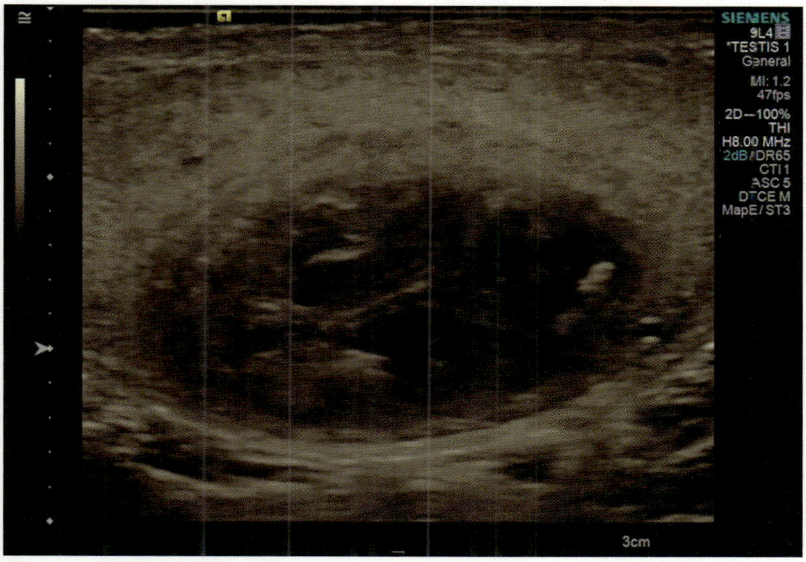

Fig. 9.83 Same patient as Fig. 9.73. Follow-up examination after 4 weeks. A 20-mm hypoechoic lesion is noted in the testicular centre

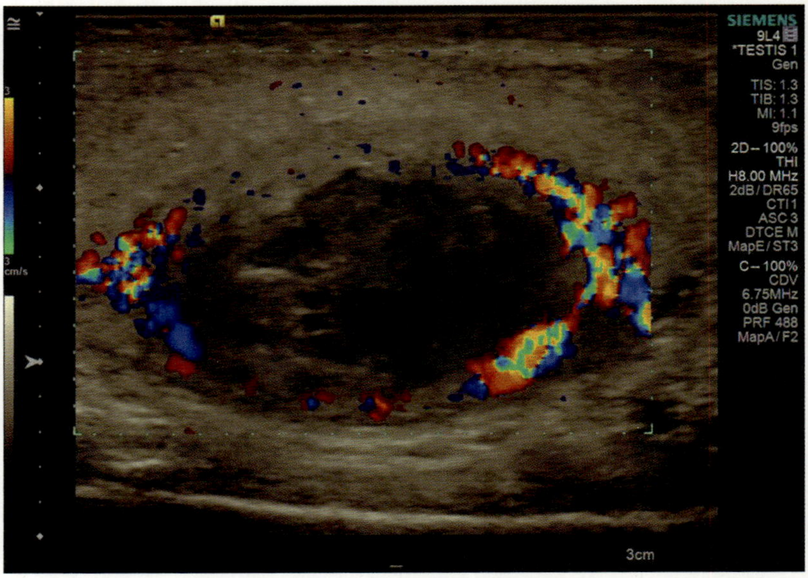

Fig. 9.84 No central vascularisation is demonstrated within the abscess, but an enlarged colour Doppler signal could be detected at the capsular of the abscess

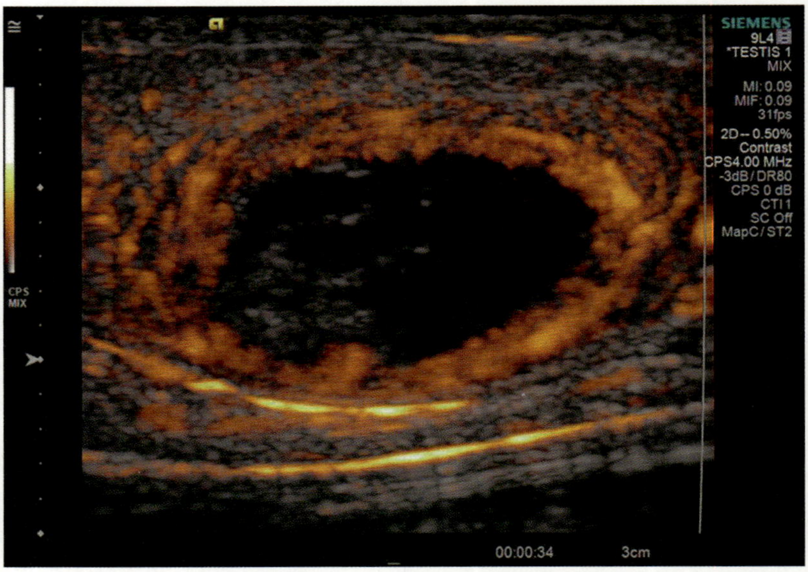

Fig. 9.85 Contrast-enhanced ultrasound confirmed no central contrast uptake of the abscess but arising peripheral contrast uptake

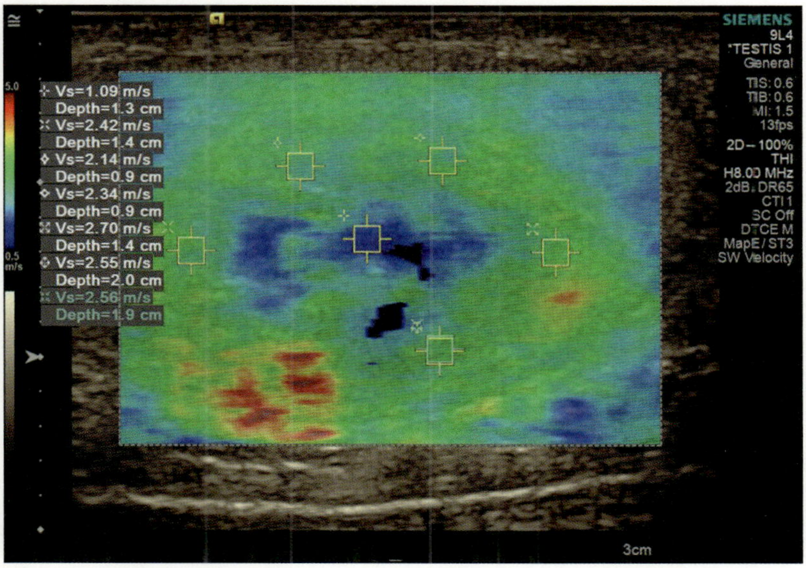

Fig. 9.86 VTIQ velocity colour overlay displayed relative shear wave velocities according to the adjacent colour spectrum, *red areas* corresponding to higher values and *blue areas* corresponding to lower values. Shear wave velocity was measured in the abscess $v = 1.09$ m/s and in the surrounding tissue level between $v = 2.14–2.70$ m/s

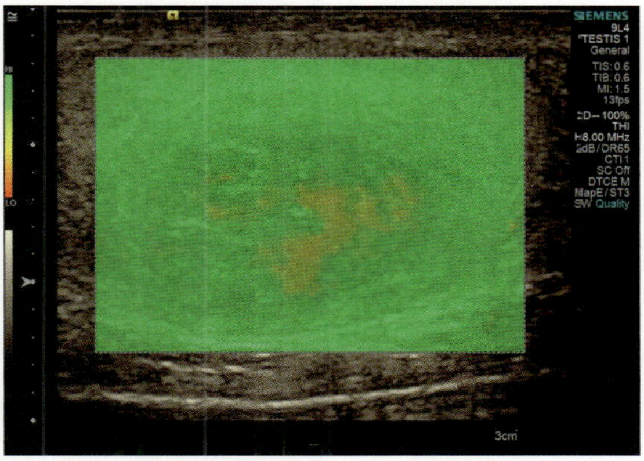

Fig. 9.87 Same lesion as Fig. 9.86. The low quality shear wave signal area representing the abscess in *yellow*, the background tissue provides a high quality signal as indicated by *green area* in the shear wave quality display in the same image

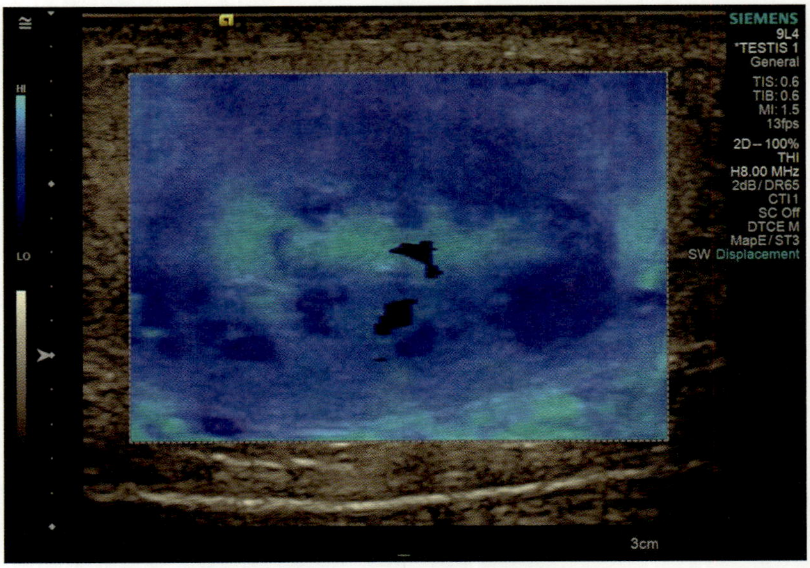

Fig. 9.88 Same lesion as Figs. 9.86 and 9.87. VTIQ displacement mode showed a low deformation of the capsule of the abscess displayed as *dark blue* in comparison to good displacement inside the abscess displayed in *bright blue*

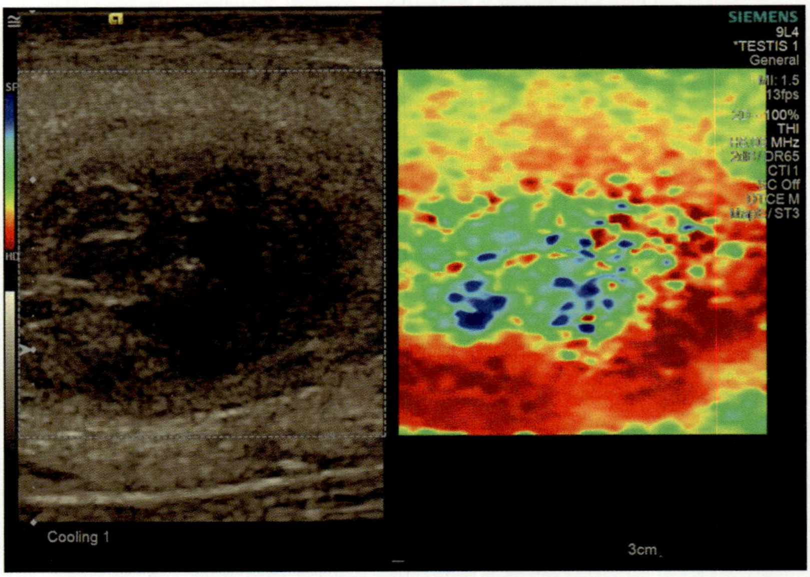

Fig. 9.89 In VTI mode elastography, the abscess appears with a stiff capsular and a more soft tissue inside the abscess

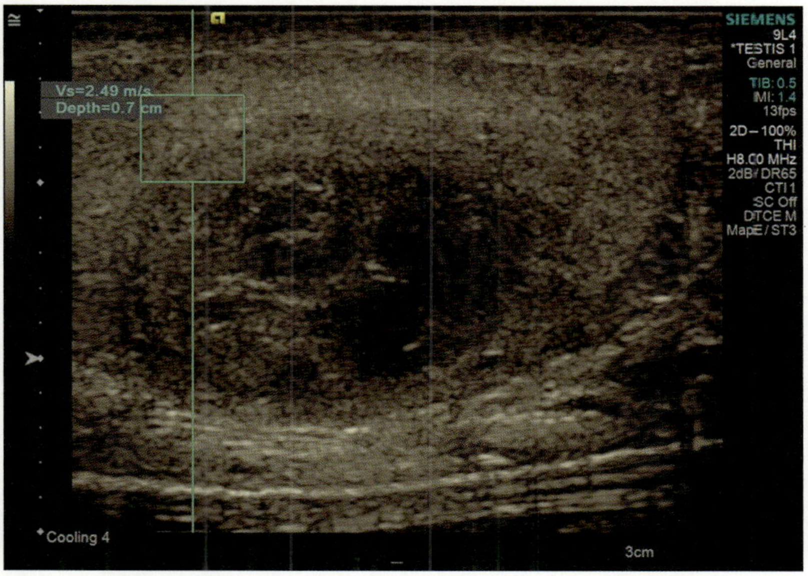

Fig. 9.90 In VTQ mode, the shear wave velocity was measured on the left side of the abscess capsular with a velocity of $v = 2.49$ m/s

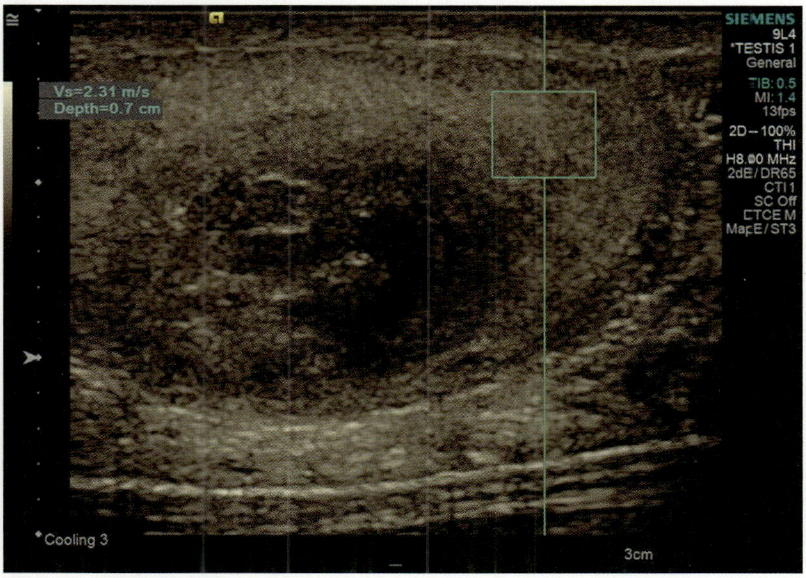

Fig. 9.91 In VTQ mode, the shear wave velocity was measured on the right side of the abscess capsular with a velocity of $v = 2.31$ m/s

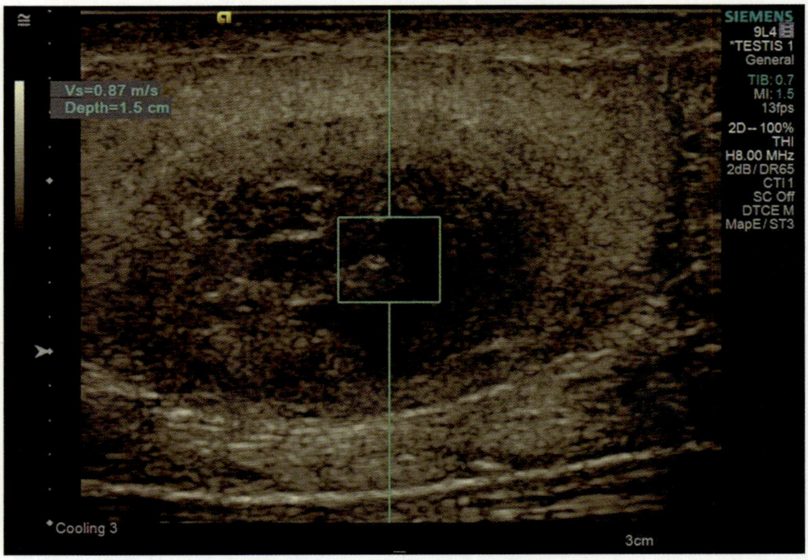

Fig. 9.92 In VTQ mode, the shear wave velocity was measured in the centre of the abscess with a velocity of $v = 0.87$ m/s

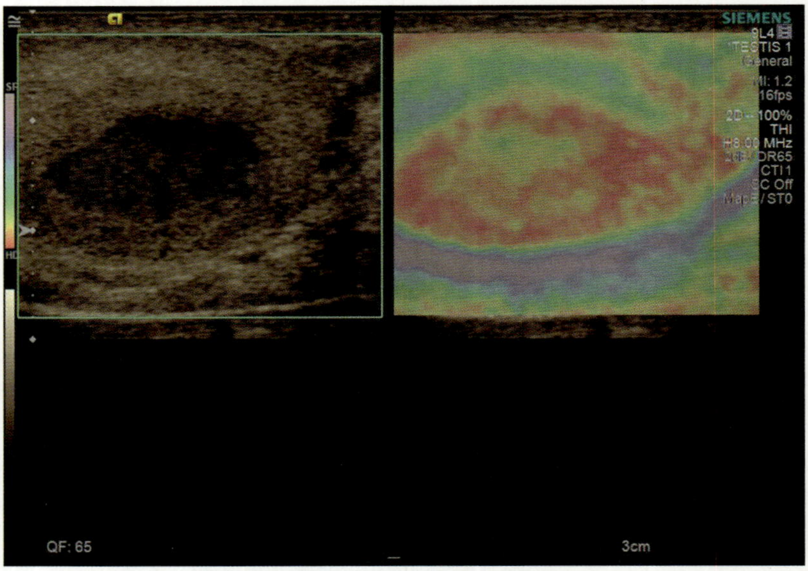

Fig. 9.93 In sonoelastography, the capsular of the abscess appears in *red* as an indicator for a very stiff tissue. The centre of the abscess is displayed *green* as an indicator for a more soft tissue

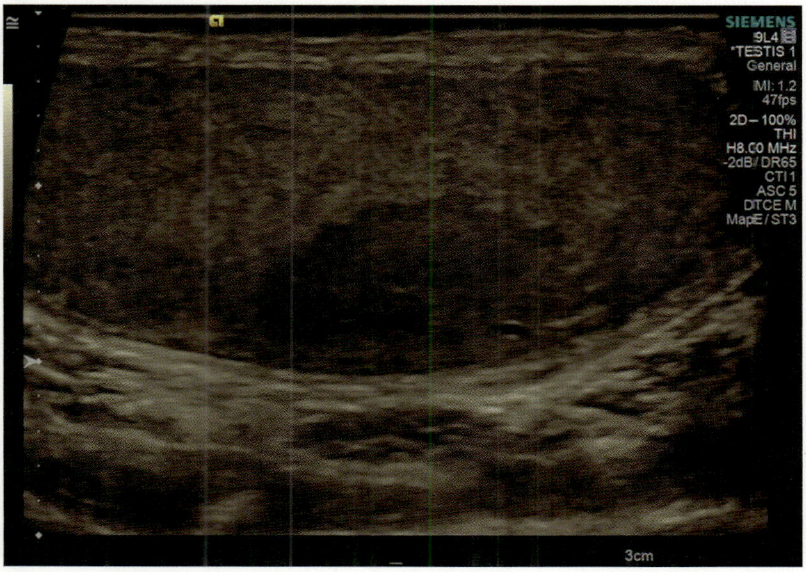

Fig. 9.94 Same patient as Fig. 9.83. Follow-up examination after 3 weeks. A 10-mm hypoechoic lesion is noted in the testicular centre

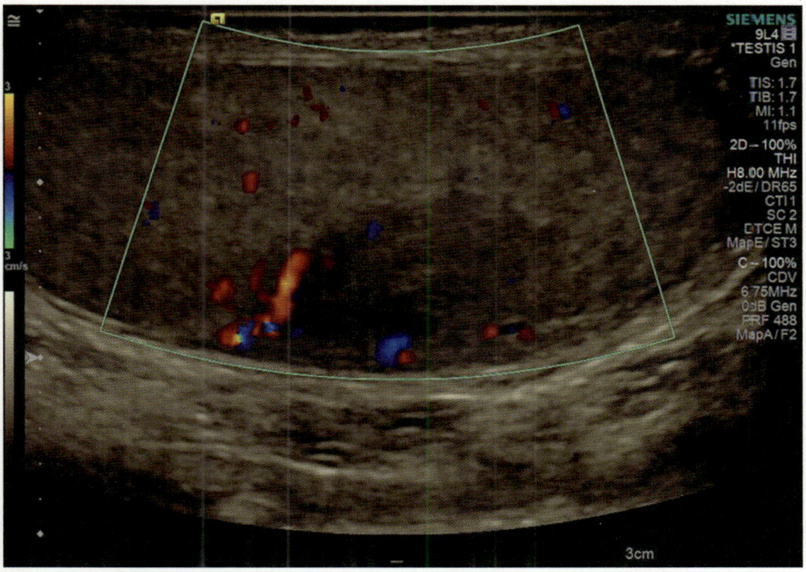

Fig. 9.95 No extended colour Doppler signal is detected in the abscess

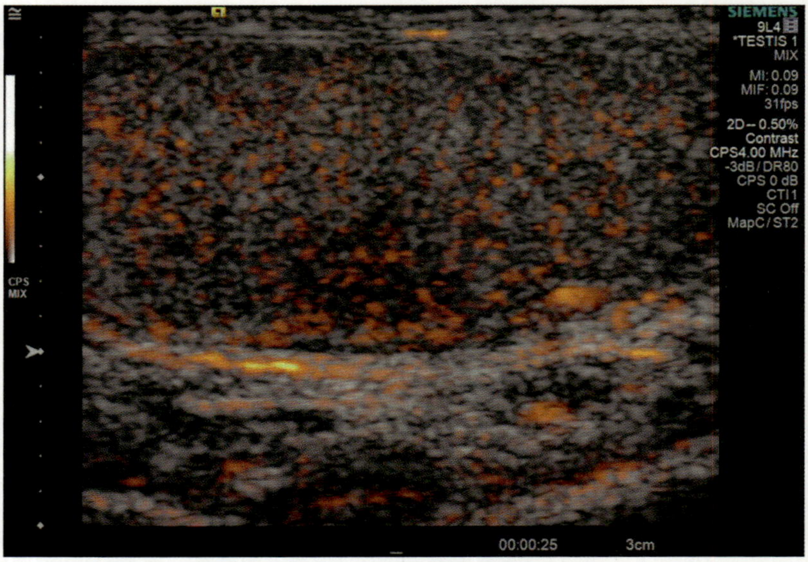

Fig. 9.96 Contrast-enhanced ultrasound confirmed a normal perfusion of the testicular tissue

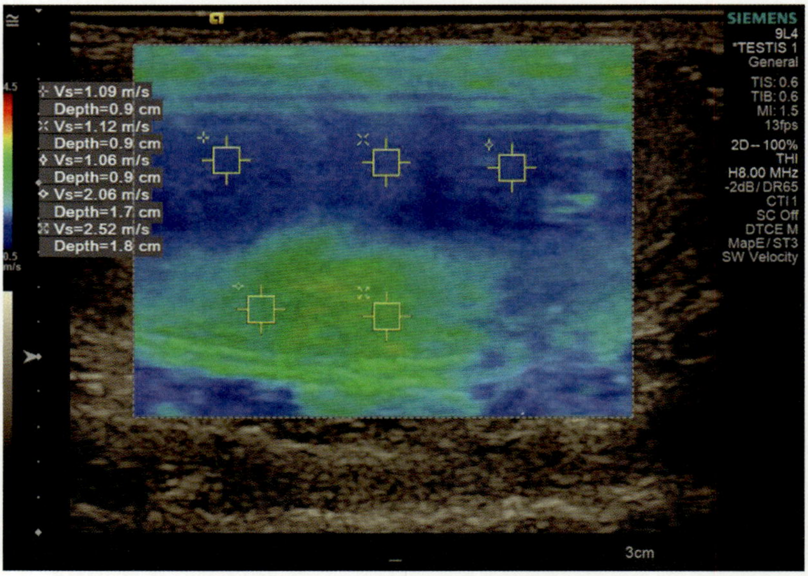

Fig. 9.97 VTIQ velocity colour overlay displayed relative shear wave velocities according to the adjacent colour spectrum, *red areas* corresponding to higher values and *blue areas* corresponding to lower values. Shear wave velocity was measured in the abscess $v = 2.06$–2.52 m/s and in the surrounding tissue level between $v = 1.06$–1.12 m/s

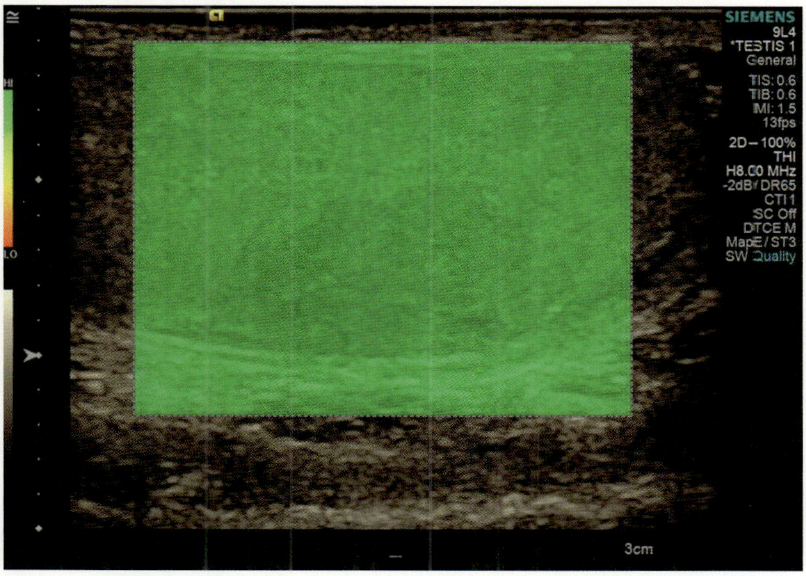

Fig. 9.98 Same lesion as Fig. 9.97. The entire testicular tissue and the lesion are coloured in *green*, as an indicator for a good quality of generated shear waves

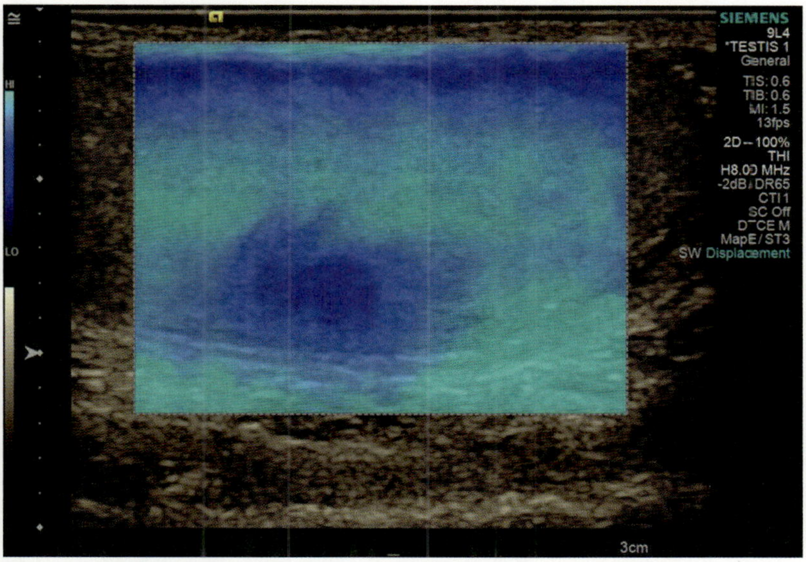

Fig. 9.99 Same lesion as Figs. 9.97 and 9.98. VTIQ displacement mode showed a low deformation of the residual abscess displayed as *dark blue* in comparison to good displacement displayed in *bright blue* of the normal testicular tissue

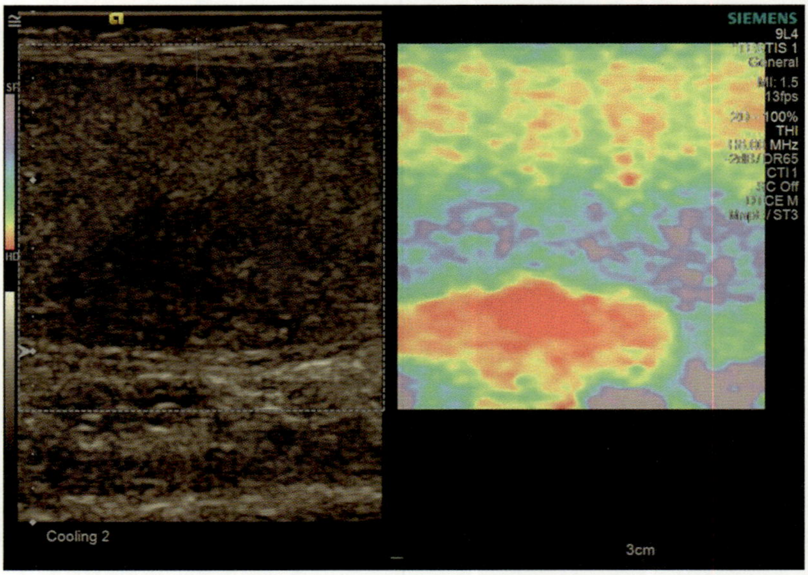

Fig. 9.100 In VTI mode elastography, the residual abscess appears in *red* as an indicator for stiff tissue, the peripheral tissue in purple as an indicator for soft tissue

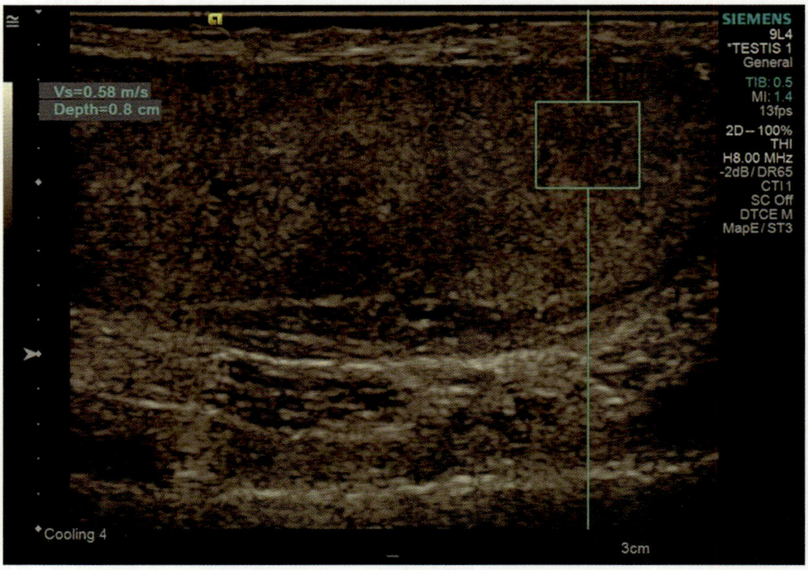

Fig. 9.101 In VTQ mode, the shear wave velocity was measured in the normal tissue with a velocity of $v = 0.58$ m/s

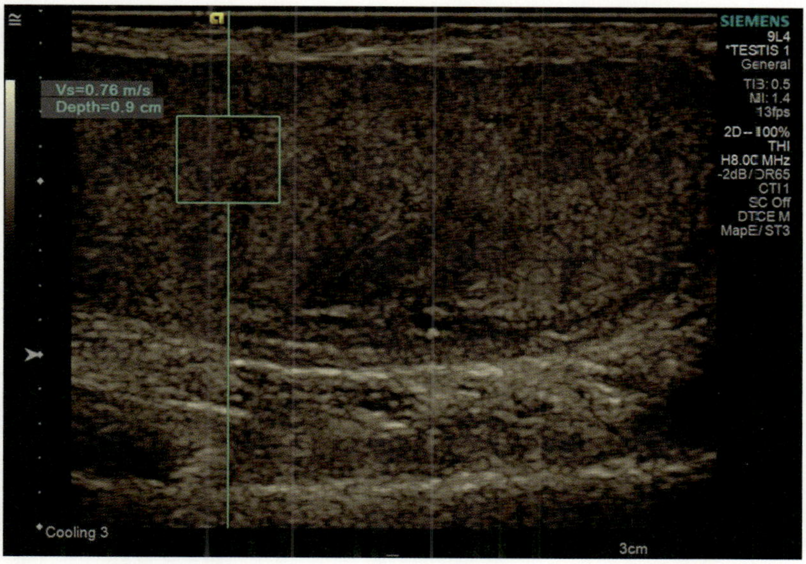

Fig. 9.102 In VTQ mode, the shear wave velocity was measured in the normal tissue with a velocity of $v = 0.76$ m/s

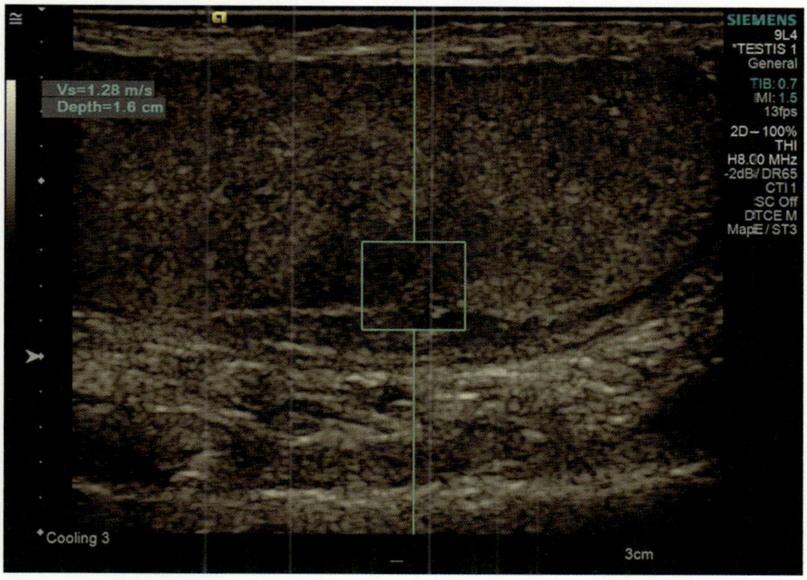

Fig. 9.103 In VTQ mode, the shear wave velocity was measured in the residual abscess with a velocity of $v = 1.28$ m/s

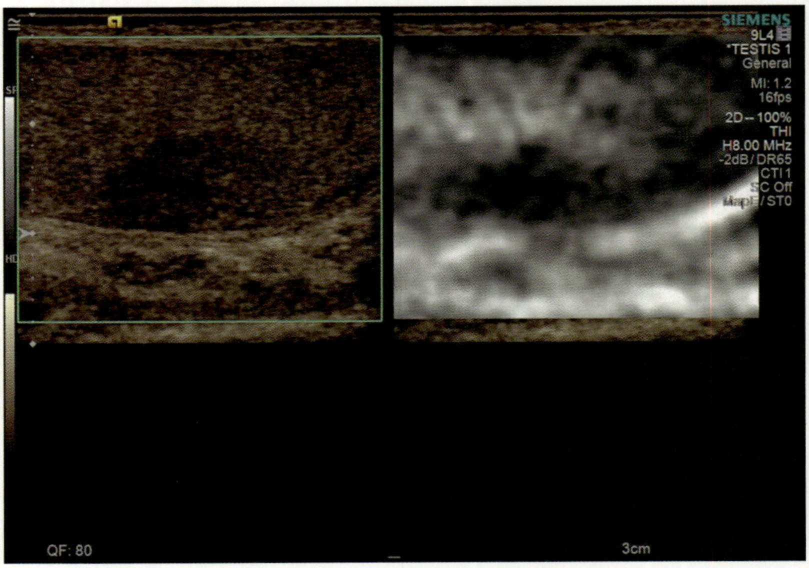

Fig. 9.104 In sonoelastography, the residual abscess appears in *black* as an indicator for a stiff tissue. The border of the lesions is displayed well in this technique

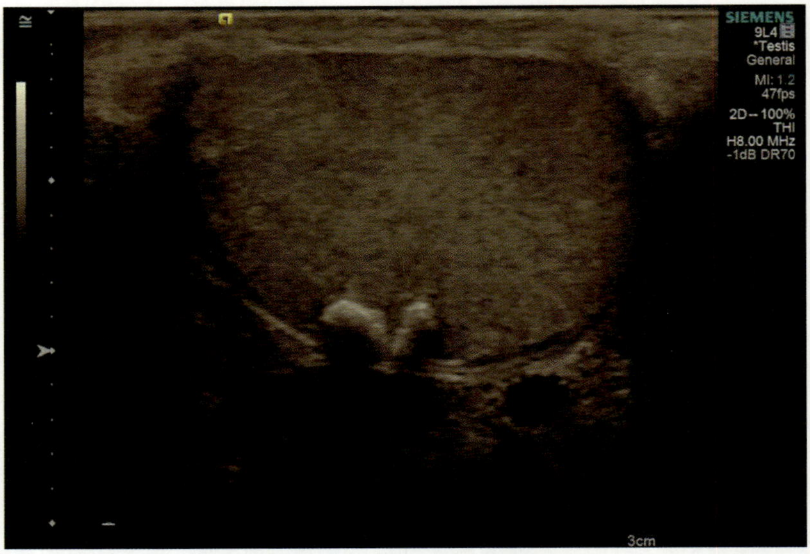

Fig. 9.105 A 47-year-old man with routine examination of the testis. A focal clump of calcification is present in the peripheral aspect of the testis on ultrasound

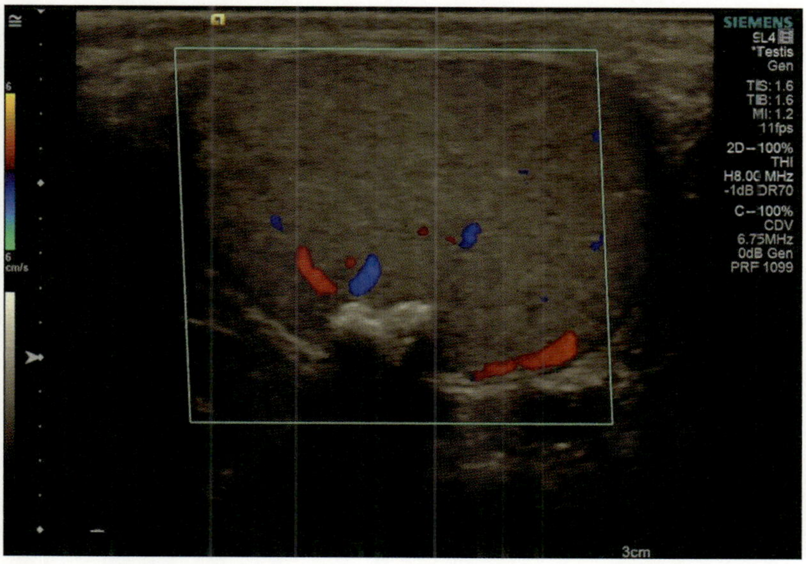

Fig. 9.106 No colour Doppler signal is detected in the calcification

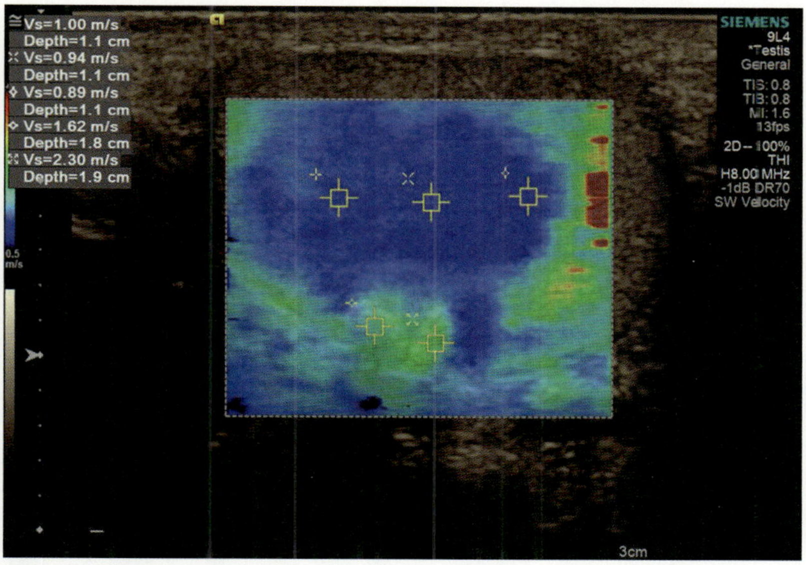

Fig. 9.107 VTIQ velocity colour overlay displayed relative shear wave velocities according to the adjacent colour spectrum, *red areas* corresponding to higher values and *blue areas* corresponding to lower values. Shear wave velocity was measured in the calcification $v = 1.62$–2.30 m/s and in the surrounding tissue level between $v = 0.89$–1.00 m/s

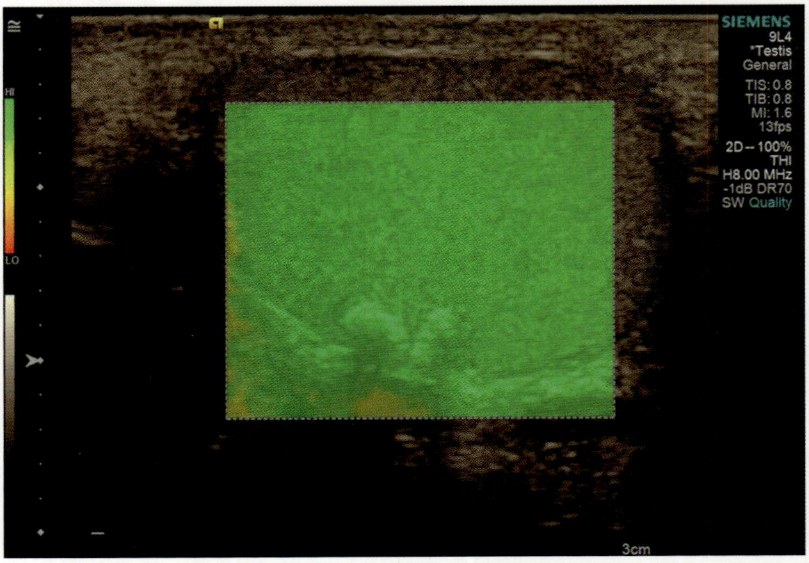

Fig. 9.108 Same lesion as Fig. 9.107. The entire testicular tissue and the lesion are coloured in *green*, as an indicator for a good quality of generated shear waves

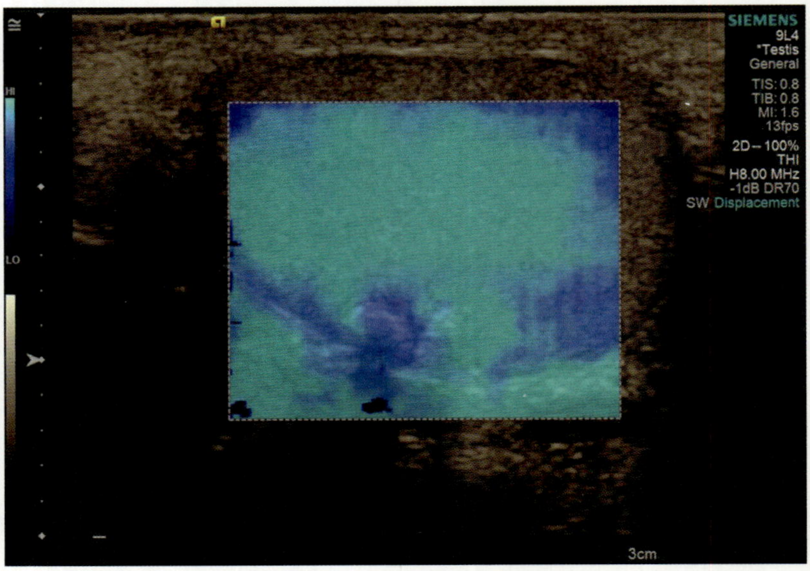

Fig. 9.109 Same lesion as Figs. 9.107 and 9.108. The *dark blue* of the VTIQ displacement mode in the region of the calcification shows a low deformation of that area in comparison to good displacement of the normal testicular tissue displayed by *bright blue*

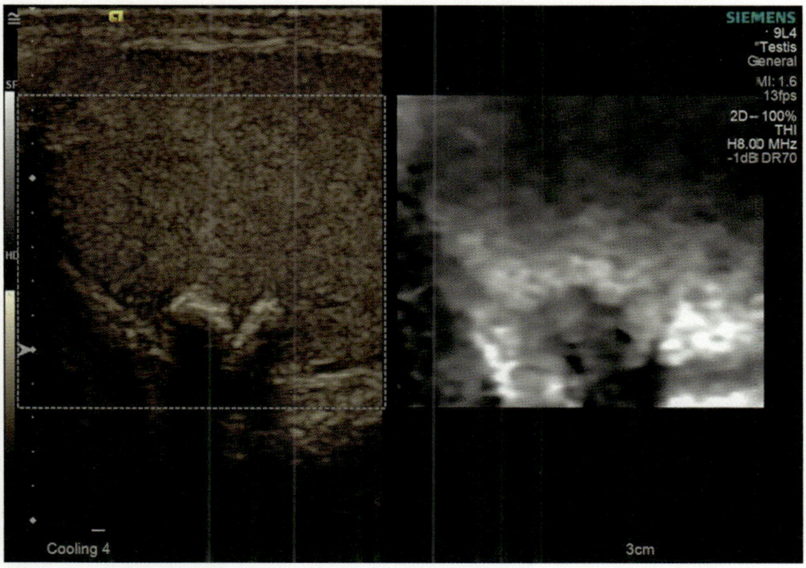

Fig. 9.110 In VTI elastography mode, the calcification appears as *black* indicating stiff tissue, whereas the peripheral tissue appears *bright grey* as an indicator of soft tissue

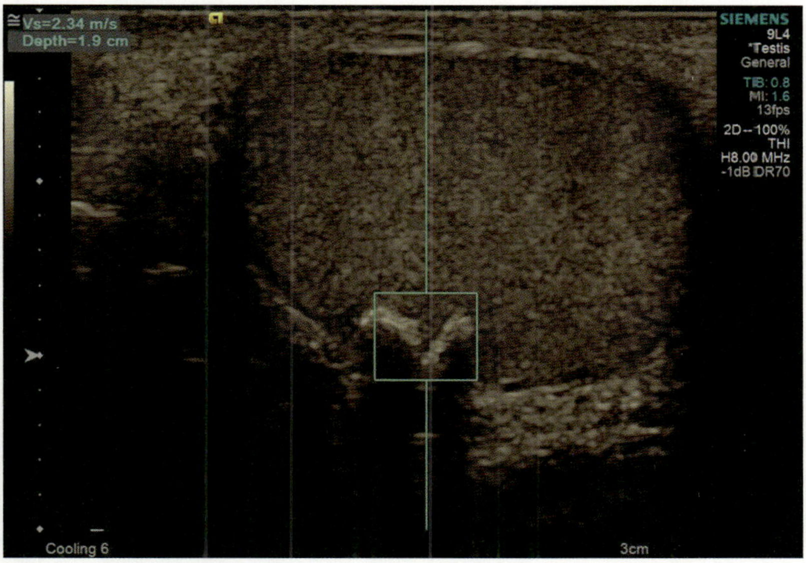

Fig. 9.111 In VTQ mode, the shear wave velocity was measured in the calcification area with a velocity of $v = 2.34$ m/s

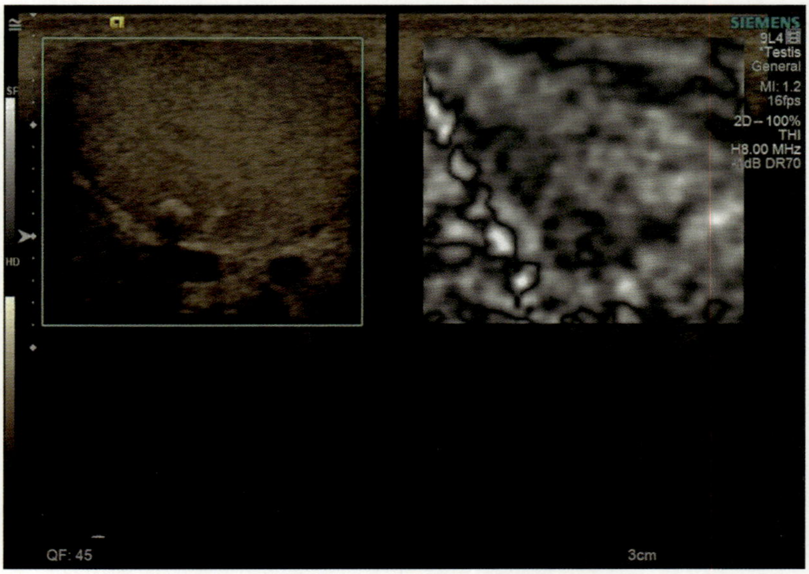

Fig. 9.112 In the strain elastogram, the calcification appears in *black* which is an indicator of stiff tissue

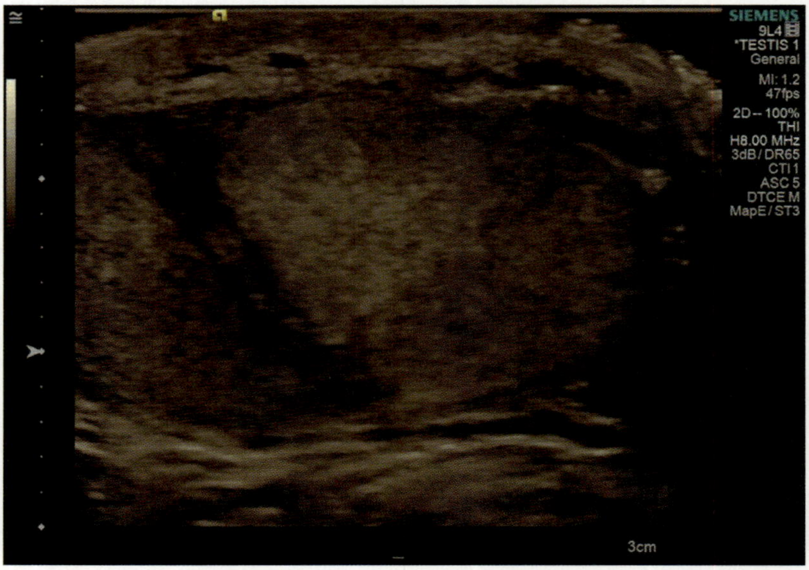

Fig. 9.113 A 52-year-old man with routine examination of the testis. The linear low-reflective structure seen bisecting the testis fits with the location of the trans-mediastinal artery and vein

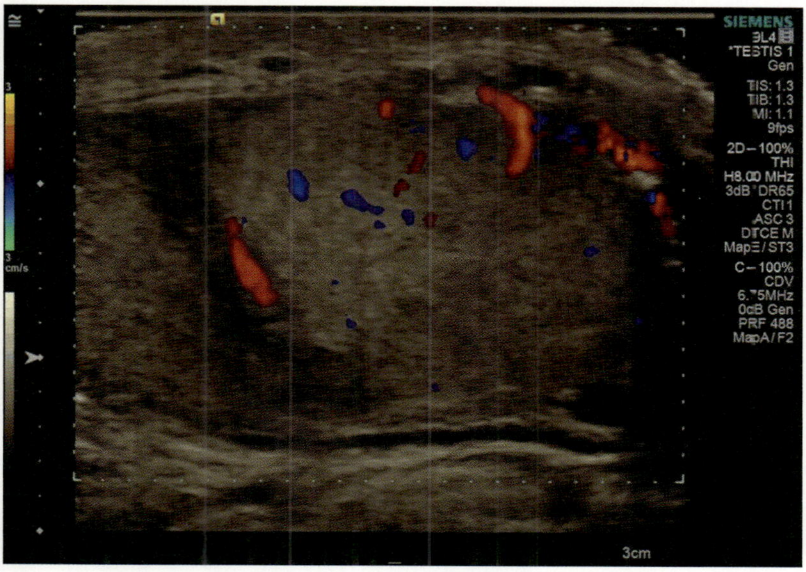

Fig. 9.114 Colour Doppler signal depicts the trans-mediastinal vessels

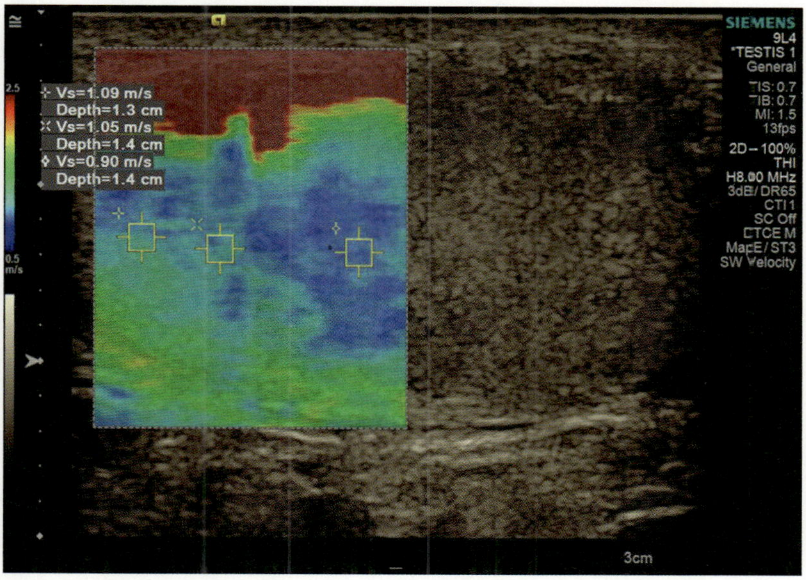

Fig. 9.115 VTIQ velocity colour overlay displayed relative shear wave velocities according to the adjacent colour spectrum, *red areas* corresponding to higher values and *blue areas* corresponding to lower values. Shear wave velocity was measured in the testis $v = 0.90–1.09$ m/s

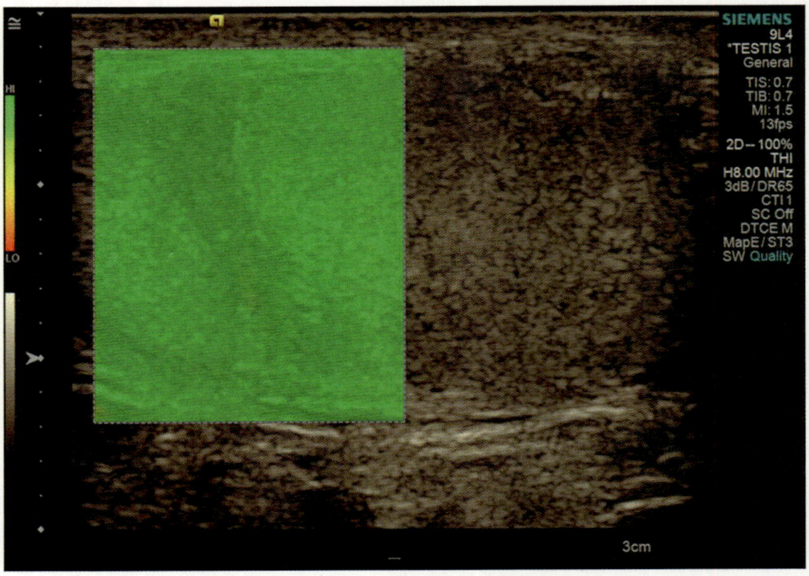

Fig. 9.116 Same lesion as Fig. 9.115. Using the VTIQ quality map the entire testicular tissue and the lesion are coloured *green*, indicating the shear waves generated are of a high

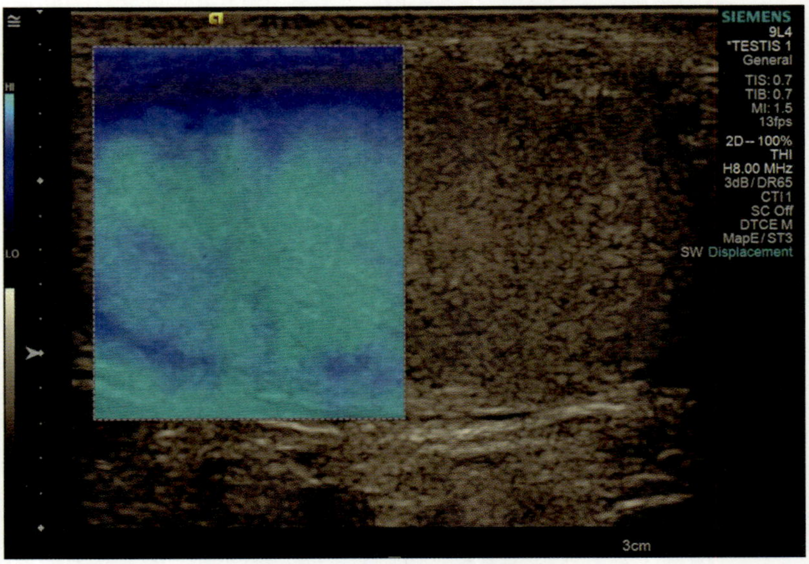

Fig. 9.117 Same lesion as Figs. 9.115 and 9.116. VTIQ displacement mode showed a normal deformation of the testicular tissue displayed in *bright blue*

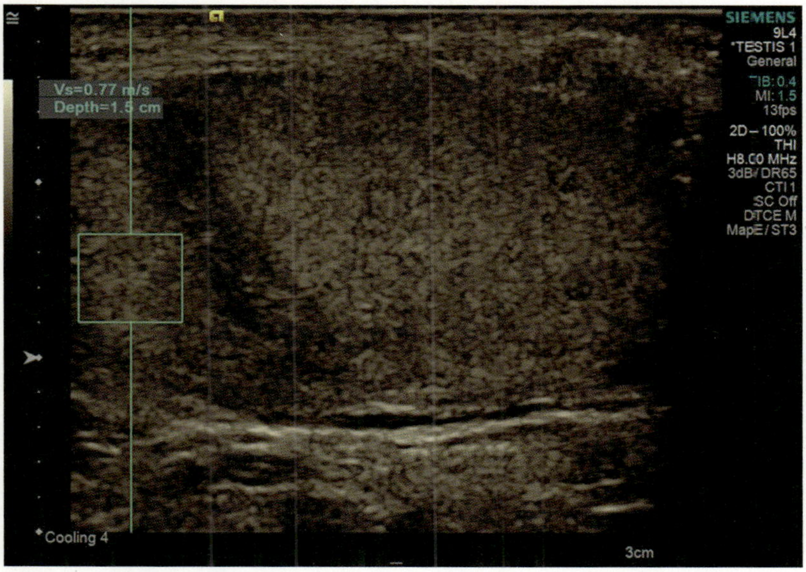

Fig. 9.118 In VTQ mode, the shear wave velocity was measured in the normal tissue with a velocity of $v = 0.77$ m/s

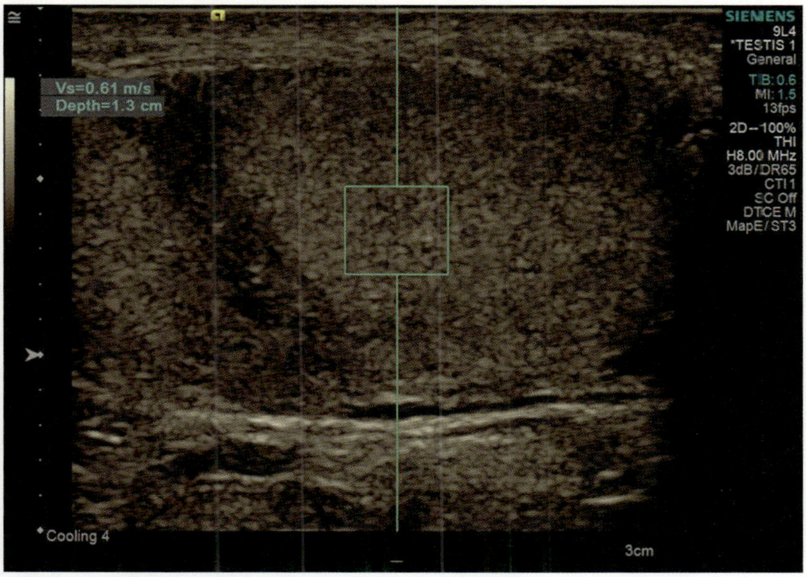

Fig. 9.119 In VTQ mode, the shear wave velocity was measured in the normal tissue with a velocity of $v = 0.61$ m/s

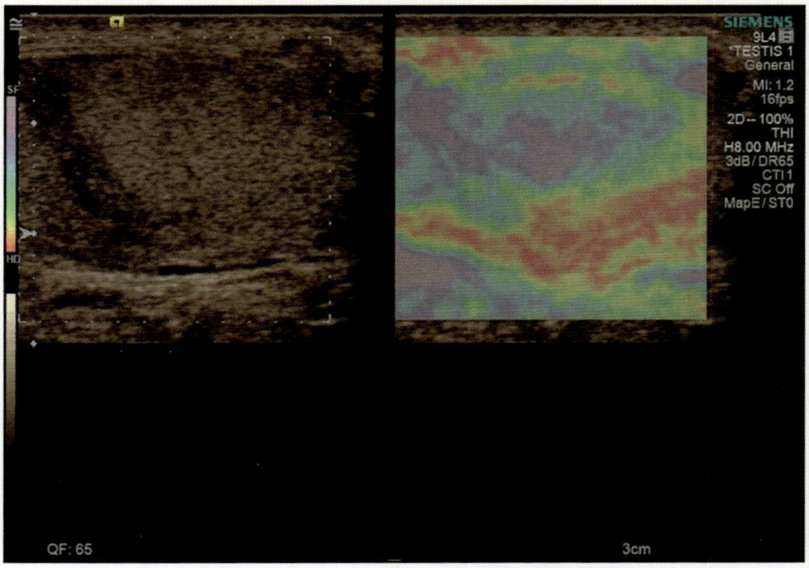

Fig. 9.120 In the strain elastogram, the trans-mediastinal vessels demonstrate a similar stiffness to the surrounding tissue

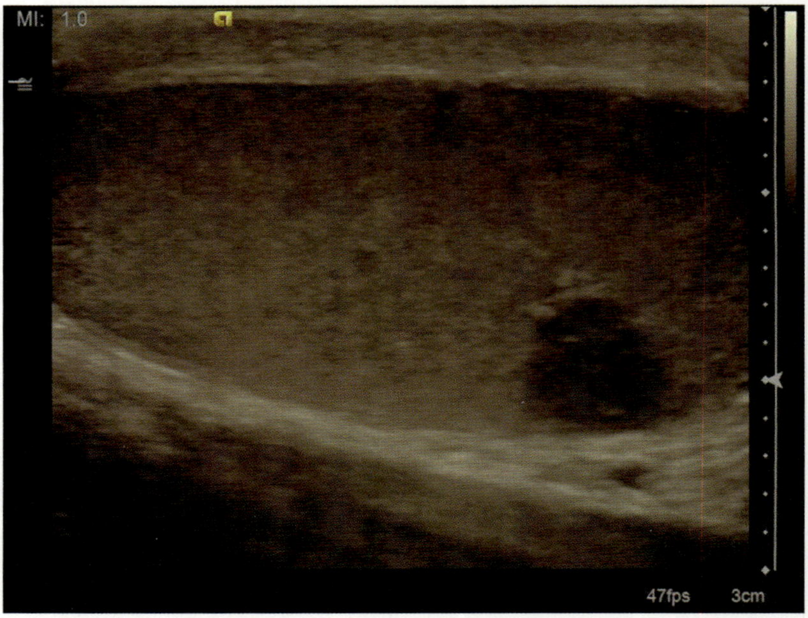

Fig. 9.121 Ultrasound images of a 43-year-old man. B-mode ultrasound demonstrates a hypoechoic lesion. The histological diagnosis, surgically proven, was that of a Leydig-Cell Tumour

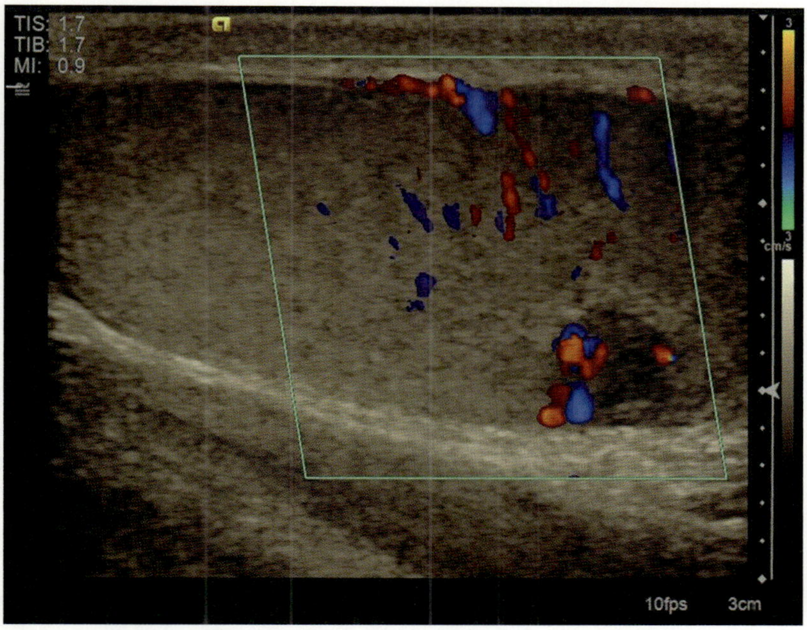

Fig. 9.122 Colour Doppler ultrasound demonstrates a high vascularity within the tumour in comparison to the surrounding tissue

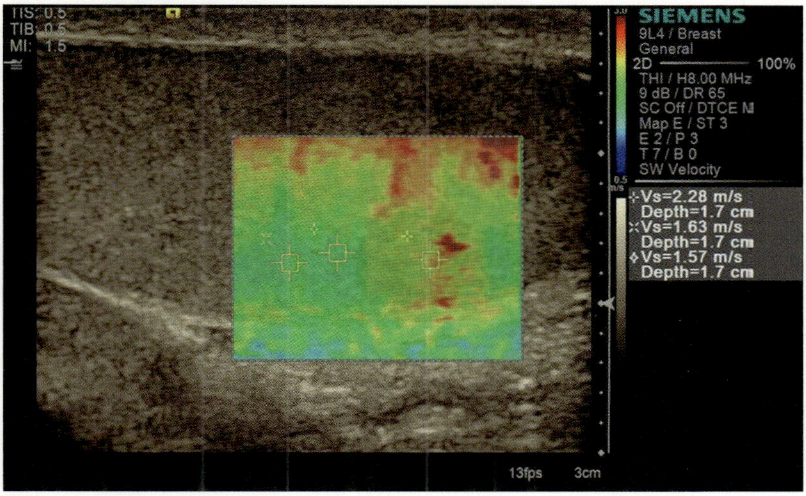

Fig. 9.123 VTIQ velocity colour overlay displayed relative shear wave velocities according to the adjacent colour spectrum, *red areas* corresponding to higher values and *blue areas* corresponding to lower values. Shear wave velocity was measured in the Leydig cell tumour $v = 2.28$ m/s and in the surrounding tissue level in the range of $v = 1.57–1.63$ m/s

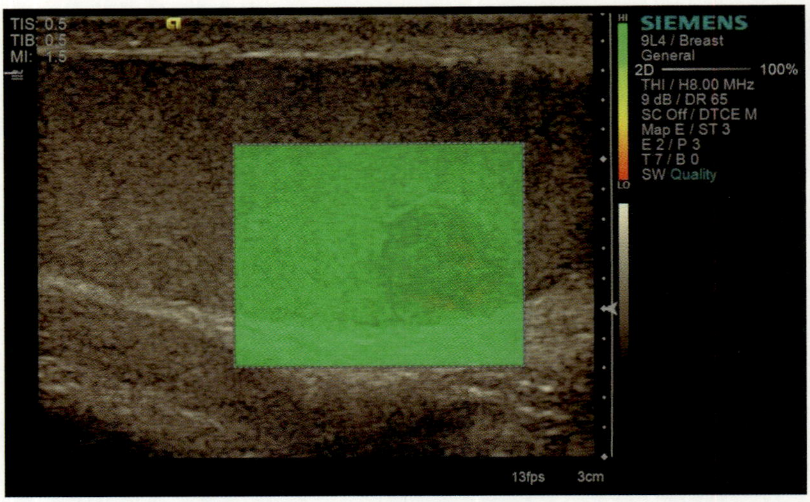

Fig. 9.124 Same lesion as Fig. 9.123. The entire testicular tissue and the lesion are coloured *green*, as an indicator of the high quality of generated shear waves

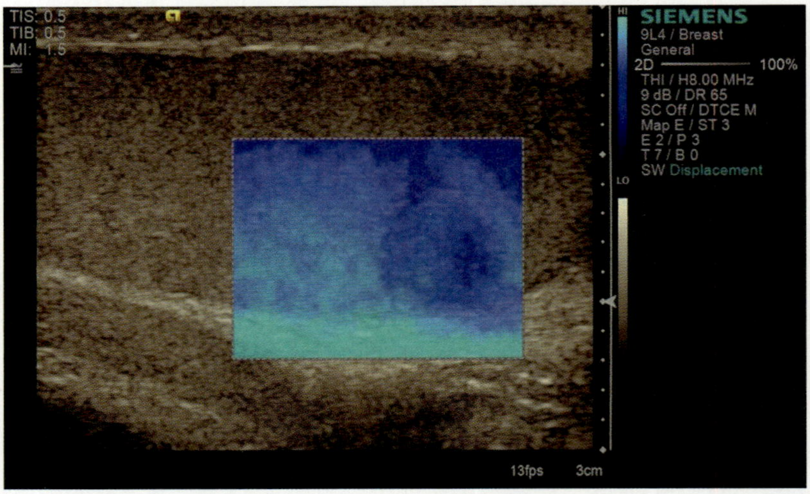

Fig. 9.125 Same lesion as Figs. 9.123 and 9.124. VTIQ displacement mode showed a low deformation of the tumour displayed as *dark blue* in comparison to good displacement of the surrounding tissue displayed in *bright blue*

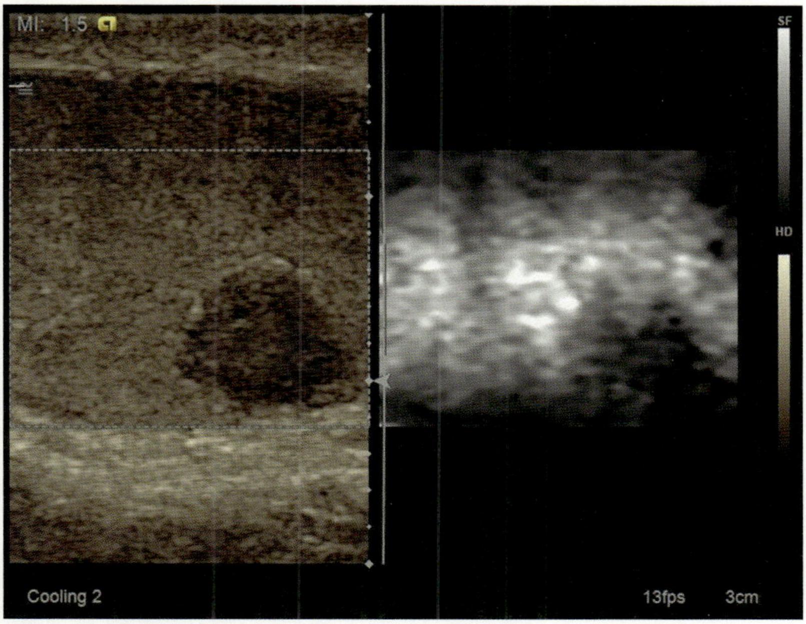

Fig. 9.126 In VTI elastography mode, the tumour appears *black* indicating stiff tissue, whereas the peripheral tissue is shown in *bright grey* as an indicator of soft tissue

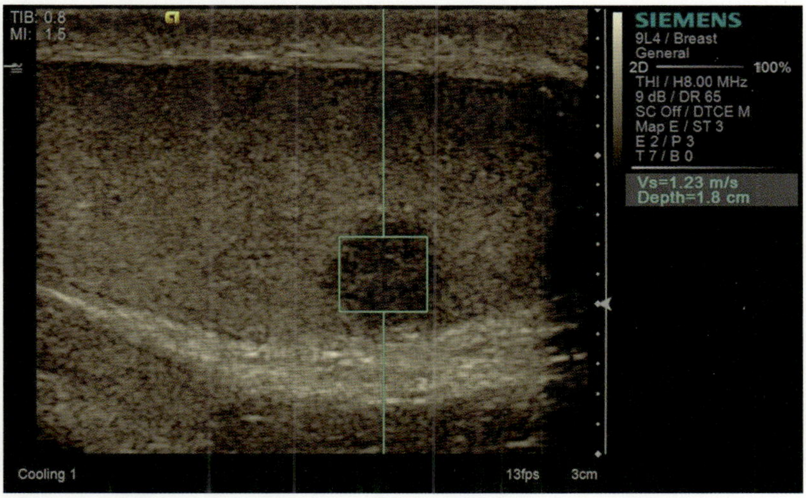

Fig. 9.127 In VTQ mode, the shear wave velocity was measured in the tumour with a velocity of $v = 1.23$ m/s

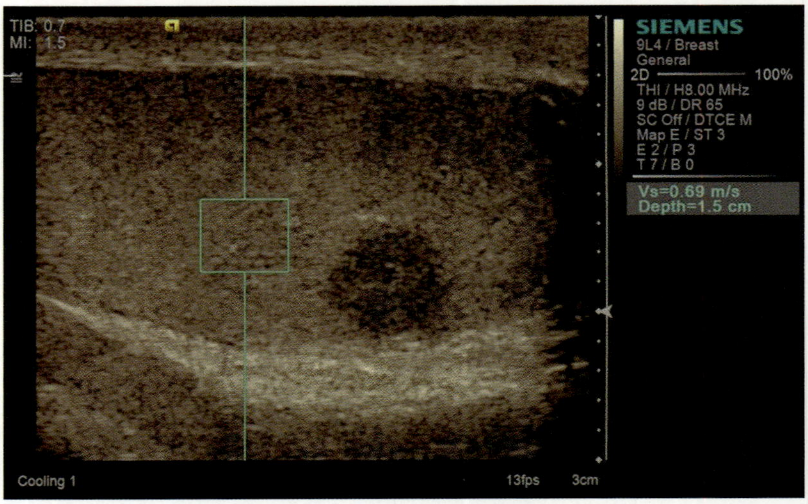

Fig. 9.128 In VTQ mode, the shear wave velocity was measured in the normal tissue with a velocity of $v = 0.69$ m/s

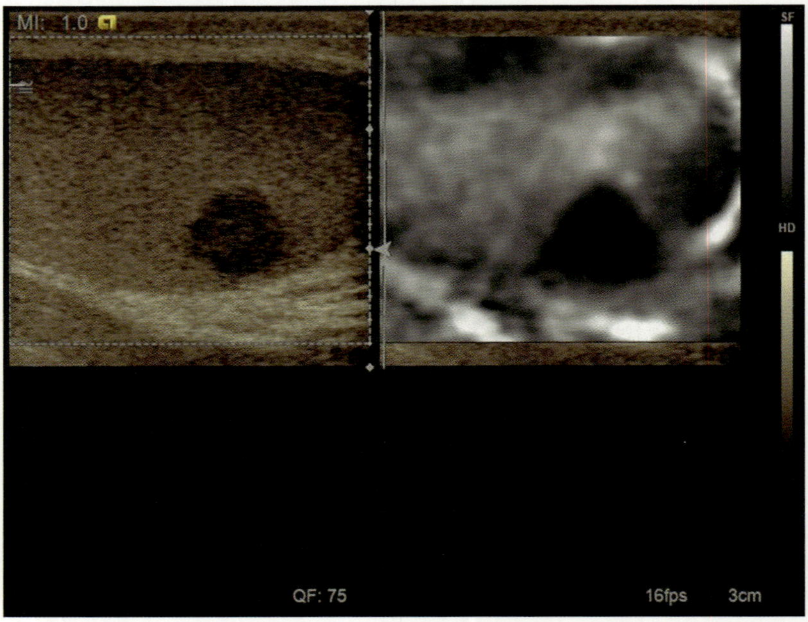

Fig. 9.129 In the strain elastogram, the tumour appears *black* as an indication of stiff tissue in comparison to the *light grey* display of the soft surrounding tissue

References

1. Huang DY, Sidhu PS. Focal testicular lesions: colour Doppler ultrasound, contrast-enhanced ultrasound and tissue elastography as adjuvants to the diagnosis. Br J Radiol. 2012;85(Spec No 1):S41–53.
2. Ragheb D, Higgins Jr JL. Ultrasonography of the scrotum: technique, anatomy and pathologic entities. J Ultrasound Med. 2002;21:171–85.
3. Mihmanli I, Kantarci F. Sonography of scrotal abnormalities in adults: an update. Diagn Interv Radiol. 2009;15:64–73.
4. Deurdulian C, Mittelstaedt CA, Chong WK, Fielding JR. US of acute scrotal trauma: optimal technique, imaging findings, and management. Radiographics. 2007;27:357–69.
5. Wöhrle NK, Hellerhoff K, Reiser MF, Clevert DA. Modern gray-scale sonography of the breast. Radiologe. 2010;50(11):964; 966–72.
6. Schlenker B, Clevert DA, Salomon G. Sonographic imaging of the prostate. Urologe A. 2014;53(7):1052–60.
7. Rjosk-Dendorfer D, Reichelt A, Clevert DA. Elastography as an additional tool in breast sonography. Technical principles and clinical applications. Radiologe. 2014;54(3):211–6.
8. Goddi A, Sacchi A, Magistretti G, Almolla J, Salvadore M. Real-time tissue for testicular lesion assessment. Eur Radiol. 2012;22(4):721–30.
9. Krouskop TA, Dougherty DR, Vinson FS. A pulsed Doppler ultrasonic system for making noninvasive measurements of the mechanical properties of soft tissue. J Rehabil Res Dev. 1987;24:1–8.
10. Ophir J, Céspedes I, Ponnekanti H, Yazdi Y, Li X. Elastography: a quantitative method for imaging the elasticity of biological tissues. Ultrason Imaging. 1991;13:111–34.
11. Miyagawa T, Tutsumi M, Matsumura T, Shimokama T, Miyanagas N, Akazas H. Real-time elastography for the diagnosis of the prostate cancer: evaluation of elastographic moving images. Jpn J Clin Oncol. 2009;39:394–8.
12. Zhi H, Ou B, Luo BM, Feng X, Wen YL, Yang HY. Comparison of ultrasound elastography, mammography, and sonography in the diagnosis of solid breast lesions. J Ultrasound Med. 2007;26:807–15.
13. Lyshchik A, Higashi T, Asato R, Tanaka S, Ito J, Mai JJ, Pellot-Barakat C, Insana MF, Brill AB, Saga T, Hiraoka M, Togashi K. Thyroid gland tumor diagnosis at US elastography. Radiology. 2007;237:202–11.
14. Lyshchik A, Higashi T, Asato R, Tanaka S, Ito J, Hiraoka M, Insana MF, Brill AB, Saga T, Togashi K. Cervical lymph node metastases: diagnosis at sonoelastography – initial experience. Radiology. 2007;243:258–67.
15. Grasso M, Blanco S, Raber M, Nespoli L. Elastosonography of the testis: preliminary experience. Arch Ital Urol Androl. 2010;82:160–3.
16. Patel K, Sellars ME, Clarke JL, Sidhu PS. Sonography and real-time tissue elastography. J Ultrasound Med. 2012;31:115–22.
17. Ianculescu V, Ciolovan LM, Dunant A, Vielh P, Mazouni C, Delaloge S, Dromain C, Blidaru A, Balleyguier C. Added value of Virtual Touch IQ shear wave elastography in the ultrasound assessment of breast lesions. Eur J Radiol. 2014;83(5):773–7.
18. Golatta M, Schweitzer-Martin M, Harcos A, Schott S, Gomez C, Stieber A, Rauch G, Domschke C, Rom J, Schütz F, Sohn C, Heil J. Evaluation of virtual touch tissue imaging quantification, a new shear wave velocity imaging method, for breast lesion assessment by ultrasound. Biomed Res Int. 2014;2014:960262.
19. Golatta M, Schweitzer-Martin M, Harcos A, Schott S, Junkermann H, Rauch G, Sohn C, Heil J. Normal breast tissue stiffness measured by a new ultrasound technique: virtual touch tissue imaging quantification (VTIQ). Eur J Radiol. 2013;82(11):e676–9.
20. Horster S, Mandel P, Zachoval R, Clevert DA. Comparing acoustic radiation force impulse imaging to transient elastography to assess liver stiffness in healthy volunteers with and without valsalva manoeuvre. Clin Hemorheol Microcirc. 2010;46(2–3):159–68.
21. Zengel P, Schrötzlmair F, Schwarz F, Paprottka P, Kramer M, Berghaus A, Clevert DA. Elastography: a new diagnostic tool for evaluation of obstructive diseases of the salivary glands; primary results. Clin Hemorheol Microcirc. 2012;50(1–2):91–9.
22. D'Anastasi M, Schneevoigt BS, Trottmann M, Crispin A, Stief C, Reiser MF, Clevert DA. Acoustic radiation force impulse imaging of the testes: a preliminary experience. Clin Hemorheol Microcirc. 2011;49(1–4):105–14.
23. Trottmann M, Marcon J, D'Anastasie M, Bruce MF, Stief CG, Reiser MF, Buchner A, Clevert DA. Shear-wave elastography of the testis in the healthy man – determination of standard values. Clin Hemorheol Microcirc. 2016;62:273–81.
24. Barr RG. Shear wave imaging of the breast: still on the learning curve. J Ultrasound Med. 2012;31(3):347–50.
25. Trottmann M, Marcon J, D'Anastasie M, Karl A, Stief CG, Reiser MF, Buchner A, Clevert DA. The role of VTIQ as a new tissue strain analytics measurement technique in testicular lesions. Clin Hemorheol Microcirc. 2014;58:195–209.

Printed by Printforce, the Netherlands